Inherited Disorders of Carbohydrate Metabolism

Previous Symposia of the Society for the Study of Inborn Errors of Metabolism*

1. Neurometabolic Disorders in Childhood. Ed. K. S. Holt and J. Milner 1963
2. Biochemical Approaches to Mental Handicap in Children. Ed. J. D. Allan and K. S. Holt 1964
3. Basic Concepts of Inborn Errors and Defects of Steroid Biosynthesis. Ed. K. S. Holt and D. N. Raine 1965
4. Some Recent Advances in Inborn Errors of Metabolism. Ed. K. S. Holt and V. P. Coffey 1966
5. Some Inherited Disorders of Brain and Muscle. Ed. J. D. Allan and D. N. Raine 1969
6. Enzymopenic Anaemias, Lysosomes and other papers. Ed. J. D. Allan, K. S. Holt, J. T. Ireland and R. J. Pollitt 1969
7. Errors of Phenylalanine Thyroxine and Testosterone Metabolism. Ed. W. Hamilton and F. P. Hudson 1970
8. Inherited Disorders of Sulphur Metabolism. Ed. N. A. J. Carson and D. N. Raine 1971
9. Organic Acidurias. Ed. J. Stern and C. Toothill 1972
10. Treatment of Inborn Errors of Metabolism. Ed. J. W. T. Seakins, R. A. Saunders and C. Toothill 1973
11. Inborn Errors of Skin, Hair and Connective Tissue. Ed. J. B. Holton and J. T. Ireland 1975
12. Inborn Errors of Calcium and Bone Metabolism. Ed. H. Bickel and J. Stern 1976
13. Medico-Social Management of Inherited Metabolic Disease. Ed. D. N. Raine 1977
14. The Cultured Cell and Inherited Metabolic Disease. Ed. R. A. Harkness and F. Cockburn 1977
15. Inborn Errors of Immunity and Phagocytosis. Ed. F. Güttler, J. W. T. Seakins and R. A. Harkness 1979

The Society exists to promote exchanges of ideas between workers in different disciplines who are interested in any aspect of inborn metabolic disorders. Particulars of the Society can be obtained from the Editors of this Symposium.

* Symposia 1–10 published by E. & S. Livingstone

Inherited Disorders of Carbohydrate Metabolism

Monograph based upon
Proceedings of the Sixteenth Symposium of
The Society for the Study of Inborn Errors of Metabolism

Edited by
D. Burman
J. B. Holton
and
C. A. Pennock

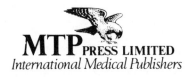

MTP PRESS LIMITED
International Medical Publishers

LSPKJ EEF

Published by
MTP Press Limited
Falcon House
Lancaster
England

British Library Cataloguing in Publication Data

Inherited disorders of carbohydrate metabolism.
 —(Society for the Study of Inborn Errors of
 Metabolism. Symposia; 16).
 1. Carbohydrate metabolism disorders
 —Congresses   2. Metabolism, Inborn errors
 of—Congresses
 I. Burman, D   II. Holton, John Bernard
 III. Pennock, C A
 616.3'99   RC632.C3

 ISBN 0–85200–267–X

Text set in 11/12 pt Photon Times, printed and bound
in Great Britain at The Pitman Press, Bath

Contents

SECTION THREE

SECTION FOUR

SECTION SEVEN

Genetic Aspects of Diabetes

List of Contributors

O. Ortved ANDERSEN
Medical Department E, Fredericksberg Hospital, Copenhagen, Denmark

K. BAERLOCHER
Children's Hospital, Claudiustrasse 6, CH-9006, St. Gallen, Switzerland

J. P. BLASS
Dementia Research Service, Burke Rehabilitation Center, 785 Mamoroneck Avenue, White Plains, New York 10605, USA

N. J. BRANDT
Section of Clinical Genetics, University Department of Paediatrics and of Obstetrics and Gynaecology, Rigshospitalet, Copenhagen, Denmark

D. BURMAN
Bristol Royal Hospital for Sick Children, Bristol

M. CHRISTY
Steno Memorial Hospital, DK-2820, Gentofte, Denmark

Th. de BARSY
Laboratoire de Chimie Physiologique, International Institute of Cellular and Molecular Pathology, U.C.L. 75.39, 75 avenue Hippocrate, B-1200 Brussels, Belgium

R. M. DENTON
Department of Biochemistry, University of Bristol Medical School, University Walk, Bristol

Th. DIAS
Laboratory of Developmental Biochemistry, Department of Paediatrics, University of Groningen School of Medicine, Groningen, The Netherlands

G. N. DONNELL
University of Southern California School of Medicine, Department of Pediatrics, Children's Hospital of Los Angeles, 4650 Sunset Boulevard, Los Angeles, California 90054, USA

J. FERNANDES
University Hospital, Groningen, The Netherlands

K. FISHLER
University of Southern California School of Medicine, Division of Medical Genetics, Children's Hospital of Los Angeles, 4650 Sunset Boulevard, Los Angeles, California 90054, USA

R. GITZELMANN
Department of Paediatrics, Division of Metabolism, University of Zurich, Children's Hospital Steinwiesstrasse 75, CH-8032, Zurich, Switzerland

A. P. HALESTRAP
Department of Biochemistry, University of Bristol Medical School, University Walk, Bristol

R. G. HANSEN
Department of Chemistry and Biochemistry, Utah State University, Logan, Utah, USA

M. J. HARRAN
Department of Child Health, University of Leicester, Leicester

J. T. HARRIES
Institute of Child Health, The Hospital for Sick Children, Great Ormond Street, London

H. G. HERS
Laboratoire de Chimie Physiologique, International Institute of Cellular and Molecular Pathology, U.C.L. 75.39, 75 avenue Hippocrate, B-1200 Brussels, Belgium

J. B. HOLTON
Department of Clinical Chemistry, Southmead Hospital, Bristol

F. A. HOMMES
Laboratory of Developmental Biochemistry, Department of Paediatrics, University of Groningen School of Medicine, Groningen, The Netherlands

G. HUG
Department of Pediatrics, University of Cincinnati College of Medicine – Division of Enzymology, The Children's Hospital Medical Center, Cincinnati, Ohio, USA

R. KOCH
University of Southern California School of Medicine – Division of Medical Genetics, Children's Hospital of Los Angeles, 4650 Sunset Boulevard, Los Angeles, California, USA

G. M. KOMROWER
Department of Medical Biochemistry, University of Manchester, Manchester

M. KROMANN
Steno Memorial Hospital, DK-2820, Gentofte, Denmark

B. LEDERER
Laboratoire de Chimie Physiologique, International Institute of Cellular

and Molecular Pathology, U.C.L. 75.39, 75 avenue Hippocrate, B-1200 Brussels, Belgium

H. L. LEVY
State Laboratory Institute, Massachusetts Department of Public Health, Department of Neurology, Harvard Medical School — Joseph P. Kennedy Jr Laboratories of the Neurology Service, Massachusetts General Hospital, Boston, USA

C. R. MADDOCK
Department of Paediatrics, King's Mill Hospital, Mansfield Road, Sutton-in-Ashfield, Nottinghamshire

D. P. R. MULLER
Institute of Child Health, The Hospital for Sick Children, Great Ormond Street, London

A. MACNAB
Department of Paediatrics, University College Hospital Medical School, London

A. S. McNEISH
Department of Child Health, University of Leicester, Leicester

J. NERUP
Steno Memorial Hospital, DK-2820, Gentofte, Denmark

W. G. NG
Division of Medical Genetics, Children's Hospital of Los Angeles, 4650 Sunset Boulevard, Los Angeles, California, USA

C. A. PENNOCK
Clinical Chemistry Department, Bristol Maternity Hospital, Bristol

P. PLATZ
Tissue Typing Laboratory, Rigshospitalet, DK-2100 Copenhagen, Denmark

C. M. RAYMONT
Department of Clinical Chemistry, Southmead Hospital, Bristol

L. P. RYDER
Tissue Typing Laboratory, Rigshospitalet, DK-2100, Copenhagen, Denmark

B. E. RYMAN
Department of Biochemistry, Charing Cross Hospital Medical School, Fulham Palace Road, London

I. B. SARDHARWALLA
Willink Biochemical Genetics Unit, Royal Manchester Children's Hospital, Pendlebury, Manchester

J. SCHRIJVER
Laboratory of Developmental Biochemistry, Department of Paediatrics, University of Groningen School of Medicine, Groningen, The Netherlands

V. SCHWARZ
Willink Biochemical Genetics Unit, Royal Manchester Children's Hospital, Pendlebury, Manchester

S. M. M. SHERIFF
Department of Ophthalmology, King's Mill Hospital, Mansfield Road, Sutton-in-Ashfield, Nottinghamshire

T. E. STACEY
Department of Paediatrics, University College Hospital Medical School, London

B. STEINMANN
Department of Paediatrics, Division of Metabolism, University of Zurich, Children's Hospital, Switzerland

L. B. STRANG
Department of Paediatrics, University College Hospital Medical School, London

A. SVEJGAARD
Tissue Typing Laboratory, Rigshospitalet, DK-2100 Copenhagen, Denmark

R. TATTERSALL
Nottingham General Hospital, Nottingham

J. G. TETLEY
Department of Haematology, King's Mill Hospital, Mansfield Road, Sutton-in-Ashfield, Nottinghamshire

M. THOMSEN
Tissue Typing Laboratory, Rigshospitalet, DK-2100 Copenhagen, Denmark

H. F. WOODS
Department of Therapeutics, University of Sheffield – The Hallamshire Hospital, Sheffield

Preface

The sixteenth annual symposium of the Society for the Study of Inborn Errors of Metabolism was held in Bristol from 12th to 14th July, 1978. About 25 invited speakers and 150 participants came from many parts of Europe and North America to consider the topic, 'Inherited Disorders of Carbohydrate Metabolism'. Although some aspects of these disorders have formed part of the programme of previous symposia organized by the Society, this was the first attempt to discuss them in a systematic manner.

The subject, carbohydrate disorders, embraces both familiar and well documented conditions and some lesser known aspects of genetic disease. In all of these there remains much to be learnt about clinical and laboratory diagnosis, treatment, biochemical screening and pathogenesis. Thus one aim of the Society, to combine clinical and scientific interest, can rarely have been better achieved in a single symposium.

Since the programme included diseases from six different areas of carbohydrate metabolism and contained so many distinguished speakers, it is impossible to highlight the more important aspects of this symposium within a short space. Each section made a notable contribution to knowledge and, when time was available, lively discussions ensued which have been recorded in the book. However, we wish to mention our two special lectures, because they recognise people to whom the Society owes a great deal.

The Milner lecture has been given for the past 6 years as a tribute to Mr J. Milner who has supported the Society in numerous ways since its beginning. This year we were honoured to have Professor Hers to give the lecture. Probably no one has added more to our understanding of carbohydrate metabolism and its inherited disorders then Professor Hers, and he contributed much to our discussions throughout the Symposium.

The F. P. Hudson Memorial Lecture is being sponsored annually by Mr J. G. Jones of Hospital Scientific Supplies. Freddie Hudson, a founder member and past chairman of the Society, contributed significantly to paediatrics, in particular the management of phenylketonuria, and was known to many members of the Society as a friend. In his introduction to the Memorial Lecture, Dr Komrower pays a full tribute to Dr Hudson and indicates how fortunate and appropriate it was that Professor Fernandes accepted our invitation to give the first lecture.

The symposium was made possible through the combined efforts of many people. We are indebted to the other Bristol members of the Society, Drs Beryl Corner, Linda Tyfield and Ian Barnes, who shared in organizing the meeting. In particular, we were very fortunate that the first of these was chosen as President of the Society for 1978 and guided our proceedings with great experience and charm. We were helped considerably by Professor Brenda Ryman and Dr George Komrower who first provided the ideas for the sections on glycogen storage diseases and galactose disorders, respectively, and then chaired the sessions. Finally, we owe much gratitude to our secretaries, Joyce Andrews and Iris Lynn, who worked so hard both during the symposium and in the preparation of these proceedings.

David Burman
John Holton
Charles Pennock

SECTION ONE

Introduction

1

Carbohydrate metabolism and its regulation

H. G. Hers

INTRODUCTION

Before discussing carbohydrate metabolism, it may be appropriate to consider why this metabolism is of primary importance and needs to be tightly regulated.

Glucose occupies a unique position in intermediary metabolism for two reasons: (1) It is the substrate of glycolysis which is the only pathway to produce ATP in anaerobic life. Although anaerobiosis is an exceptional condition in mammals, it is important to recall that erythrocytes, because they are deprived of mitochondria, are entirely dependent upon glycolysis for their supply of adenosine triphosphate (ATP). (2) Glucose is the major substrate of brain metabolism; indeed, fatty acids are bound to albumin and cannot penetrate the blood–brain barrier. Ketone bodies are easily utilized by the brain but their concentration in the blood is normally very low and increases only upon fasting. A significant decrease in the level of glycaemia could therefore cause major damage to the brain. This in itself is a justification for the rather elaborate and sometimes expensive mechanisms of control that the liver has developed to maintain a constant level of glycaemia.

A SUMMARY OF CARBOHYDRATE METABOLISM

Figure 1.1 shows a brief summary of carbohydrate metabolism. The main

3

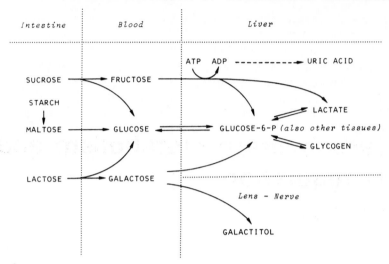

Figure 1.1 A summary of carbohydrate metabolism

dietary carbohydrates are starch, sucrose and lactose which are hydrolytically degraded into the free sugars, glucose, fructose and galactose. Hydrolysis of the oligosaccharides occurs through the action of oligosaccharidases located in the intestinal wall. This specific location prevents the accumulation of free sugars in the intestinal lumen and their utilization by microorganisms.

Fructose is very rapidly utilized by the liver and converted to glucose and lactate. When fructose is given intravenously, its utilization may be so intense that lactic acidosis may occur. Furthermore, fructose-1-phosphate accumulates in the liver causing depletion of P_i and ATP, followed by conversion of adenine nucleotides to uric acid and resulting in hyperuricaemia[1].

Galactose is also rapidly utilized by the liver and its metabolism normally causes no problem. It is only in congenital galactosaemia that the galactose concentration in the blood increases. Under these conditions, galactose can be converted to galactitol by aldose reductase, the activity of which is approximately proportional to substrate concentration; this enzyme is present in several tissues, including lens and nerve, in which the accumulation of galactitol may cause various types of damage, particularly cataract. The metabolism of fructose and of galactose is not subject to regulation.

Glucose is utilized by all tissues in the body and its penetration into muscle and adipose tissue is controlled by insulin. One important function of the liver is to control the level of glycaemia. When this level is elevated, as is the case after a meal, the liver takes up glucose and converts it mostly to glycogen; little of this glucose is utilized for the energy needs of the liver, which consumes mostly fatty acids. When the level of glycaemia is low, as for instance during fasting, the liver delivers a large amount of glucose to the blood for the benefit of the brain, erythrocytes and other tissues. This glucose is provided by the breakdown of glycogen and by gluconeogenesis.

Soskin[2] has emphasized that the concentration of glucose in the blood is the primary stimulus that elicits glucose uptake or glucose output by the liver and he compared this homeostatic control of the level of glycaemia to a thermostat system in a furnace. He defined the hepatic threshold of glucose as the glucose concentration at which the liver is converted from an organ of glucose output to an organ of glucose uptake. This threshold corresponds to the level of glycaemia that the animal usually maintains, which may vary according to hormonal conditions. In the following paragraphs, we describe the biochemical mechanisms by which these homeostatic and hormonal controls occur.

CONTROL OF GLYCOGEN METABOLISM IN THE LIVER

As explained in detail in recent reviews[3,4], the rate limiting steps of glycogen synthesis and breakdown in the liver are catalysed by glycogen synthetase and glycogen phosphorylase. Each of these enzymes exists in two forms: *a*, which is active, and *b*, which is inactive in the ionic conditions that prevail in the hepatocytes. The *a* and *b* forms are interconvertible through phosphorylation by kinases and dephosphorylation by phosphatases as indicated in Figure 1.2, which also shows the point of control by cyclic AMP and glucose.

Control by glucose

Glucose transport across the membrane of the hepatocyte is an efficient carrier mediated process which is not influenced by insulin; the concentrations of hexose in the liver cell and in the blood are always approximately equal. As shown in Figure 1.2, the primary effect of glucose in the hepatocyte is to bind to phosphorylase *a*, which may be considered the glucose receptor of the liver[5]. Phosphorylase *a* is inhibited by glucose and, more importantly, the glucose-bound phosphorylase *a* is rapidly converted to phosphorylase *b* by phosphorylase phosphatase. This first effect of glucose is to decrease and eventually to arrest glycogen degradation in the liver.

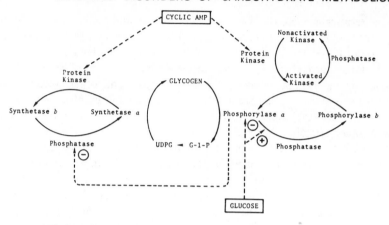

Figure 1.2   The control of glycogen metabolism in the liver

Glucose also stimulates glycogen synthesis by allowing the activation of glycogen synthetase. Indeed, synthetase phosphatase, which is the synthetase activating enzyme, is strongly inhibited by phosphorylase a[6]. This mechanism prevents synthetase from being activated when phosphorylase is active. Consequently, the activation of glycogen synthetase by glucose occurs only after a latency period which corresponds to the time required for the conversion of phosphorylase a into phosphorylase b (see Figure 1.3B).

A glucose load may also cause marked inactivation of phosphorylase which, however, is not sufficient to release synthetase phosphatase from inhibition. Under these circumstances, the glucose load diminishes glycogen breakdown without stimulating glycogen synthesis (see Figure 1.3A). These two types of response have been observed in the liver of anaesthetized rats[7], and in isolated hepatocytes[8].

Ionic effects

Glycogen synthesis in isolated hepatocytes is greatly increased when Na^+ is replaced by K^+ as the predominant cation in the incubation medium. As illustrated in Figure 1.3, this effect is also related to a faster and more complete inactivation of phosphorylase in a K^+ medium and, again, the activation of glycogen synthetase occurs only when the concentration of phosphorylase a falls below the threshold value at which it ceases to inhibit synthetase phosphatase completely[8]. A similar effect was also obtained by removing Ca^{++} from the external medium. The molecular mechanisms of these ionic effects are poorly understood.

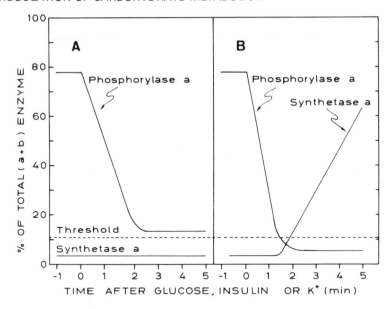

Figure 1.3 Sequential inactivation of glycogen phosphorylase and activation of glycogen synthetase[3]. This schematic representation illustrates that glycogen synthetase is activated only when the concentration of phosphorylase is lowered below a threshold value (dotted line), equal approximately to 10% of total ($a + b$) phosphorylase. This sequence has been observed in anesthetized rats[7], primates[23], and rabbits[24] following the administration of glucose or of insulin. In normal rats, the response to insulin, when detectable, was shown in A; in primates and rabbits, an activation of glycogen synthetase has been observed, as in B. The same kind of A or B response was observed in isolated hepatocytes by varying either glucose or K^+ concentration in the incubation medium[8]

Hormonal control

Figure 1.2 illustrates the classical mechanism by which cyclic adenosine monophosphate (AMP), in activating protein kinase, arrests glycogen synthesis and initiates glycogen breakdown[9]. Indeed, cyclic AMP dependent protein kinase acts both as a synthetase kinase and as a phosphorylase kinase kinase; it therefore activates phosphorylase which in turn converts phosphorylase b into phosphorylase a. Glucagon and β-adrenergic agents are known to increase the concentration of cyclic AMP in the liver, whereas insulin is able to decrease the cyclic AMP concentration after it has been elevated by small concentrations of these effectors[10]. Figure 1.4 shows a parallel dose-dependent activation of protein kinase (measured with histone

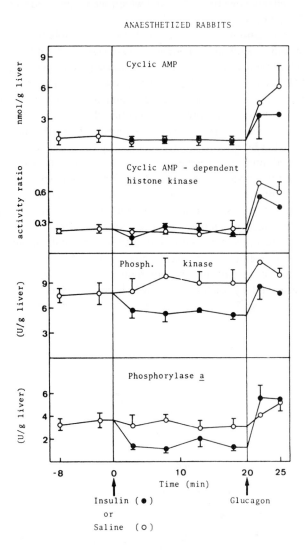

Figure 1.6 Effect of the successive administration of insulin (2 U/kg) and glucagon (0.5 mg) on the concentration of cyclic AMP and on the activities of cyclic AMP dependent histone kinase, of phosphorylase kinase, and of phosphorylase in the liver of anaesthetized rabbits[24]

activation of glycogen synthetase was very striking (see Figure 8 in reference 22). In the livers of normal monkeys[23], of rabbits[24], and less regularly of rats[7], the administration of insulin caused an immediate inactivation of phosphorylase. In a second step, which occurs only after a pronounced inactivation of phosphorylase, glycogen synthetase becomes activated. This secondary effect was observed in monkeys and rabbits although not in rats (see Figure 1.3).

In rabbits, it has been shown that the inactivation of phosphorylase was parallel to an inactivation of phosphorylase kinase, although not of protein kinase, and was not accompanied by a change in the concentration of cyclic AMP (Figure 1.6). These observations suggest that insulin acts on phosphorylase kinase through a messenger different from cyclic AMP, possibly a cation; an ionic change may influence the activity of phosphorylase kinase kinase (cyclic AMP dependent protein kinase, or maybe a different kinase) or of phosphorylase kinase phosphatase. The different regulation mechanisms discussed above are summarized in Figure 1.7.

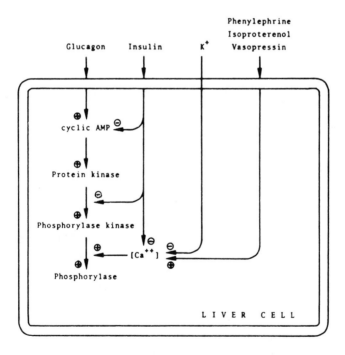

Figure 1.7 The ionic and hormonal control of glycogen metabolism in the liver[11]

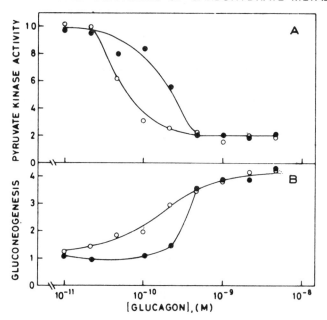

Figure 1.9 Effect of various concentrations of glucagon on the activity of pyruvate kinase (U/g of cells) and the rate of gluconeogenesis (μmol pyruvate converted to glucose + glycogen per 20 min/g of cells) of hepatocytes incubated with (●) or without (○) 10 nmol/l insulin[29]

The recycling between fructose-6-phosphate and fructose diphosphate

The operation of this cycle in the liver can be studied by the release of ^3H_2O from glucose labelled with ^3H in various positions and by the randomization of carbon between C1 and C6 of the glucose formed from [1-^{14}C]galactose. Both methods fail to reveal an important recycling at the level of fructose diphosphate in the rat or mice *in vivo*[30, 31]. Some recycling, however, occurs in isolated rat hepatocytes and is cancelled by glucagon[32]. The mechanism of this glucagon effect is at present unknown; it might be related to the tendency of hexose diphosphatase to be phosphorylated and simultaneously activated by cyclic AMP dependent protein kinase[33].

Recycling between glucose and glucose-6-phosphate

Recycling at this level has been shown by investigations with doubly labelled glucose. Indeed, it appears that [^3H]glucose decays faster than [^{14}C]glucose in isolated hepatocytes[34], in intact animals[35], and in children, although not in patients deficient in glucose-6-phosphate[36]. The recycling system consists of two high K_m enzymes for which there is no rapid mechanism of control other than substrate concentration[37]. It has been calculated that at the level of glycaemia equal to 5.7 mmol/l, the activity of glucokinase balances that of glucose-6-phosphatase, both of them allowing the conversion of 0.9 μmol of substrate/min per g of liver, so that there is no net flux of metabolites through the system.

Increasing the concentration of substrate of one of the two reactions will increase its rate of conversion to a product of which a higher level will favour the reverse reaction. Therefore, little or no change in the net flux of metabolites is expected. It is remarkable, however, that increasing the concentration of glucose causes a very temporary increase in the level of glucose-6-phosphate and is followed by a marked decrease as soon as the metabolites are rapidly utilised for the synthesis of glycogen. This occurs because glycogen synthesis is stimulated by the mechanism described above. As a result, the activity of glucose-6-phosphatase is decreased and there is now a large difference between the rate of glucose phosphorylation and the rate of glucose phosphate hydrolysis. The net uptake approaches 1 μmol/min which corresponds to a very fast rate of glycogen synthesis. Conversely, when glycogenolysis is intense, for instance after the administration of glucagon, there is a several-fold increase of the concentration of glucose-6-phosphate in the liver and therefore of its rate of conversion to glucose. The glucose, however, diffuses freely out of the liver cells and is dispersed in the body, so that the change in concentration will be relatively small.

The main advantage of the recycling system is to allow very large changes in glucose uptake and output to be controlled only by substrate concentration. An increase in glucose concentration influences, in a coordinated manner, the phosphorylase synthetase system and the recycling of glucose and glucose-6-phosphate, allowing the second system to keep pace with the first. An alternative mechanism for the control of glucose uptake or output would be to switch glucokinase or glucose-6-phosphatase on and off simultaneously with glycogen synthetase or phosphorylase. Such a system would be complicated by the fact that glucose-6-phosphate is used not only for glycogen synthesis but also for glycolysis and for the pentose phosphate pathway; it is formed by glucokinase, by glycogenolysis and by gluconeogenesis. The control of an on/off mechanism would therefore be exceedingly complex, whereas the control by substrate concentration may operate whatever the source or the fate of glucose-6-phosphate. The expenditure of energy by the glucose–glucose-6-phosphate cycle has been estimated to be 15 kcal/(d kg of liver)[37]. This seems negligible in comparison to the importance of this regulatory mechanism for the control of the level of glycaemia.

Inborn errors of gluconeogenesis

In both type I glycogenosis (glucose-6-phosphatase deficiency) and hexose diphosphatase deficiency, there is a complete block of gluconeogenesis. In both diseases, there is a marked hypoglycaemia and lactic acidosis. A remarkable observation is that in type I glycogenosis there is no increase in the concentration of glucose-6-phosphate in the liver[38]. This indicates that gluconeogenesis has been inhibited by a feedback mechanism that remains to be discovered.

References

1. Van den Berghe, G. (1978). Metabolic effects of fructose in the liver. *Curr. Top. Cell. Regul.,* **13,** 97
2. Soskin, S. (1940). The liver and carbohydrate metabolism. *Endocrinology,* **26,** 297
3. Hers, H. G. (1976). The control of glycogen metabolism in the liver. *Annu. Rev. Biochem.,* **45,** 167
4. Stalmans, W. (1976). The role of the liver in the homeostasis of blood glucose. *Curr. Top. Cell. Regul.,* **11,** 51
5. Stalmans, W., Laloux, M. and Hers, H. G. (1974). The interaction of liver phosphorylase *a* with glucose and AMP. *Eur. J. Biochem.,* **49,** 415
6. Stalmans, W., De Wulf, H. and Hers, H. G. (1971). Control of liver glycogen synthetase phosphatase by phosphorylase. *Eur. J. Biochem.,* **18,** 582
7. Stalmans, W., De Wulf, H., Hue, L. and Hers, H. G. (1974). The sequential inactivation of glycogen phosphorylase and activation of glycogen synthetase in the liver after the administration of glucose to mice and rats: The mechanism of the hepatic threshold. *Eur. J. Biochem.,* **41,** 127
8. Hue, L., Bontemps, F. and Hers, H. G. (1975). The effect of glucose and of potassium ions on the interconversion of the two forms of glycogen phosphorylase and glycogen synthetase in isolated rat liver preparations. *Biochem. J.,* **152,** 105
9. Robison, G. A., Butcher, R. W. and Sutherland, E. W. (1971). *Cyclic AMP.* (New York: Academic Press)
10. Exton, J. H., Lewis, S. B., Ho, R. J., Robison, G. A. and Park, C. R. (1971). The role of cyclic AMP in the interaction of glucagon and insulin in the control of liver metabolism. *Ann. N.Y. Acad. Sci.,* **185,** 85
11. van de Werve, G., Hue, L. and Hers, H. G. (1977). Hormonal and ionic control of the glycogenolytic cascade in rat liver. *Biochem. J.,* **162,** 135
12. Sherline, P., Lynch, A. and Glinsmann, W. H. (1972). Cyclic AMP and adrenergic receptor control of rat liver glycogen metabolism. *Endocrinology,* **91,** 680

13. Exton, J. H. and Harper, S. C. (1975). Role of cyclic AMP in the actions of catecholamines on hepatic carbohydrate metabolism. In G. I. Drummond, P. Grungaard and G. A. Robison (eds.). *Advances in Cyclic Nucleotide Research*, **5**, pp. 519–532. (New York: Raven Press)

14. Hems, D. A. and Whitton, P. D. (1973). Stimulation by vasopressin of glycogen breakdown and gluconeogenesis in the perfused rat liver. *Biochem. J.*, **136**, 705

15. Kirk, C. J. and Hems, D. A. (1974). Hepatic action of vasopressin: lack of a role for adenosine-3',5'-cyclic monophosphate. *FEBS Lett.*, **47**, 128

16. Keppens, S. and De Wulf, H. (1975). The activation of liver glycogen phosphorylase by vasopressin. *FEBS Lett.*, **51**, 29

17. Keppens, S. and De Wulf, H. (1976). The activation of liver glycogen phosphorylase by angiotensin. *FEBS Lett.*, **68**, 279

18. De Wulf, H. and Keppens, S. (1976). Is calcium the second messenger in liver for cyclic AMP-independent glycogenolytic hormones? *Arch. Int. Physiol. Biochim.*, **84**, 159

19. Keppens, S., Vandenheede, J. R. and De Wulf, H. (1977). On the role of calcium as second messenger in liver for the hormonally induced activation of glycogen phosphorylase. *Biochim. Biophys. Acta*, **496**, 448

20. Foden, S. and Randle, P. J. (1978). Calcium metabolism in rat hepatocytes. *Biochem. J.*, **170**, 615

21. Bishop, J. S., Goldberg, N. D. and Larner, J. (1971). Insulin regulation of hepatic glycogen metabolism in the dog. *Am. J. Physiol.*, **220**, 499

22. Stalmans, W. and Hers, H. G. (1973). Glycogen synthesis from UDPG. In P. D. Boyer (ed.) *The Enzymes*, **9**, pp. 309–361. (New York: Academic Press)

23. Curnow, R. T., Rayfield, E. J., George, D. T., Zenser, T. V. and De Rubertis, F. (1975). Control of hepatic glycogen metabolism in the rhesus monkey: effect of glucose, insulin, and glucagon administration. *Am. J. Physiol.*, **228**, 80

24. van de Werve, G., Stalmans, W. and Hers, H. G. (1976). The effect of insulin on the glycogenolytic cascade and on the activity of glycogen synthetase in the liver of anaesthetized rabbits. *Biochem. J.*, **162**, 143

25. Exton, J. H. and Park, C. R. (1972). Interaction of insulin and glucagon in the control of liver metabolism. In: *Handbook of Physiology*, **7**, *Endocrinology*, *1*. D. F. Steiner and N. Frenkel (eds.). (Washington: The American Physiological Society)

26. Friedmann, B., Goodman, E. H. and Saunders, H. L. (1971). An estimation of pyruvate recycling during gluconeogenesis in the perfused rat liver. *Arch. Biochem. Biophys.*, **143**, 566

27. Ljungström, O., Hjehlmquist, G. and Engström, L. (1974). Phosphorylation of purified rat liver pyruvate kinase by cyclic 3',5'-AMP-stimulated protein kinase. *Biochim. Biophys. Acta*, **358**, 289

28. Titanji, V. P. K., Zetterqvist, O. and Engström, L. (1976). Regulation *in vitro* of rat liver pyruvate kinase by phosphorylation-dephosphorylation reactions, catalyzed by cyclic-AMP dependent protein kinases and a histone phosphatase. *Biochim. Biophys. Acta*, **422**, 98

29. Feliu, J. E., Hue, L. and Hers, H. G. (1976). Hormonal control of pyruvate kinase activity and of gluconeogenesis in isolated hepatocytes. *Proc. Nat. Acad. Sci. USA*, **73**, 2762

2

Basic causes of carbohydrate malabsorption

J. T. Harries and D. P. R. Muller

INTRODUCTION

Carbohydrates are important constituents of the diet of man throughout the world and, following intestinal hydrolysis and absorption, provide a critical source of metabolic energy. Defects in hydrolysis and/or absorption result in retention of residues within the intestinal tract, and gastrointestinal symptoms, i.e. carbohydrate or sugar 'intolerance'. Sugar intolerance is a common clinical problem and may have serious consequences, particularly when it occurs in early life.

The major carbohydrates ingested by man are starch, lactose and sucrose, and the physiological mechanisms involved in their absorption will be reviewed to provide a background for considering the defects which result in malabsorption and disease. Other carbohydrates such as raffinose and stachyose are consumed in small amounts in legumes (e.g. lentils and beans) but are of no nutritional importance since they cannot be hydrolysed by pancreatic or mucosal enzymes.

PHYSIOLOGY

Intraluminal hydrolysis

Starch is a glucose polymer composed of two moieties, amylopectin and amylose. Amylopectin constitutes 80–90% of starch. It is a branched polymer which contains glucose residues linked by α 1–4 glucosidic bonds with the branching points resulting from α 1–6 glucosidic links. Amylose is a straight-chain polymer of glucose residues linked by α 1–4 bonds (Figure 2.1).

Hydrolysis is initiated by salivary α-amylase and completed by the pancreatic enzyme. Both enzymes hydrolyse only α 1–4 bonds, and have a low affinity for terminal links as well as those immediately adjacent to α 1–6 links. Amylose is therefore hydrolysed to maltose and maltotriose, and amylopectin to maltose, maltotriose and α-limit dextrins (glucose polymers containing five to eight monomers linked by both α 1–4 and α 1–6 bonds). Pancreatic α-amylase is found principally within the small intestinal lumen, although Ugolev[1] has provided evidence that some amylase is adsorbed to the mucosa where it can exert its catalytic effect at a locus adjacent to mucosal hydrolytic and translocation systems.

Mucosal hydrolysis

Prior to translocation of monosaccharides across the brush border membrane of the mucosal absorptive cell (enterocyte), hydrolysis of maltose, maltotriose, α-linked dextrins, sucrose and lactose to glucose, galactose and fructose is necessary. In contrast to oligopeptides, only minute amounts of oligosaccharides can enter the enterocyte intact. Hydrolysis is achieved by the oligosaccharidases lactase, maltase and sucrase-isomaltase. These enzymes are large glycoproteins, with pH optima of approximately 6.0, and are superficially located with their active sites orientated towards the intestinal lumen[2]. Peak oligosaccharidase activities are found in the proximal jejunum and are much lower in the duodenum and distal ileum[3].

In the rat oligosaccharidase activities have been shown to undergo circadian rhythms in relation to food intake[4]; activities began to rise prior to food intake suggesting that the triggering factor was anticipation of food.

The rate limiting step for lactose absorption is hydrolysis whereas translocation of the monomer products of hydrolysis is rate limiting for the other oligosaccharides[5]. Hydrolysis is an extremely rapid and efficient process, and if allowed to proceed in an uncontrolled fashion the concentrations of monomer products would rapidly exceed the T_{max} of the membrane carriers resulting in back-diffusion of monosaccharides into the lumen and osmotic diarrhoea[6]. This is prevented by a negative feedback system whereby there is product inhibition of oligosaccharidase activity[2,6].

Three distinct lactases (β-galactosidases) have been identified[7–11], a neutral brush border lactase, a neutral cytoplasmic hetero β-galactosidase and an acid lysosomal β-galactosidase. Only the brush border enzyme is of

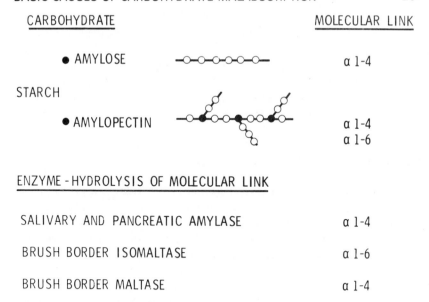

Figure 2.1   Structure of components of starch and enzymes responsible for their hydrolysis

importance in the physiology of lactose absorption.

All the α-glucosidases, except trehalase, hydrolyse maltose and thus can be considered as maltases; indeed as much as 75% of mucosal maltase activity can be accounted for by sucrase. The maltases hydrolyse α 1–4 glucosidic bonds sequentially from the non-reducing end of the oligosaccharide. Sucrase-isomaltase is a hybrid molecule made up of two non-identical subunits joined by one or more disulphide bonds[12]. The sucrase and isomaltase subunits have molecular weights of 130 000 and 120 000 respectively. As the molecular weight of the whole complex was found to be 280 000, it was postulated that the additional 30 000 daltons could be largely accounted for by a polypeptide involved in linking the two enzymes. The isomaltase subunit appears to be particularly labile when separated from sucrase. Utilising artificial liposome membranes Brunner *et al.*[13] have provided evidence that the sucrase–isomaltase complex is 'anchored' to the lipid membrane by hydrophobic interactions between the isomaltase subunit and the membrane. The α-limit dextrins, not isomaltose, are physiological substrates for isomaltase and it is likely that sucrase and isomaltase act in concert in the hydrolysis of α-limit dextrins to glucose, sucrase hydrolysing α 1–4 bonds and isomaltase cleaving the α 1–6 links of the molecule.

Electronmicroscopic and immunological studies indicate that with the exception of trehalase, the oligosaccharidases are superficially located on the luminal surface of the brush border[14, 15]; trehalase appears to be deeply embedded in the lipid rich membrane.

Brush border membrane translocation

It has been postulated that surface oligosaccharidases are located immediately adjacent to brush border membrane monosaccharide 'carriers' (Figure 2.2). Such a system would be biologically advantageous in presenting high concentrations of released monosaccharides to specific high affinity transport systems, as well as minimising back diffusion of monomers into the intestinal lumen.

Glucose and galactose   Glucose and galactose share the same sodium coupled energy-dependent transport system which is electrogenic[2]. This system has a structural requirement for a five carbon pyranose ring with the hydroxyl group at carbon two being positioned below the horizontal plane of the ring. Glucose and galactose are transported more rapidly than the pentose xylose because presence of a sixth carbon markedly enhances absorption. Transport systems display saturation kinetics analogous to enzyme reactions. It has been assumed that the monosaccharides bind to specific receptor sites on carriers followed by translocation across the brush border membrane into the enterocyte. To date, no such carrier has been isolated from mammalian brush borders.

In 1965, Crane[16] proposed a model to describe glucose transport across the enterocyte, and several subsequent studies have provided strong evidence in support[17]. Crane suggested that the carrier has two binding sites, one for glucose and galactose and one for the monovalent cations sodium and potassium. Sodium binding increases affinity for glucose whereas potassium exerts the reverse effect. Intracellular concentration of sodium is kept low as a result of active extrusion of sodium from the enterocyte across the lateral membrane into the intercellular spaces; energy results from the hydrolysis of adenosine triphosphate by membrane-bound (Na^+–K^+)-ATPase (i.e. the 'sodium pump'). The net result is generation of a sodium gradient between the intestinal lumen and the enterocyte interior. Thus, carrier bound sodium enters the enterocyte by a process of simple passive

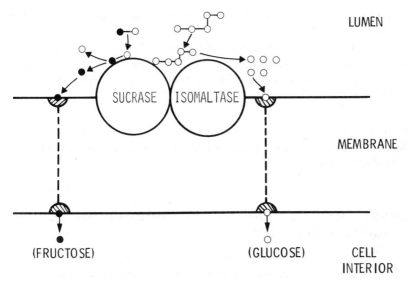

LUMEN

MEMBRANE

(FRUCTOSE)   (GLUCOSE)   CELL
                                                INTERIOR

Figure 2.2   Membrane orientation of sucrase–isomaltase complex to the glucose and fructose carriers

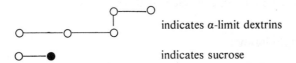

indicates α-limit dextrins

indicates sucrose

diffusion down an electrochemical gradient, and it is the energy inherent in this gradient which allows active translocation of glucose into the enterocyte against a concentration gradient.

The accumulated glucose enters the lateral intercellular spaces by simple diffusion down a concentration gradient, probably by a carrier mediated system. Since there is an inverse relationship between the intracellular and luminal concentrations of sodium and potassium, there is an asymmetrical distribution of the two cations across the brush border. Such an arrangement will favour binding of glucose to the carrier at the luminal surface of the brush border membrane, and release at the intracellular surface due to competition by the cations for their binding site.

Recent studies suggest that two or more transport systems participate in the absorption of glucose and its analogues, each having different kinetic constants[18,19]. Animal work has demonstrated an 'hydrolase related' transport (HRT) system by which active glucose absorption occurs only when glucose is presented to the mucosa as a constituent of an oligosaccharide[20-22].

In contrast to Crane's classical sodium coupled transport system, absorption of glucose from this HRT system is independent of the presence of sodium. It remains to be established whether these transport systems are nutritionally important in man.

Fructose   Current evidence suggests that absorption of fructose is carrier mediated and, in contrast to glucose and galactose, transport is independent of sodium and energy[2, 23-25].

GENETICALLY DETERMINED DISORDERS OF CARBO- HYDRATE ABSORPTION

Four genetically determined disorders of carbohydrate transport are recognised: lactase, sucrase-isomaltase and trehalase deficiency, and congenital glucose-galactose malabsorption. The disorders are specific absorptive defects and the small intestinal mucosa is morphologically normal. They are probably all inherited as autosomal recessives.

Lactase deficiency

In man lactase deficiency may be congenital or acquired.

Congenital lactase deficiency   This entity is a rare disorder and was first described in 1959 by Holzel *et al*[26]. Patients present with profuse watery diarrhoea soon after the introduction of milk feeds, and the condition is fatal unless an early diagnosis is established and lactose withdrawn from the diet. A presumptive diagnosis can be made on the basis of a careful clinical history, but a definitive diagnosis rests on the demonstration of a specific deficiency or absence of lactase activity in mucosa[27].

Asp and Dahlqvist[11] have studied the enzymatic activities of the three β-galactosidases present in normal intestinal mucosa (i.e. lactase, acid β-galactosidase and hetero β-galactosidase) in four children with congenital lactase deficiency. In three of the patients no activity of brush border lactase could be detected and in the fourth there was only a trace. The activity of the other two β-galactosidases was normal. Freiburghaus *et al*.[28] have used polyacrylamide gel electrophoresis of brush border fragments to study lactase in four patients. They found traces of lactase activity with reduced amounts of protein in the lactase position in three patients and lactase completely absent in the fourth; no evidence for abnormal protein was found. On the basis of their results Freiburghaus et al.[28] suggested that the congenital disorder is due to a defect in protein regulation with a very early 'switch off' of lactase biosynthesis (see below).

Acquired (ontogenetic late onset) lactase deficiency In most mammals the activity of intestinal lactase is maximal in the perinatal period, decreasing during weaning to reach low levels (10% of maximal activity) in the adult. In certain species of sea lions, lactase activity is absent at birth and, as might be anticipated, the mother's milk contains no lactose[29].

In the human most adults have low lactase activity, but in some it remains high throughout life. Many population studies of different ethnic groups have now been carried out[30] and these have revealed that in most non-Caucasian races the prevalence of low lactase levels is extremely high (50–90%) whereas in Caucasians the prevalence is much lower (2–30%). Thus, the majority of human adults are lactase deficient and malabsorb lactose. It would appear that the capacity of some adults to be able to digest lactose represents a deviation from both the typical human and mammalian pattern of lactase activity.

Gastrointestinal symptoms are relatively mild in subjects with acquired lactase deficiency, and appear between the ages of one and five years. Asp et al.[31] have studied the activities of the β-galactosidases in a large number of affected individuals and found lactase activities to be approximately 5–10% of controls, whereas the activities of the acid and hetero β-galactosidases were normal. The properties of this residual lactase were similar to those of the normal brush border enzyme. Following gel filtration β-galactosidase activity was found in the expected position for brush border lactase with an apparent molecular weight of 40 000; the K_m of this residual activity against both a synthetic substrate (p-nitrophenyl β-galactoside) and lactose, and its pH optimum against lactose (5.5–6.0), were in agreement for those of the 'normal' brush border lactase. The residual activity also showed a normal distribution from the crypt to the villus tip[32]. On polyacrylamide gel electrophoresis, reduced amounts of protein in the lactase region have been detected by both Crane et al.[33] and Freiburghaus et al.[28]

Two theories have been proposed to explain the differences in adult lactase activities in different populations: first, an adaptive response to dietary lactose; and second, a genetic mechanism[34]. The adaptive theory is based on the observation that an increase in total and specific lactase activities can be induced by prolonged feeding of lactose rich diets to rats[35]. In these experiments, unphysiological amounts of lactose were required to produce an effect, and the observed differences in lactase activities in the two groups of rats were relatively small. There is convincing evidence that human lactase activity is not dependent on dietary lactose intake. Kogut et al.[36] studied a group of patients with galactosaemia who had received a lactose restricted diet for periods of up to 17 years, and found that all the Caucasian subjects hydrolysed and tolerated a lactose load normally. The group of Pima Indians studied by Johnson et al.[39] consume reasonable quantities of milk from an early age, and yet virtually all have lactose malabsorption from the age of four.

A genetic basis is now generally accepted, and recent studies using both ethnically pure and mixed families are consistent with the hypothesis that high lactase levels are inherited as an autosomal dominant trait whereas reduced lactase activity is inherited in an autosomal recessive manner[37–39].

Sucrase–isomaltase deficiency

Congenital sucrase–isomaltase (S–I) deficiency was first described in 1960 by Weijers et al.[40] and, although it is generally believed to be a very rare condition, it may occur in as many as 0.2% of North Americans[41] and 10% of Greenland Eskimos[42]. This means that the prevalence of the heterozygous state may vary from 9–43%.

There is a wide spectrum in the severity of symptoms ranging from severe diarrhoea in infancy to intermittent bothersome symptoms in the older child[43,44]. As a result the correct diagnosis may be missed, symptoms being attributed to conditions such as 'irritable colon' or 'maternal anxiety'. The definitive diagnosis requires the demonstration of deficiency of sucrase and isomaltase activities. Maltase (a-glucosidase) activity is also reduced in this condition since sucrase, which also splits the a 1–4 glucosidic links of maltose and other straight chain polymers of glucose, accounts for up to 75% of the total maltase activity. Elimination of sucrose from the diet results in prompt symptomatic improvement.

In recent years increasing interest has been focussed on the molecular level in an attempt to understand the nature of the defect in S–I deficiency. As previously discussed, Conklin et al.[12] have separated the sucrase and isomaltase moieties of the complex and found isomaltase to be labile in the absence of its partner. On this basis they suggested that in S–I deficiency it was the sucrase moiety which was deleted or defective, and that isomaltase deficiency was a secondary event.

Using an immunofluorescent technique, Dubs et al.[45] have reported varying quantities of sucrase–isomaltase protein in enzymatically inactive jejunal mucosa from six affected patients. This suggests a discrete structural alteration of the sucrase affecting the catalytic site. The same group[46], using polyacrylamide gel electrophoresis of membrane fractions, could not detect normal S–I protein but observed an abnormal protein band. They suggested that the latter band could be the protein identified by immunofluorescence, but insufficient biopsy material was available to confirm this.

Using similar electrophoretic techniques other workers[47, 48] were also unable to find a normal S–I band, but in contrast to Freiburghaus et al.[46] they were unable to detect an abnormal protein. These results suggest that the enzyme protein is absent. Similar findings were reported by Gray et al.[49] who analysed the protein quantitatively by radioimmunoassay as well as the hydrolytic activity. The protein was undetected in seven patients, but present in trace amounts in two. Thus, either the protein was absent or had undergone major conformational changes affecting both the antigenic and catalytic sites.

These studies suggest the existence of two or more variants, but the precise nature of the molecular defect in S–I deficiency has not yet been defined.

Trehalase deficiency

Trehalose (α-D-glucopyranosil-α-D-glucopyranoside) is a non-reducing disaccharide which occurs in most lower plants, some microorganisms, many insects, and in *Ascaris lumbricoides* and *Artenia salina*. It is a curious paradox that although the young growing mushroom is the only known source of trehalose for man, trehalase is a well established member of the human brush border oligosaccharidases. Trehalase deficiency has only once been well documented in a family who developed symptoms following the ingestion of mushrooms[50]. It is suggested that an autosomal dominant type of inheritance is likely.

Congenital glucose–galactose malabsorption

This disorder is now a well established entity and was first described in 1962 by Lindquist and Meeuwisse[51].

Severe gastrointestinal symptoms follow the ingestion of milk in the neonatal period and unless glucose and/or galactose containing foods are withdrawn from the diet, the condition can be fatal. Since its original description several studies have been directed towards defining the basic defect and these are summarized in Table 2.1. *In vitro* and *in vivo* studies

TABLE 2.1   **Studies in congenital glucose–galactose malabsorption**

Authors	Findings
[52]Schneider, Kinter and Stirling (1966)	Absent binding of galactose and phlorizin to mucosa
[57]Eggermont and Loeb (1966)	No active mucosal uptake of glucose L-leucine mucosal uptake normal
[56]Meeuwisse and Dahlqvist (1968)	No active mucosal uptake of glucose L-alanine mucosal uptake normal Mucosal $(Na^+–K^+)$-ATPase normal Impaired glucose absorption* Impaired glucose uptake in father
[58]Elsas et al. (1970)	No active mucosal uptake of glucose Reduced V_{max} ; K_m normal Impaired renal reabsorption of glucose* Impaired mucosal uptake in both parents
[53]Phillips and McGill (1973)	No active glucose absorption* Na^+-coupled glucose absorption absent*
[54]Wimberley, Harries and Burgess (1974)	Na^+-coupled glucose uptake absent L-leucine uptake normal
[55]Hughes and Senior (1975)	No HRT† or glucose* Reduced number of carriers not demonstrated*
[59]Fairclough et al. (1978)	No active glucose absorption* No HRT† of glucose* Reduced number of carriers not demonstrated*

* Indicates *in vivo* studies; all other studies perform *in vitro* on biopsy material.
† Denotes hydrolase related transport

have demonstrated defective or completely absent sodium coupled mucosal uptake of glucose in affected cases, and two studies reported impaired uptake in one or both parents. Absorption of fructose, xylose, and the amino acids leucine and alanine is intact[52–55]. As previously discussed $(Na^+–K^+)$-ATPase provides the driving force to maintain the sodium gradient across the brush border membrane of the enterocyte; this gradient permits active absorption of glucose, galactose and amino acids into the cell. The fact that amino acid absorption and $(Na^+–K^+)$-ATPase activity is normal argues strongly against diminution of the sodium gradient as the basic defect in this condition. The studies shown in Table 2.1 strongly suggest that the defect lies at the brush border level of the cell, but the precise molecular defect has not been defined. *In vitro* studies have suggested a reduced number of normal affinity glucose–galactose carriers, but two *in vivo* perfusion studies have failed to substantiate this[55, 59]. It seems more likely that an absent or defective carrier is the basic cause of glucose–galactose malabsorption, and the application of techniques such as SDS polyacrylamide gel electrophoresis to brush border preparations obtained from patients with glucose–galactose malabsorption should resolve this intriguing question.

Mucosal disaccharidase activities are normal[53, 54, 56] and, on the basis of *in vitro* animal work[20–22], absorption of glucose and galactose from disaccharides by HRT might be expected to occur in glucose–galactose malabsorption. As shown in Table 2.1, two independent groups of workers have failed to demonstrate this, casting doubt on the nutritional importance of HRT in man.

SECONDARY CARBOHYDRATE MALABSORPTION

Secondary carbohydrate malabsorption results from histological damage to the small intestinal mucosa and disruption of normal absorption systems. In contrast to the genetically determined disorders, mucosal damage may be accompanied by malabsorption of a wide variety of other nutrients depending on the extent of the lesion along the small intestine.

Causes

Numerous causes of secondary sugar malabsorption have been described and the better recognised ones are listed in Table 2.2. The severity of the clinical manifestations in these conditions is much greater in newborns and young infants than in adults.

Intolerance of lactose is by far the most important in clinical practice, particularly in young infants following an episode of acute gastroenteritis. This may be due to the fact that hydrolysis is the rate limiting step in absorption of lactose but not of other disaccharides. Depression of lactase activity is of particular clinical importance since its activity is normally considerably less than that of other disaccharidases. It may also explain why intolerance to maltose and sucrose is uncommon.

Lactulose is a non-reducing disaccharide composed of galactose and fructose and cannot be hydrolysed by the small intestinal mucosa. It is formed from lactose during the processing of milk products. Its presence may simulate lactose intolerance in infants returning to milk feeds following an episode of gastroenteritis[60].

Pancreatic α-amylase activity is extremely low or even absent at birth, particularly in premature infants[61]. A dramatic increase to optimum levels

TABLE 2.2   **Causes of secondary carbohydrate malabsorption**

Disaccharides:

Gastroenteritis
Cow's milk protein intolerance
Malnutrition
Coeliac disease
Tropical sprue
Following surgery to the gastrointestinal tract
Phototherapy in newborns
Immune deficiency syndromes
Necrotizing enterocolitis

Monosaccharides:

Gastroenteritis
Malnutrition
Staphylococcal pneumonia

(600-fold in premature and 200-fold in full term infants) occurs by the age of 9 months to 13 years. Starch feeding in early infancy may therefore result in diarrhoea, but this is not severe since the osmotic effect of intraluminal starch is relatively small. Approximately 30% of starch is normally hydrolysed to α-limit dextrins[62] which cannot be absorbed without further hydrolysis by isomaltase. Ingestion of starch may therefore produce diarrhoea in patients with secondary depression of mucosal isomaltase, but again symptoms are mild because of the higher molecular weight of α-limit dextrins which, per unit weight, have only 10–20% of the osmotic effect of disaccharides.

Secondary malabsorption of one or all three of the important dietary monosaccharides (glucose, galactose and fructose) is uncommon but has been reported[63–65] and in one infant appeared to be secondary to staphylococcal pneumonia[63].

Mechanisms

Reduction of mucosal disaccharidase activities in an enteropathy is multifactorial. Structural damage to enterocyte brush border membrane coupled with a reduction in the absorptive surface area of the small intestine could reduce the hydrolytic capacity of the mucosa.

The degree of maturity of the surface epithelial cells may also be important. Disaccharidase activities are low in undifferentiated crypt cells, and increase to reach maximal activity when these cells have differentiated to mature enterocytes at about the mid-villous region of the mucosa[2]. In conditions where the rate of turnover of surface cells is increased (e.g. coeliac disease and viral enteritis) the population of immature cells in the epithelium increases and the capacity to hydrolyse disaccharides decreases. A similar relationship between crypt and villous cells exists for (Na^+-K^+)-ATPase, the enzyme which provides the driving force for active sodium coupled absorption of monosaccharides and amino acids. Thus, increased numbers of immature cells may also impede the absorption of monosaccharides and amino acids.

It should be stressed that gastrointestinal symptoms (i.e. clinical 'intolerance') occur only when there is extensive disruption of the small intestinal mucosa. The enteropathy seen in coeliac disease, for example, is a predominantly proximal lesion and clinical intolerance to ingested sugars is rare in our experience, presumably because the more distal region of the small intestine is able to compensate. This is particularly important in the interpretation of disaccharidase activities assayed in mucosa obtained from the proximal small intestine with respect to management of the patient; reduced enzyme activities are not synonymous with clinical intolerance.

PATHOPHYSIOLOGY OF GASTROINTESTINAL SYMPTOMS

Whether carbohydrate malabsorption is primary or secondary the pathophysiological mechanisms responsible for gastrointestinal symptoms are similar. Unabsorbed sugars accumulate in the lumen of the small intestine creating an osmotic gradient which results in bulk movement of fluid and electrolytes from plasma to lumen. In addition the physiological drive which glucose and galactose provide for absorption of fluid and electrolytes is lost. As a result excessive amounts of fluid and sugars enter the large intestine where bacterial metabolism of sugars generates volatile short chain organic acids (e.g. acetic, butyric, propionic, lactic acids), carbon dioxide and hydrogen. This results in a second osmotic gradient between plasma and lumen with further movement of fluid into the lumen. These pathophysiological events lead to colicky abdominal pain and distention, watery acid stools containing increased amounts of electrolytes and sugars, and perianal excoriation due to increased concentration of H^+ ion. Body losses of fluid and electrolytes, particularly in young infants, may be such as to lead to severe dehydration, neurological complications and even death.

The need for early diagnosis and prompt treatment in such cases cannot be emphasized enough.

References

1. Ugolev, A. M. (1965). Membrane (contact) digestion. *Physiol. Rev.*, **45**, 555
2. Gray, G. M. (1975). Carbohydrate digestion and absorption. Role of the small intestine. *N. Engl. J. Med.*, **292**, 1225
3. Newcomer, A. D. and McGill, D. B. (1966). Distribution of disaccharidase activity in the small bowel of normal and lactase deficient subjects. *Gastroenterology*, **51**, 481
4. Saito, M., Murakami, E. and Suda, M. (1976). Circadian rhythms in disaccharidases of rat small intestine and its relation to food intake. *Biochim. Biophys. Acta*, **421**, 177
5. Gray, G. M. and Santiago, N. A. (1966). Disaccharide absorption in normal and diseased human intestine. *Gastroenterology*, **51**, 489
6. Alpers, D. H. and Cote, M. N. (1971). Inhibition of lactose hydrolysis by dietary sugars. *Am. J. Physiol.*, **221**, 865
7. Asp, N-G., Dahlqvist, A. and Koldovsky, O. (1969). Human small intestinal β-galactosidases. Separation and characterization of one lactase and one hetero β-galactosidase. *Biochem. J.*, **114**, 351
8. Gray, G. M. and Santiago, N. A. (1969). Intestinal β-galactosidases. I. Separation and characterization of three enzymes in normal human intestine. *J. Clin. Invest.*, **48**, 716
9. Asp, N.-G. (1971). Human small intestinal β-galactosidases. Separation and characterization of three forms of an acid β-galactosidase. *Biochem. J.*, **121**, 299
10. Lojda, Z., Fric, P. and Jode, J. (1972). Histochemische Befunde in der Dünndarmschleimhaut bei Störungen der Kohlenhydratabsorption. *Dtsch. Z. Verdau. Stoffwechselkr.*, **32**, 163
11. Asp, N.-G. and Dahlqvist, A. (1974). Intestinal β-galactosidases in adult low lactase activity and in congenital lactase deficiency. *Enzyme*, **18**, 84
12. Conklin, K. A., Yamashiro, K. M. and Gray, G. M. (1975). Human intestinal sucrase-isomaltase. Identification of free sucrase and isomaltase and cleavage of the hybrid into active distinct subunits. *J. Biol. Chem.*, **250**, 5735
13. Brunner, J., Hauser, H., Semenza, G. and Wacker, H. (1977). Incorporation of pure hydrolases isolated from brush border membranes in single-bilayer lecithin vesicles. In *Biochemistry of Membrane Transport, FEBS Symposium No. 42*, p. 105. (Berlin: Springer-Verlag)
14. Maestracci, D. (1976). Enzymic solubilisation of the human intestinal brush border membrane enzymes. *Biochim. Biophys. Acta*, **433**, 469
15. Alpers, D. H. and Seetharam, B. (1977). Pathophysiology of diseases involving intestinal brush-border proteins. *N. Engl. J. Med.*, **296**, 1047
16. Crane, R. K. (1965) Na^+-dependent transport in the intestine and other animal tissues. *Fed. Proc.*, **24**, 1000
17. Kimmich, G. A. (1973). Coupling between Na^+ and sugar transport in small intestine. *Biochim. Biophys. Acta*, **300**, 31

18. Honegger, P. and Semenza, G. (1973). Multiplicity of carriers for free glucalogues in hamster small intestine. *Biochim. Biophys. Acta,* **318,** 390
19. Debnam, E. S. and Levin, R. J. (1976). Influence of specific dietary sugars on the jejunal mechanisms for glucose, galactose, and α-methyl glucoside absorption: evidence for multiple sugar carriers. *Gut,* **17,** 92
20. Malathi, P., Ramaswamy, K., Caspary, W. F. and Crane, R. K. (1973). Studies on the transport of glucose from disaccharides by hamster small intestine *in vitro.* I. Evidence for a disaccharidase-related transport system. *Biochim. Biophys. Acta,* **307,** 613
21. Ramaswamy, K., Malathi, P., Caspary, W. F. and Crane, R. K. (1974). Studies on the transport of glucose from disaccharides by hamster small intestine *in vitro.* II. Characteristics of the disaccharidase-related transport system. *Biochim. Biophys. Acta,* **345,** 39
22. Ramaswamy, K., Malathi, P. and Crane, R. K. (1976). Demonstration of hydrolase-related glucose transport in brush border membrane vesicles prepared from guinea pig small intestine. *Biochem. Biophys. Res. Commun.,* **68,** 162
23. Annegers, J. H. (1964). Intestinal absorption of hexoses in the dog. *Am. J. Physiol.,* **206,** 1095
24. Holdsworth, C. D. and Dawson, A. M. (1965). Absorption of fructose in man. *Proc. Soc. Exp. Biol. Med.,* **118,** 142
25. Schultz, S. G., and Strecker, C. K. (1970). Fructose influx across the brush border of rabbit ileum. *Biochim. Biophys. Acta,* **211,** 586
26. Holzel, A., Schwarz, V. and Sutcliffe, K. W. (1959). Defective lactose absorption causing malnutrition in infancy. *Lancet,* **1,** 1126
27. Levin, B., Abraham, J. M., Burgess, E. A. and Wallis, P. G. (1970). Congenital lactose malabsorption. *Arch. Dis. Child.,* **45,** 173
28. Freiburghaus, A. U., Schmitz, J., Schindler, M., Rotthauwe, H. W., Kuitunen, P., Launiala, K. and Hadorn, B. (1976). Protein patterns of brush border fragments in congenital lactose malabsorption and in specific hypolactasia of the adult. *N. Engl. J. Med.,* **294,** 1030
29. Sunshine, P. and Kretchmer, N. (1964). Intestinal disaccharidases. Absence in two species of sea lions. *Science,* **144,** 850
30. Gray, G. M. (1978). Intestinal disaccharidase deficiencies and glucose galactose malabsorption. In J. B. Stanberg, J. B. Wyngaarden and D. S. Fredrickson (eds). *The Metabolic Basis of Inherited Disease,* 4th Ed. pp. 1526–1536. (New York: McGraw Hill Book Company)
31. Asp, N.-G., Berg, N. O., Dahlqvist, A., Jassila, J. and Salmi, H. (1971). The activity of three different small intestinal β-galactosidases in adults with and without lactase deficiency. *Scand. J. Gastroenterol.,* **6,** 755
32. Nordstrom, C. and Dahlqvist, A. (1973). Quantitative distribution of some enzymes along the villi and crypts of human small intestine. *Scand. J. Gastroenterol.,* **8,** 407
33. Crane, R. K., Menard, D., Preiser, H. and Cerda, J. J. (1976). The molecular basis of brush border membrane disease. In L. Botz, J. F. Hoffman and A. Leaf (eds), *Membranes and Diseases: International Conference on Biological Membranes,* pp. 229–241. (New York: Raven Press)
34. Rosensweig, N. S. (1971). Adult lactase deficiency – genetic control or adaptive response? *Gastroenterology,* **60,** 464

35. Bolin, T. D., Pirola, R. C. and Davis, A. E. (1969). Adaptation of intestinal lactase in the rat. *Gastroenterology*, **57**, 406
36. Kogut, M. D., Donnell, G. N. and Shaw, K. N. F. (1967). Studies of lactose absorption in patients with galactosemia. *J. Pediatr.*, **71**, 75
37. Ransome-Kuti, O., Kretchmer, N., Johnson, J. D. and Gribble, J. T. (1975). A genetic study of lactose digestion in Nigerian families. *Gastroenterology*, **68**, 431
38. Newcomer, A. D., Gordon, H., Thomas, P. J. and McGill, D. B. (1977). Family studies of lactase deficiency in the American Indian. *Gastroenterology*, **73**, 985
39. Johnson, J. D., Simoons, F. J., Hurwitz, R., Grange, A., Mitchell, C. H., Sinatra, F. R., Surchin, P., Robertson, W. V., Bennett, P. H. and Kretchmer, N. (1977). Lactose malabsorption among the Pima Indians of Arizona. *Gastroenterology*, **73**, 1299
40. Weijers, H. A., van de Kramer, J. H., Mossel, D. A. A. and Dicke, W. K. (1960). Diarrhoea caused by a deficiency of sugar-splitting enzymes. *Lancet*, **2**, 296
41. Peterson, M. L. and Herber, R. (1967). Intestinal sucrase deficiency. *Trans. Assoc. Am. Physicians*, **80**, 275
42. McNair, A., Gudmand-Høyer, E., Jarnum, S. and Orrild, L. (1972). Sucrose malabsorption in Greenland. *Br. Med. J.*, **2**, 19
43. Antonowicz, I., Lloyd Still, J. D., Khaw, K. T. and Shwachman, H. (1972). Congenital sucrase-isomaltase deficiency. Observations over a period of six years. *Pediatrics*, **49**, 847
44. Ament, M. E., Perera, D. R. and Esther, L. J. (1973). Sucrase-isomaltase deficiency – a frequently misdiagnosed disease. *J. Pediatr.*, **83**, 721
45. Dubs, R., Steinmann, B. and Gitzelmann, R. (1973). Demonstration of an inactive enzyme antigen in sucrase-isomaltase deficiency. *Helv. Paediatr. Acta*, **28**, 187
46. Freiburghaus, A. U., Dubs, R., Hadorn, B., Gaze, H., Hauri, H. P. and Gizelmann, R. (1977). The brush border membrane in hereditary sucrase-isomaltase deficiency – abnormal protein pattern and presence of immunoreactive enzyme. *Eur. J. Clin. Invest.*, **7**, 455
47. Preiser, H., Menard, D., Crane, R. K. and Cerda, J. J. (1974). Deletion of enzyme protein from the brush border membrane in sucrase-isomaltase deficiency. *Biochim. Biophys. Acta*, **363**, 279
48. Schmitz, J., Conmegrain, C., Maestracci, D. and Rey, J. (1974). Absence of brush border sucrase-isomaltase complex in congenital sucrose intolerance. *Biomedicine*, **21**, 440
49. Gray, G. M., Conklin, K. A. and Townley, R. R. W. (1976). Sucrase-isomaltase deficiency. Absence of an inactive enzyme variant. *N. Engl. J. Med.*, **294**, 750
50. Madzarovová-Nohejlova, J. (1973). Trehalase deficiency in a family. *Gastroenterology*, **65**, 130
51. Lindquist, B. and Meeuwisse, G. W. (1962). Chronic diarrhoea caused by monosaccharide malabsorption. *Acta Paediatr.*, **51**, 674
52. Schneider, A. J., Kinter, W. B. and Stirling, C. E. (1966). Glucose-galactose malabsorption. *N. Engl. J. Med.*, **274**, 305
53. Phillips, S. F. and McGill, D. B. (1973). Glucose-galactose malabsorption in

an adult: perfusion studies of sugar, electrolyte, and water transport. *Am. J. Dig. Dis.*, **18**, 1017

54. Wimberley, P. D., Harries, J. T. and Burgess, E. A. (1974). Congenital glucose-galactose malabsorption. *Proc. R. Soc. Med.*, **67**, 755

55. Hughes, W. S. and Senior, J. R. (1975). The glucose-galactose malabsorption syndrome in a 23 year old woman. *Gastroenterology*, **68**, 142

56. Meeuwisse, G. W. and Dahlqvist, A. (1968). Glucose-galactose malabsorption. A study with biopsy of the small intestinal mucosa. *Acta Paediatr. Scand.*, **57**, 273

57. Eggermont, E. and Loeb, H. (1966). Glucose-galactose intolerance. *Lancet*, **2**, 343

58. Elsas, L. J., Hillman, R. E., Patterson, J. H. and Rosenberg, L. (1970). Renal and intestinal hexose transport in familial glucose-galactose malabsorption. *J. Clin. Invest.*, **49**, 576

59. Fairclough, P. D., Clark, M. L., Dawson, A. M., Silk, D. B. A., Milla, P. J. and Harries, J. T. (1979). Absorption of glucose and maltose in congenital glucose-galactose malabsorption. *Pediatr. Res.* (In press)

60. Hendrickse, R. G., Wooldridge, M. A. W. and Russell, A. (1977). Lactulose in baby milks causing diarrhoea simulating lactose intolerance. *Br. Med. J.*, **1**, 1194

61. Zoppi, G., Andreotti, G., Pajno-Ferrara, F., Njai, D. M. and Gaburro, D. (1972). Exocrine pancreas function in premature and full term neonates. *Pediatr. Res.*, **6**, 880

62. Roberts, P. J. P. and Whelan, W. J. (1960). The mechanism of carbohydrase action. 5. Action of human salivary α-amylase on amylopectin and glycogen. *Biochem. J.*, **76**, 246

63. Harries, J. T. and Francis, D. E. M. (1968). Temporary monosaccharide intolerance. *Acta Paediatr. Scand.*, **57**, 505

64. Lifshitz, F., Coello-Ramirez, P. and Guttierrez-Toppette, G. (1970). Monosaccharide intolerance and hypoglycaemia in infants with diarrhoea. I. Clinical course in 23 infants. *J. Pediatr.*, **77**, 595

65. Lifshitz, F., Coello-Ramirez, P. and Guttierrez-Toppette, G. (1970). Monosaccharide intolerance and hypoglycaemia in infants with diarrhoea. II. Metabolic studies in 23 infants. *J. Pediatr.*, **77**, 604

3

Clinical aspects of disordered carbohydrate absorption

A. S. McNeish and M. J. Harran

INTRODUCTION

Carbohydrate malabsorption can arise from derangement of any part of the digestive or absorptive processes that have been described in the preceding paper by Harries and Muller. In practice it is mainly disorders of the mucosal phase of carbohydrate hydrolysis and transport that give rise to clinical disease.

These disorders may be genetic or acquired, temporary or permanent. With the exception of late onset lactose intolerance, which affects older children and adults, the majority of severe clinical problems arise in the paediatric age range, and especially in infancy.

GENERAL FEATURES OF CARBOHYDRATE MALABSORPTION AND INTOLERANCE

It is important to differentiate these two terms which can cause confusion if used synonymously. Carbohydrate malabsorption arises from impairment of the normal absorptive processes in the intestine. It is essentially a laboratory diagnosis, reached as a result of, for example, oral loading tests, perfusion studies or identification of unabsorbed substrate in the stools. Carbohydrate intolerance is the clinical syndrome with prominent intestinal symptoms which may arise following the ingestion of a sugar that is poorly absorbed. All intolerant subjects have evidence of malabsorption of that sugar, but the converse is not true.

The predominant symptoms and signs in a patient with sugar intolerance are intestinal. They are the result of the osmotic effects of unabsorbed carbohydrate in the lumen of the small bowel and of the products of bacterial fermentation in the large intestine. The osmotic pressure of the unabsorbed carbohydrate in the small intestine leads to a secretion of water and electrolytes into the lumen until osmotic equilibrium is reached[1]. A proportion of the carbohydrate may be excreted unchanged in the stools, but the majority is hydrolysed by ileal and especially colonic bacteria to small carbohydrate molecules, short chain organic acids, hydrogen, carbon dioxide, and other fermentative products[2]. The organic acids lower the stool pH, inhibit water absorption from the colon[3], and contribute to the increased intestinal motility that follows increased intraluminal volume[1].

The severity of the resulting symptoms varies with age, the extent and severity of bowel disease (in secondary disorders of absorption), the dietary load of the offending carbohydrate, the capacity of the colon to absorb the excess fluid that is delivered from the small intestine, and the nature of any underlying disorder.

In general, watery acid diarrhoea with excoriated buttocks is the hallmark of sugar intolerance in the young infant; fluid losses may be profound and lifethreatening. In the older child, loose stools may be mild or intermittent only, and in the adult there may be little diarrhoea, but rather, cramping abdominal pains, borborygmi and bloating. Abdominal distension may be prominent, especially in infants, who may also have recurring vomiting. Weight loss in infants is usual.

Complications

The risk of further sequelae varies with age, and is especially important under the age of one year. Dehydration may be complicated by a metabolic acidosis which is caused by several mechanisms. Large quantities of bicarbonate are secreted into the intestinal lumen to neutralise the contents. Hydrogen ions produced by bacterial fermentation of the carbohydrate in the lower bowel are absorbed into the body fluids[4].

Untreated lactose intolerance in infancy can lead to a more generalised malabsorption of other sugars[5], nitrogenous compounds[6] and fats[7], with further impairment of nutrition. The frequency with which these complications arise varies with age, the state of nutrition before the onset of diarrhoea, and the delay in beginning adequate therapy[8]. In practice, severe complications occur more commonly in the developing world than in the UK, especially those following acute gastroenteritis. These sequelae may also contribute to the development of 'intractable diarrhoea in infancy'[9].

The interrelated mechanisms underlying the above sequence of events are incompletely understood, and there are discrepancies between experimental and clinical observations. Luminal bacteria can proliferate in a milieu of unabsorbed carbohydrate and fermentation products[10]. Such bacteria may inhibit the absorption of sugars, fluid and electrolytes in the small intestine directly[11, 12], or indirectly through deconjugated bile acids[13], short chain fatty acids[14] or other metabolic products. The possible relationship between lactose intolerance, bacteria and acquired food protein intolerance will be discussed below[15,16].

In some studies there has been a good correlation between intestinal bacterial overgrowth and sugar (especially monosaccharide) intolerance[10, 17], and between the concentration of unconjugated bile acids and impaired glucose transport[18]. Others have failed to detect significant amounts of deconjugated bile acids in the duodenum in infants with diarrhoea, sugar intolerance and bacterial overgrowth[19]. The severity of the primary illness and the intolerance, and the numbers and species of bacteria may be important in determining the outcome.

Lastly, pneumatosis intestinalis has been described as a rare complication of severe carbohydrate intolerance[20].

CLINICAL SYNDROMES OF DISORDERED CARBOHYDRATE ABSORPTION

These are summarized in Tables 3.1 and 3.2.

Primary absorptive defects

These conditions are congenital, and result from a permanent absence in the small intestine of a specific oligosaccharidase activity or of a specific transport pathway in glucose–galactose malabsorption.

Sucrase–isomaltase deficiency These enzyme activities reside within a complex protein molecule in the intestinal brush border[35]. Absence of the protein[36] is inherited as an autosomal recessive[37]. The homozygous condition is uncommon, although its exact incidence is not known. It is much commoner in Greenland Eskimos, in whom 10% may have the disorder[38].

Symptoms begin when sucrose is added to the diet. Some proprietory infant milks contain sucrose, so that in artificially fed infants, there may be an onset of watery diarrhoea within a day or two of birth. Breastfed babies are

TABLE 3.1   Classification of clinical disorders of carbohydrate absorption

Primary:

(a) Deficiency of mucosal oligosaccharidases
    Sucrase
    Lactase
    Trehalase
(b) Defective mucosal transport
    Glucose–galactose

Ontogenetic:
    Late onset lactase deficiency

Secondary:

    Disaccharide malabsorption
    Monosaccharide malabsorption

symptom free until sucrose containing weaning foods are introduced. Some infants fail to thrive but many grow normally. A mild degree of steatorrhoea has been reported[39].

For a reason that is not clear, some cases of this enzyme deficiency do not present until later childhood or even adulthood[37, 40]. In those patients, symptoms are milder and often intermittent, with a variable degree of loose stools, abdominal cramps and intestinal gas.

Heterozygotes may develop intestinal symptoms after a large oral load, and may present with 'irritable bowel syndrome'[41].

Sucrase–isomaltase also hydrolyses maltose, but there is usually sufficient maltase activity in the other brush border maltases, and therefore starch intolerance is uncommon.

The diagnosis is established by demonstrating absent or minimal sucrase and isomaltase activity, and normal lactase activity, in a biopsy of small intestine that is structurally normal. Lowered ratios of sucrase to lactase are useful in identifying the heterozygote trait[37].

The degree of dietary restriction of sucrose that is required to treat these patients varies from case to case. In infancy it is advisable to eliminate sucrose completely from the diet. Details are outlined in Dorothy Francis' excellent book[42]. Older children and adults with the disorder often become expert at adjusting their own diets to avoid symptoms.

Congenital lactase deficiency   This is a very rare inborn error of metabolism, in which the brush border β-galactosidase, lactase, is absent. Its mode of inheritance is not completely understood.

Congenital lactose intolerance was first described in 1959[43]; mucosal disaccharidase assays were not available at that time. In the literature of the next few years, the condition was probably overdiagnosed, because at that time it was not realised that secondary lactase deficiency could be found in a mucosa that had only minor histological abnormalities, as luctase is the most vulnerable enzyme.

Nevertheless, there are a few cases described of primary lactase deficiency that withstand close scrutiny[44-46]. These infants develop severe watery diarrhoea within a day or two of birth, as soon as milk feeding is established. For reasons of practicality and safety, investigations at that time may have to be confined to examination of the stools (see below) and the observation of response to a lactose free milk. Attempts to perform lactose tolerance tests in these young infants can lead to dangerous fluid losses, and therefore should be avoided.

The hallmark of diagnosis of lactase deficiency is demonstration of an isolated absence of brush border lactase in a mucosa that is structurally normal. There are two other β-galactosidases in the enterocytes, and one of these, lysosomal acid β-galactosidase, can hydrolyse lactose. If the assay for lactase is made on a conventional mucosal homogenate[47], residual weak 'lactase' activity will be found in the absence of brush border lactase[48].

In 1958, Durand[49] described a form of congenital lactose intolerance in infants with vomiting, failure to thrive, acidosis, lactosuria and aminoaciduria. Some children died, while others appeared to recover and to tolerate lactose after a few months. It has been shown that this is a different condition from congenital alactasia, since lactase activity is present in the mucosa[50]. The aetiology is unknown. Berg et al.[51] have postulated that there might be an abnormal permeability of the gastric mucosa to lactose and other oligosaccharides.

Trehalase deficiency Trehalose is a disaccharide that is found in some insects, worms, bacteria and plants. The only known dietary source for humans is young mushrooms.

A single family has been described in which at least two members had intolerance to mushrooms, and mucosal trehalase deficiency[52].

Congenital glucose–galactose malabsorption This rare condition, first described in 1962[53, 54], has attracted much attention because of the information that it yields about basic absorptive mechanisms. Harries and Muller have reviewed these in the previous paper.

Clinically, this is a recessive disorder, characterised by explosive watery diarrhoea within 48 hours of birth. Renal tubular reabsorption of glucose is also impaired, with resulting glycosuria[55]. These infants are able to tolerate and absorb fructose, and a proprietory milk with fructose as the only carbohydrate forms a satisfactory basis of early dietary treatment. An adult with this condition has been described[56].

As in some other congenital disorders of sugar intolerance, a limited dietary tolerance to offending carbohydrates develops with increasing age, but some form of lifelong dietary restriction is required.

Ontogenetic late onset (acquired) lactase deficiency

Among many animal species, the pattern of intestinal lactase development is similar: peak levels are found in the neonatal animal, and after weaning enzyme activity falls to low levels[57]. Within the past 12 years it has become apparent that this pattern of lactase activity is commonly found in man. First described in Africa[58] and the Americas[59], it has now been observed in many parts of the world. It is now considered that this pattern of enzyme activity, with variable adult lactose intolerance, is the normal, and that persistence of lactase activity in the adult is the result of a genetic mutation[60]. Genetic studies in Nigeria[61] have indicated that the capacity to digest lactose is a Mendelian dominant, while lactose non-digestion is recessive.

It is not known what causes lactase levels to fall in the adult. There is no evidence in man that lactase levels are substrate dependent[62,63]. Kretchmer[60] has postulated that there is a regulatory gene that controls the developmental pattern of lactase synthesis and that mutation of this gene gave rise to the less common lactase persistence.

The patterns of adult human lactase activity throughout the world fall broadly into three classes[64]. Firstly, there are those who live in a classical non-milking zone and are non-digestors of lactose; this includes all the aboriginal peoples of Americas and Oceania, together with East Asians and many Africans. Secondly, there are those who live in a milking zone and cannot digest lactose; for example, many people from the Mediterranean and Near East, several African tribes and the majority of American Blacks. Thirdly, there are those who live in a milking zone and can digest lactose; this includes North Europeans, the inhabitants of West Pakistan and the Punjab, and three African groups (Fulani, Tussi, Masai). Simoons[65] has postulated that the pattern of development of dairying was closely related to those peoples with genetic lactase persistence.

There is considerable variation in the symptoms that milk will induce in these lactase deficient subjects. Certainly, many live in an area where milk is not consumed, so that no practical problem exists. The common symptoms previously described can of course be induced by drinking milk, but there are many lactase deficient adults who appear to be able to 'adapt' to milk drinking after weeks or months[66]. This is not the result of induction of lactase activity[67]; the mechanism is unknown.

Lactase deficiency of this type may be an aggravating problem in treating infectious diarrhoea or protein–energy malnutrition in many parts of the world and it is advisable to use a lactose free milk during the period of treatment and convalescence[68]. But milk products can be useful in these children, even if diarrhoea is provoked by their use[6]. The Food and Agriculture Organisation have stated that it would be wrong to discourage programmes to improve milk supplies and increase milk consumption among children because of a fear of milk intolerance[69].

Secondary absorptive disorders

Collectively, these disorders are much more frequent than the primary malabsorptive states. In oversimplified terms, many of them can be thought of as secondary to 'mucosal damage'. In some cases, the pathogenic mechanisms are complex, with contributions from mucosal injury, subnutrition, luminal metabolites, bacterial overgrowth and immunopathological processes. Age is again important so that secondary sugar intolerances are seen most frequently as temporary disorders in infants.

In reviewing the literature of these conditions it is clearly necessary to distinguish between sugar malabsorption and sugar intolerance. The references cited in Table 3.2 should be consulted for details of each disorder. The following paragraphs consider some aspects of clinically important intolerances.

Gastroenteritis   Bacterial and viral gastroenteritis may be complicated by sugar intolerance[12]. This is especially important if infection occurs under the age of 3 months, when up to 20% may have sugar intolerance[70]. Gastroenteritis superimposed on malnutrition is also very likely to be complicated by carbohydrate intolerance[22]. In most cases the aetiology is considered to be secondary to mucosal lesion[71], but overgrowth of luminal bacteria may play a part in severe cases. Coello-Ramirez and colleagues[10] found that the frequency of carbohydrate malabsorption was closely related to the abnormal numbers of bacteria that were cultured from the upper small intestine.

Lactose is most frequently the offending sugar, and lactase is the most readily depressed of the mucosal disaccharidases following mucosal injury[72]. Lactase is also the last to recover to normal values after mucosal healing[21]. Intolerance to sucrose and polysaccharides may be found in the most severe cases. Intolerance to all monosaccharides may complicate

TABLE 3.2   Secondary carbohydrate malabsorption (with references)

Disaccharide Malabsorption:

Coeliac disease[21]
Protein–energy malnutrition[22]
Gastroenteritis[12]
Giardiasis[23]
Tropical sprue[24]
Cystic fibrosis[25]
Immune deficiency states[26]
Cow's milk protein intolerance[15]
Inflammatory bowel disease[27]
Abetalipoproteinaemia[28]
Drugs[29]
Intestinal resection[30]
After intestinal surgery in neonates[3]
Phototherapy[31]
Hypoxia[32]
Prematurity[33]

Monosaccharide Malabsorption:

Gastroenteritis[12]
Intractable diarrhoea[9]
Gastrointestinal surgery in neonates[30]
Necrotising enterocolitis[34]
Protein–energy malnutrition[22]

---

gastroenteritis in neonates and young infants. It is more common in those cases where there is also severe lactose intolerance[5].

Details of therapy are beyond the scope of this review but it should be noted that iatrogenic factors can inadvertently play a part in causing all these post-enteritis problems. In the past, physicians have stopped all milk feeds for 24 to 48 h in infants with gastroenteritis followed by cautious reintroduction of dilute feeds. A return of diarrhoea has been the signal to stop feeds again, with perhaps a later trial of another dilute formula. Some infants with persisting diarrhoea have been treated in this way for many weeks[73] with grossly inadequate energy intake. This iatrogenic malnutrition has been proposed as an important factor in causing persistence of intestinal dysfunction[73].

Cow's milk protein intolerance   This condition is seen in infants, and is a temporary disorder[16, 74] that may follow acute gastroenteritis. There is usually a moderate enteropathy with depressed disaccharidase levels[75]. Liu *et al.*[15] showed that such infants are tolerant of lactose while on a milk-protein free diet, but quickly become intolerant of lactose if cow's milk protein is introduced. This lactose intolerance does not always correlate well with lactase levels in a jejunal biopsy specimen[76]. Whether this lactose intolerance with apparently normal lactase levels is a reflection of biopsy sampling error in a patchy mucosal lesion is not known.

The important practical point is that detection of lactose intolerance in an infant with gastroenteritis may be a clue that there is also an underlying food protein intolerance.

Coeliac disease The hallmark of untreated coeliac disease is a severe enteropathy with subtotal villous atrophy in the proximal small intestine. Depression of mucosal disaccharidases, especially lactase, is almost invariable[21], and lactose malabsorption can be demonstrated by various techniques[21]. This led to the recommendation that all newly diagnosed coeliac patients should be treated with a lactose-free (as well as a gluten-free) diet[77]. In practice, less than 5% of coeliac children have clinically important lactose intolerance[78]. The great majority thrive on a diet that contains lactose, again underlining the important distinction between biochemical malabsorption and clinical intolerance.

Intestinal surgery in neonates Burke and Anderson[30] described disaccharide and monosaccharide intolerance following intestinal surgery in neonates. In some, there had been partial resection of the small intestine, and loss of surface area for absorption was presumed to be the main cause. In other infants, the surgical procedures involved only the large intestine (for example, fashioning a colostomy in Hirschprung's disease); here the aetiology is less clear. Possible mechanisms involving stasis, overgrowth of bacteria, bile acids and other luminal metabolites have been discussed.

Secondary monosaccharide malabsorption This can arise in young infants as an accompaniment to disaccharide intolerance from many causes listed in Table 3.2. In addition, there are a group of young infants who have 'protracted'[9] or 'intractable'[79] diarrhoea, with multiple defects including monosaccharide malabsorption. In some of these infants, a post-enteritis aetiology is proposed[80] but seldom proven. There is occasionally a family history[9]. Some infants are intolerant of all monosaccharides, while others can tolerate fructose. The disorder may be temporary, but is frequently fatal[9]. Much needs to be learned about its basic causes.

DIAGNOSIS OF CARBOHYDRATE ABSORPTIVE DISORDERS

In primary disorders there may be a positive family history or symptoms suggesting one of the conditions that underlie a secondary malabsorption. Undoubtedly the most important information is obtained from a detailed dietary history, linking symptoms to ingestion of particular sugars. For infants, this requires a full knowledge of the composition of infant milks and weaning foods[42]. In older children and adults with intermittent symptoms, a dietary aetiology is not at all obvious. Table 3.3 outlines circumstances when the diagnosis of sugar intolerance should be considered.

Clinical response to dietary exclusion

The clinical response to dietary exclusion is sometimes listed as the last confirmatory evidence of sugar intolerance. In practice many infants with intolerance are too ill to justify formal challenges or even to have detailed invasive investigations. An empirical diagnosis, based on the history, clinical features and stool examination (see below) leads to the prescribing of lactose free, disaccharide free or even carbohydrate free diets[70]. The diagnosis can be confirmed later, after clinical recovery. In secondary disorders, even this confirmation is not always possible. The initial empirical treatment is continued for weeks or months[70]; during this period spontaneous recovery may occur so that subsequent investigation is unable to confirm beyond doubt the original diagnosis[81].

Examination of stools

This includes measurement of reducing substances, sugar chromatography, pH and organic acid content. In general these tests are more useful in infants than in older subjects.

TABLE 3.3   Clinical features that may suggest sugar intolerance

Infant:	Post infectious diarrhoea
	Relapse of diarrhoea when milk reintroduced
	Failure to thrive
	Family history of milk intolerance
	Chronic diarrhoea with abdominal distortion
	Irritable bowel syndrome
Older child and adult:	Abdominal cramps or loose stools after meals
	Irritable bowel syndrome
	Failure to thrive
	Recurring abdominal pain
	Coeliac disease ⎫ with persistent symptoms
	Inflammatory bowel disease ⎭

All tests must be performed on the liquid portion of fresh specimens, collected on polythene or other non-absorbent material[82]. Formed stools are unlikely to contain significant amounts of sugars[83]. It is necessary to perform the tests immediately or to freeze the specimen for later analysis. Faecal bacteria hydrolyse sugars very rapidly at room temperature[84] and pH and lactic acid content change quickly[85]. All stools must be tested, because some specimens may be sugar free even in patients with severe intolerance[5].

Tests for reducing substances[86] are very useful particularly if used serially through an illness. False positives can arise. Non-absorbable sugars (lactulose, plant hexoses), oligosaccharides of bacterial origin and non-carbohydrate substances may be present without any sugar intolerance[82, 83, 87, 88]. Sugars (mainly lactose, sucrose, glucose, galactose) may be found in healthy neonates and in older children and adults with diarrhoea that is not caused by sugar intolerance. For these reasons, sugar chromatography may be necessary to assess the significance of the stool reducing substances. With added knowledge of the detailed dietary intake, the type of sugar malabsorption can be accurately determined[83].

Faecal pH is influenced by the degree of colonic fermentation of unabsorbed carbohydrate, and reports differ about the diagnostic usefulness of measuring stool pH[83, 89]. A pH of less than 6 is frequently found in infants with fermentative diarrhoea but higher values do not exclude the diagnosis. Holzel[50] found that elevated faecal lactic acid was an aid to diagnosis, but it is not widely used.

Oral sugar loading tests

The observed response to an oral sugar load is one of the standard tests of carbohydrate absorption. The result can be interpreted in two ways. The shape of the blood sugar curve after ingestion is a measure of absorption: the observed symptoms after ingestion (coupled with stool examination, discussed above) may indicate clinical intolerance.

False positive and false negative blood sugar curves can occur[40, 62, 90]. 'Flat' blood glucose curves after oral lactose have been reported in up to 30% of normal subjects[62], probably as a result of delayed gastric emptying.

Ethanol given before oral lactose inhibits the hepatic metabolism of absorbed galactose. Isokoski et al.[91] showed that a failure of blood galactose to rise after lactose–ethanol identified accurately subjects with lactase deficiency. Newcomer et al.[92] confirmed the usefulness of this test, which gave only occasional false negative results. However, it is unethical for use in children.

Some eminent workers[85, 93] have found that the alteration in the water and sugar content of the stools after oral challenge is a very useful diagnostic aid. However there has been little attempt to standardise the techniques, and the tests are probably most useful if performed serially through an illness. On occasion, diarrhoea may be produced in normal subjects by the dose of sugar (2 g/kg) that is commonly used[62].

Perfusion studies of the intestine to examine carbohydrate absorption[94] are powerful research techniques reserved for special centres; they have great potential.

Radiology

Laws and Neale[95] reported that a barium-lactose meal gave a characteristic and diagnostic radiological appearance in lactase deficient subjects, with dilatation of the small bowel, dilution of contents and a rapid transit time. These findings have been confirmed[96, 97], though in the latter series there were 10–15% false positive results.

The test has been modified for use in children[78, 98]. Disadvantages include the need for a preliminary film using barium alone[78], and occasional unpleasant side effects. It is not widely used, but may have a place in the diagnosis of hypolactasia or hyposucrasia in the older child.

Mucosal enzyme assay

The development of an accurate assay for mucosal disaccharidases[47] in peroral biopsy specimens was the major stimulus to the understanding of the disorders that are summarized in this chapter.

In interpreting the results, several points need to be considered. Normal values for disaccharidase activities vary slightly with any modification of the original assay[99, 100]. They also vary with the population from which the control values were derived. The exact anatomical site of the biopsy is important and should be standardized, because disaccharidase levels vary throughout the small intestine[101].

In primary disorders of disaccharide absorption assay of enzyme levels is rightly regarded as the definitive test, with the finding of an isolated disaccharidase deficiency in an otherwise normal intestinal biopsy. In secondary disorders an intestinal biopsy can give information only about the structure and enzyme levels in a very small area of the intestinal mucosa. In these circumstances, there may be a poor correlation between disaccharidase levels and evidence of sugar intolerance.

Specimens of intestinal mucosa can also be used for *in vitro* studies of monosaccharide transport[102] but they are research tools beyond the scope of this review.

Breath tests

$^{14}CO_2$ If $^{14}CO_2$ is recovered in the breath after oral ingestion of a ^{14}C-labelled compound, it can be concluded that at least a proportion of the compound has been absorbed and metabolized. This principle has been applied to assess the absorption of $[1-^{14}C]$lactose[103, 104]. Newcomer et al.[92] observed a better correlation between $^{14}CO_2$ exhalation and lactase activity in small intestinal biopsies than by measured blood glucose after oral intake of lactose. The $^{14}CO_2$ breath test gave complete separation between lactase deficient and normal individuals, with no false positive or negative results. These results have been confirmed by others[105].

Though these results are encouraging there are some theoretical disadvantages. The test will be affected by gastric emptying and glucose intermediary metabolism. It depends on the proportion of sugar that is absorbed, whereas the clinically important measurement is of the excreted amount. $^{14}CO_2$ may be produced by fermentation in the colon of unabsorbed ^{14}C-sugar, and this could contribute to a false negative result. Lastly ^{14}C is unacceptable for use in children because of its radioactivity. ^{13}C-labelled sugars are available in special centres[106, 107] and are non-radioactive, but have the other disadvantages of ^{14}C-labelling discussed above.

H_2 The amount of hydrogen (H_2) excreted in the breath correlates well with the amount that is produced in the intestine by fermentation of luminal carbohydrates[108]. This principle can be used to study the delivery of digestible or absorbable substrates (e.g. lactose, D-glucose, D-xylose) or undigestible (e.g. lactulose) substrates to the colon[109] which contains bacteria capable of H_2 production[2]. The proximal small intestine is the site of carbohydrate absorption, and is not normally colonized by H_2 producing bacteria. Breath H_2 concentration after an oral load of sugar is therefore a measure of the degree of malabsorption. It is independent of gastric emptying and intermediary metabolism, and does not involve the use of radio-istopes. Technical details are available elsewhere[110].

Current data suggest that breath H_2 measurement is the most accurate indirect method of detecting lactase deficiency[110, 111]. It can also be used for population screening for lactase deficiency[112] and has great potential in paediatric gastroenterology[113]. Misleading results could occur in the rare instance that there is absence of H_2 producing bacteria in the colon[114], or if there is bacterial contamination of the small intestine.

SUMMARY

Delineation of the disorders of carbohydrate metabolism has been possible only to the extent that the underlying physiology has been understood. New techniques of investigation will undoubtedly illuminate areas presently obscured. There is much still to challenge the physician, clinical physiologist, biochemist, epidemiologist, geneticist and molecular biologist.

Acknowledgements

A. S. McNeish is grateful to Professor Charlotte Anderson for many stimulating discussions. The authors thank Miss S. Mangal for secretarial assistance.

References

1. Launiala, K. (1968). The effect of unabsorbed sucrose and mannitol on the small intestinal flow rate and mean transit time. *Scand. J. Gastroenterol.*, **39,** 655

2. Calloway, D. H., Colasito, D. J. and Mathews, R. D. (1966). Gases produced by human intestinal microflora. *Nature*, **212,** 1238

3. Bayless, T. M. and Christopher, N. L. (1969). Disaccharidase deficiency. *Am. J. Clin. Nutr.*, **22,** 181

4. Lugo-de-Rivera, C., Rodriguez, H. and Torres-Pinedo, R. (1972). Studies on the mechanism of sugar malabsorption in infantile infectious diarrhoea. *Am. J. Clin. Nutr.*, **25,** 1248

5. Lifshitz, F., Coello-Ramirez, P., Gutierrez-Topete, G. and Cornado-Cornet, M. C. (1971). Carbohydrate intolerance in infants with diarrhoea. *J. Pediatr.,* **79,** 760

6. Bowie, M. D. (1975). Effect of lactose-induced diarrhoea on absorption of nitrogen and fat. *Arch. Dis. Child.*, **50,** 363

7. Anderson, C. M. and Burke, V. (1975). *Paediatric Gastroenterology*, p. 201. (Oxford: Blackwell Scientific Publications)

8. Lifshitz. F., Coello-Ramirez, P. and Gutierrez-Topete, G. (1970). Monosaccharide intolerance and hypoglycaemia in infants with diarrhoea. 1) Clinical course of 23 cases. *J. Pediatr.*, **77,** 595

9. Larcher, V. F., Shepherd, R., Francis, D. E. M. and Harries, J. T. (1977). Protracted diarrhoea in infancy: analysis of 82 cases with particular reference to diagnosis and management. *Arch. Dis. Child.*, **52,** 597

10. Coello-Ramirez, P., Lifshitz. F. and Zanuga, V. (1972). Enteric microflora and carbohydrate intolerance in infants with diarrhoea. *Pediatrics*, **49,** 233

11. Field, M. (1974). Intestinal secretion. *Gastroenterology*, **66,** 1063

12. Barnes, G. L., Bishop, R. F. and Townley, R. R. W. (1974). Microbial flora and disaccharidase depression in infantile gastroenteritis. *Acta Paediatr. Scand.*, **63,** 423

13. Harries, J. T. and Sladen, G. E. (1972). The effects of different bile salts on the

absorption of fluid, electrolytes and monosaccharides in the small intestine of the rat *in vivo. Gut*, **13,** 596

14. Ammon, H. V., Thomas, P. J. and Phillips, S. F. (1974). Effects of oleic and ricinoleic acids on net jejunal water and electrolyte movement. *J. Clin. Invest.*, **53,** 374

15. Liu, H.-Y., Tsao, M. U., Moore, B. and Giday, Z. (1968). Bovine milk protein-induced malabsorption of lactose and fat in infants. *Gastroenterology*, **62,** 227

16. Harrison, B. M., Kilby, A., Walker-Smith, J. A., France, N. E., and Wood, C. B. S. (1976). Cows' milk protein intolerance: a possible association with gastroenteritis, lactose intolerance and IgA deficiency. *Br. Med. J.*, **1,** 1501

17. Gracey, M., Burke, V. and Anderson, C. M. (1969). Association of monosaccharide malabsorption with abnormal small-intestinal flora. *Lancet*, **2,** 384

18. Rodriguez, J. T., Huang, T. L., Alvarado, J., Klish, W. J., Darby, W. E., Flores, N. and Nicols, B. L. (1974). Role of free bile acids in acquired monosaccharide intolerance. *Pediatr. Res.*, **8,** 385

19. Challacombe, D. N., Richardson, J. M., Rowe, B. and Anderson, C. M. (1974). Bacterial microflora of the upper gastrointestinal tract in infants with protracted diarrhoea. *Arch. Dis. Child.*, **49,** 270

20. Coello-Ramirez, P., Gutierrez-Topete, G. and Lifshitz, F. (1970). Pneumatosis intestinalis. *Am. J. Dis. Child.*, **120,** 3

21. Plotkin, G. R. and Isselbacher, K. J. (1964). Secondary disaccharidase deficiency in adult celiac disease (non-tropical sprue) and other malabsorption states. *N. Engl. J. Med.*, **271,** 1033

22. Bowie, M. D., Barbezat, G. O. and Hansen, J. D. L. (1967). Carbohydrate absorption in malnourished children. *Am. J. Clin. Nutr.*, **20,** 89

23. Hoskins, L. C., Winawer, S. J., Broitman, S. A., Gottlieb, L. S. and Zamchick, N. (1967). Clinical giardiasis and intestinal malabsorption. *Gastroenterology*, **53,** 265

24. Bayless, T. M. (1964). Tropical sprue: a comparison with celiac disease. *Am. J. Dig. Dis.*, **9,** 779

25. Cozzetto, F. J. (1963). Intestinal lactase deficiency in a patient with cystic fibrosis. *Pediatrics*, **32,** 228

26. Dubois, R. S., Roy, C. C., Fulginiti, V. A., Merrill, D. A. and Murray, R. L. (1970). Disaccharidase deficiency in children with immunological defects. *J. Pediatr.*, **76,** 377

27. Cavell, B. Hildebrand, H., Meeuwisse, G. W. and Lindquist, B. (1977). Chronic inflammatory bowel disease. *Clin. Gastroenterol.*, **6,** 481

28. Anderson, C. M. (1966). Malabsorption in childhood. *Arch. Dis. Child.*, **41,** 571

29. Paes, I. G., Searl, P. and Rubert, M. W. (1967). Intestinal lactase deficiency and saccharide malabsorption during oral neomycin administration. *Gastroenterology*, **53,** 49

30. Burke, V. and Anderson, C. M. (1966). Sugar intolerance as a cause of protracted diarrhoea following surgery of the gastrointestinal tract in neonates. *Aust. Paediatr. J.*, **2,** 219

31. Bakken, A. F. (1976). Intestinal lactase deficiency as an aetiology factor in the diarrhoea of jaundiced infants treated with phototherapy. *Acta Paediatr. Belg.*, **29,** 205

32. Lifshitz, F., Wapnir, R. A., Pergolizzi, R. and Teichberg, S. (1976). Hypoxia (HY) effects on carbohydrate (CHO) transport. *Pediatr. Res.*, **10**, 356

33. Boellner, S. W., Beard, A. G. and Panos, T. C. (1965). Impairment of intestinal hydrolysis of lactose in newborn infants. *Pediatrics*, **36**, 542

34. Book, L. S., Herbst, J. J. and Jung, A. L. (1976). Carbohydrate malabsorption in necrotising enterocolitis. *Pediatrics*, **57**, 201

35. Gray, G. M. (1975). Carbohydrate digestion and absorption. Role of the small intestine. *N. Engl. J. Med.*, **292**, 1225

36. Preiser, H., Menard, D., Crane, R. K. and Cerda, J. J. (1974). Deletion of enzyme protein from the brush border membrane in sucrase–isomaltase deficiency. *Biochim. Biophys. Acta*, **363**, 279

37. Kerry, K. R. and Townley, R. R. W. (1965). Genetic aspects of intestinal sucrase-isomaltase deficiency. *Aust. Paediatr. J.*, **1**, 223

38. McNair, A., Hyer, E. G., Jarnum, S. and Orrild, L. (1972). Sucrose malabsorption in Greenland. *Br. Med. J.*, **2**, 19

39. Holzel, A. (1967). Sugar malabsorption due to deficiencies of disaccharidase activities and of monosaccharide transport. *Arch. Dis. Child.*, **42**, 341

40. Neale, G., Clark, M. and Levin, B. (1965). Intestinal sucrase deficiency presenting as sucrose intolerance in adult life. *Br. Med. J.*, **2**, 1223

41. McNeish, A. S. (1976). Unpublished observations.

42. Francis, D. E. M. (1974). *Diets for sick children*, 3rd Ed. p. 434. (Oxford: Blackwell Scientific Publications)

43. Holzel, A., Schwarz, V. and Sutcliffe, K. W. (1959). Defective lactose absorption causing malnutrition in infancy. *Lancet*, **1**, 1126

44. Launiala, K. (1967). Intestinal betagalactosidase and betaglucosidase activities in congenital and acquired lactose malabsorption. *Scand. J. Clin. Lab. Invest.*, **19**, suppl. 95, 69

45. Levin, B., Abraham, S. M., Burgess, E. A. and Wallis, P. G. (1970). Congenital lactose malabsorption. *Arch. Dis. Child.*, **45**, 173

46. Launiala, K., Kuitunen, P. and Visakorpi, J. K. (1977). Cited by Dahlqvist, A. In D. Barltrop (Ed.). *Paediatric implications for some adult disorders*, p. 60. London: Fellowship of Postgraduate Medicine

47. Dahlqvist, A. (1964). Method for assay of intestinal disaccharidases. *Anal. Biochem.*, **7**, 18

48. Dahlqvist, A. (1977). The basic aspects of the chemical background of lactase deficiency. In D. Barltrop (ed.). *Paediatric implications for some adult disorders*, p. 60 (London: Fellowship of Postgraduate Medicine)

49. Durand, P. (1958). Lattosuria idiopatica in una paziente con diarrea cronica et acidosis. *Minerva Pediatr.*, **10**, 706

50. Holzel, A. (1968). Disaccharide intolerance. In K. S. Holt and V. P. Coffey (eds.). *Some recent advances in inborn errors of metabolism*, p. 101. (Edinburgh: Livingstone)

51. Berg, N. O., Dahlqvist, A., Lindberg, T. and Studnitz, W. (1969). Severe familial lactose intolerance – a gastrogen disorder? *Acta Paediatr.*, **58**, 525

52. Madzarovova-Nohejlova, J. (1973). Trehalase deficiency in a family. *Gastroenterology*, **65**, 130

53. Laplane, R., Polonovski, C., Etienne, M., Debray, P., Lods, J. C. and Pisarro, B. (1962). L' intolerance aux sucres à transport-intestinal actif (ses rapports avec l'intolerance au lactose et le syndrome coeliaque). *Arch. Fr. Pediatr.*, **19**, 895

54. Lindquist, B. and Meeuwisse, G. W. (1962). Chronic diarrhoea caused by monosaccharide malabsorption. *Acta Paediatr.*, **51**, 674

55. Meeuwisse, G. W. (1970). Glucose-galactose malabsorption studies in renal glycosuria. *Helv. Paediatr. Acta*, **25**, 13

56. Phillips, S. F. and McGill, D. B. (1973). Glucose-galactose malabsorption in an adult: perfusion studies of sugar, electrolyte and water transport. *Am. J. Dig. Dis.*, **18**, 1017

57. Rubino, A., Zimbalatti, F. and Auricchio, S. (1964). Intestinal disaccharidase activities in adult and suckling rats. *Biochim. Biophys. Acta*, **92**, 305

58. Cook, G. C. and Kajubi, S. K. (1966). Tribal incidence of lactase deficiency in Uganda. *Lancet*, **1**, 725

59. Bayless, T. M. and Rosensweig, N. S. (1966). A racial difference in the incidence of lactase deficiency. *J. Am. Med. Assoc.*, **197**, 968

60. Kretchmer, N. (1972). Lactose and lactase. *Sci. Am.*, **227**, 70

61. Ransome-Kuti, O., Kretchmer, N., Johnson, J. D. and Gribble, J. T. (1975). A genetic study of lactose digestion in Nigerian families. *Gastroenterology*, **68**, 431

62. Newcomer, A. D. and McGill, D. B. (1967). Disaccharidase activity in the small intestine: prevalence of lactase deficiency in 100 healthy subjects. *Gastroenterology*, **53**, 881

63. Knudson, K. B., Welsh, J. D., Kronenberg, R. S., Vanderveen, J. E. and Heidelbaugh, N. D. (1968). Effect of a non-lactose diet on human intestinal disaccharidase activity. *Am. J. Dig. Dis.*, **13**, 593

64. Johnson, J. D., Kretchmer, N. and Simoons, F. J. (1974). Lactose malabsorption: its biology and history. *Adv. Pediatr.*, **21**, 197

65. Simoons, F. J. (1970). Primary adult lactose intolerance and the milking habit: a problem in biological and cultural interrelations. II. A culture historical hypothesis. *Am. J. Dig. Dis.*, **15**, 695

66. Cook, G. C., Asp, N. G. and Dahlqvist, A. (1973). Activities of brush border lactase, acid betagalactosidase and hetero-betagalactosidase in the jejunum of the Zambian African. *Gastroenterology*, **64**, 405

67. Keusch, G. T., Troncale, F. J., Thavaramara, B., Prinyanout, P., Anderson, P. R. and Bhamarapravathian, N. (1969). Lactase deficiency in Thailand: Effect of prolonged lactose feeding. *Am. J. Clin. Nutr.*, **22**, 638

68. Wharton, B., Howells, G. and Phillips, I. (1968). Diarrhoea in kwashiorkor. *Br. Med. J.*, **4**, 608

69. Protein Advisory Group, United Nations Organisation (1972). Low lactase activity and milk intake. *PAG Bulletin.* Vol. II, No 2. (New York: United Nations)

70. Walker-Smith, J. A. (1975). *Diseases of the small intestine in childhood.*, p. 174, (Tonbridge Wells, Kent: Pitman Medical)

71. Barnes, G. L. and Townley, R. R. W. (1973). Duodenal mucosal damage in 31 infants with gastroenteritis. *Arch. Dis. Child.*, **48**, 343

72. McNeish, A. S. (1968). The diagnosis of coeliac disease in retrospect. *Arch. Dis. Child.*, **43**, 362

73. Anderson, C. M. and McNeish, A. S. (1976). In *Acute diarrhoea in childhood. Ciba Foundation Symposium*, **42**, p. 20. (Amsterdam: Ciba Foundation)

74. Iyngkaran, N., Robinson, M. J., Sumithran. E., Lam, S. K., Puthucheary, S. D. and Yadav, M. (1978). Cows' milk protein-sensitive enteropathy: An important factor in prolonging diarrhoea of acute infective enteritis in early

infancy. *Arch. Dis. Child.*, **53**, 150

75. Walker-Smith, J., Harrison, M., Kilby, A., Phillips, A. and France, N. (1978). Cows' milk sensitive enteropathy. *Arch. Dis. Child.*, **53**, 375

76. Harrison, B. M. and Walker-Smith, J. A. (1977). Reinvestigation of lactose intolerant children: lack of correlation between continuing lactose intolerance and small intestinal morphology, disaccharidase activity and lactose tolerance tests. *Gut*, **18**, 48

77. Arthur, A. B., Clayton, B. E., Cottom, D. G., Seakins, J. W. T. and Platt, J. W. (1966). Importance of disaccharide intolerance in the treatment of coeliac disease. *Lancet*, **1**, 172

78. McNeish, A. S. and Sweet, E. M. (1968). Lactose intolerance in coeliac disease: assessment of its incidence and importance. *Arch. Dis. Child.*, **43**, 433

79. Sunshine, P., Sinatra, F. R. and Mitchell, C. H. (1977). Intractable diarrhoea of infancy. *Clin. Gastroenterol.*, **6**, 445

80. Lloyd-Still, J. D., Shwachman, H. and Filler, R. (1973). Protracted diarrhoea of infancy treated by intravenous alimentation 1) Clinical Studies of 16 infants. *Am. J. Dis. Child.*, **125**, 358

81. McNeish, A. S. and Rolles, C. J. (1976). Criteria for the diagnosis of temporary gluten intolerance. *Arch. Dis. Child.*, **51**, 275

82. Davidson, A. F. G. and Mullinger, M. (1970). Reducing substances in neonatal stools detected by Clinitest. *Pediatrics*, **46**, 632

83. Soeparto, P., Stobo, E. A. and Walker-Smith, J. A. (1972). Role of chemical examination of the stool in the diagnosis of sugar malabsorption in children. *Arch. Dis. Child.*, **47**, 56

84. Lindquist, B. and Wranne, L. (1976). Problems in analysis of faecal sugar. *Arch. Dis. Child.*, **51**, 319

85. Lifshitz, F. (1977). Carbohydrate problems in paediatric gastroenterology. *Clin. Gastroenterol.*, **6**, 415

86. Kerry, K. R. and Anderson, C. M. (1964). A ward test for sugar in faeces. *Lancet*, **1**, 981

87. Ford, J. D. and Haworth, J. C. (1963). The faecal excretion of sugars in children. *J. Pediatr.*, **63**, 988

88. Gryboski, J. D., Zillis, J. and Ma, O. H. (1964). A study of faecal sugars by high voltage electrophoresis. *Gastroenterology*, **47**, 26

89. McMichael, H. B., Webb, J. and Dawson, A. M. (1965). Lactase deficiency in adults: a cause of 'functional' diarrhoea. *Lancet*, **1**, 717

90. Krasilnikoff, P. A., Gudmand-Hoyer, E. and Moltke, H. H. (1975). Diagnostic value of disaccharide tolerance tests in children. *Acta Paediatr. Scand.*, **64**, 693

91. Isokoski, M., Jussila, J. and Sarna, S. (1972). A simple screening method for lactose malabsorption. *Gastroenterology*, **62**, 28

92. Newcomer, A. D., McGill, D. B., Thomas, P. J. and Hofmann, A. F. (1975). Prospective comparison of different methods for detecting lactase deficiency. *N. Engl. J. Med.*, **293**, 1232

93. Burke, V., Kerry, K. R. and Anderson, C. M. (1965). The relationship of dietary lactose to refractory diarrhoea in infancy. *Aust. Paediatr. J.*, **1**, 147

94. Read, N. W., Holdsworth, C. D. and Levin, R. J. (1974). Electrical measurements of intestinal absorption of glucose in man. *Lancet*, **2**, 624

95. Laws, J. W. and Neale, G. (1966). Radiological diagnosis of disaccharidase deficiency. *Lancet*, **2**, 139

96. Rosenquist, C. J., Heaton, J. W., Gray, G. R. and Zboralske, F. F. (1972). Intestinal lactase deficiency: diagnosis by routine upper gastrointestinal radiography. *Radiology*, **102**, 275

97. Morrison, W. J., Christopher, N. L., Bayless, T. M. and Dana, E. A. (1974). Low lactase levels: evaluation of the radiologic diagnosis. *Radiology*, **111**, 513

98. Bowdler, J. D. and Walker-Smith, J. A. (1969). Le rôle de la radiologie dans le diagnostic de l'intolerance au lactose chez l'enfant. *Ann. Radiol.*, (Paris), **12**, 467

99. Townley, R. R. W., Khaw, K.-T. and Shwachman, H. (1965). Quantitative assay of disaccharidase activities of small intestinal mucosal biopsy specimens in infancy and childhood. *Pediatrics*, **36**, 911

100. Haemmerli, U. P., Kistler, H., Ammann, R., Marthalar, T., Semenza, G., Auricchio, S. and Prader, A. (1965). Acquired milk intolerance in the adult caused by lactose malabsorption due to a selective deficiency of intestinal lactase activity. *Am. J. Med.*, **38**, 7

101. Newcomer, A. D. and McGill, D. B. (1966). Distribution of disaccharidase activity in the small bowel of normal and lactase deficient subjects. *Gastroenterology*, **51**, 481

102. Meeuwisse, G. and Dahlqvist, A. (1968). Glucose – galactose malabsorption. A study with biopsy of the small intestinal mucosa. *Acta Paediatr.*, (Stockholm), Suppl **188**, 19

103. Salmon, P. R., Read, A. E. and McCarthy, C. F. (1969). An isotope method for measuring lactose absorption. *Gut*, **10**, 685

104. Sasaki, Y., Iio, M., Kamed, H., Neda, H., Aoyagi, T., Christopher, N. L., Bayless, T. M. and Wagner, N. H. (1970). Measurements of ^{14}C-lactose absorption in the diagnosis of lactase deficiency. *J. Lab. Clin. Med.*, **76**, 824

105. Bond, J. H. and Levitt, M. D. (1976). Quantitative measurement of lactose absorption. *Gastroenterology*, **70**, 1058

106. Shreeve, W. W., Shoop, J. D., Ott, D. G. and McInteer, B. B. (1976). Test for alcoholic cirrhosis by conversion of ^{14}C or ^{13}C galactose to expired air. *Gastroenterology*, **71**, 98

107. Hofmann, A. F. and Lauterberg, B. H. (1977). Breath test with isotopes of carbon: progress and potential. *J. Lab. Clin. Med.*, **90**, 405

108. Levitt, M. D. (1969). Production and excretion of hydrogen gas in man. *N. Engl. J. Med.*, **281**, 122

109. Caspary, W. F. (1978). Breath tests. *Clin. Gastroenterol.*, **7**, 351

110. Metz, G., Gassull, M. A., Leeds, A. R., Blendis, L. M. and Jenkins, D. J. A. (1976). A simple method of measuring breath hydrogen in carbohydrate malabsorption by end-expiratory sampling. *Clin. Sci. Mol. Med.*, **50**, 237

111. Maffei, H. V. L., Metz, G. L. and Jenkins, D. J. A. (1976). Hydrogen breath test: adaptation of a simple technique to infants and children. *Lancet*, **1**, 1110

112. Newcomer, A. D., Thomas, P. J., McGill, D. B. and Hofmann, A. F. (1977). Lactase deficiency: a common genetic trait of the American Indian. *Gastroenterology*, **72**, 234

113. Douwes, A. C., Fernandes, J. and Rietveld, W. (1978). Hydrogen breath test in infants and children: sampling and storing expired air. *Clin. Chim. Acta*, **82**, 293

114. Levitt, M. D. and Donaldson, R. M. (1970). Use of respiratory hydrogen (H_2) excretion to detect carbohydrate malabsorption. *J. Lab. Clin. Med.*, **75**, 937

SECTION THREE

Disorders of Galactose Metabolism

4

Galactose metabolism, hereditary defects and their clinical significance
R. Gitzelmann and R. G. Hansen

THE METABOLISM OF LACTOSE AND GALACTOSE

Most galactose in the diet is in the form of the disaccharide lactose, which is synthesized in the mammary gland, mainly from glucose. Lactose is the primary carbohydrate source for nursing mammals and it provides about 40% of the energy in human milk. Why lactose evolved as the unique carbohydrate of milk is unclear, especially since most individuals can meet their galactose needs by biosynthesis from glucose. The simultaneous occurrence of calcium and lactose in milk may be of evolutionary significance. Lactose, in contrast to other saccharides, appears to enhance the absorption of calcium[1, 2]. In man, calcium absorption may be associated with the hydrolysis of lactose[3].

Lactose catabolism

In mammals, lactose digestion is initiated by hydrolysis of the disaccharide into absorbable monosaccharides. Mammalian β-galactosidase activity is localized in the brush border fraction of the mucosal cells of the small intestine[4]. The ability to hydrolyze lactose, present during infancy, disappears in many adults who become lactose intolerant. Whether 'adult type' β-galactosidase is induced or constitutive in man has not been clearly established, but in populations that traditionally depend on milk as a significant source of energy throughout life, most adults retain the ability to hydrolyze lactose. In populations where lactose is not a significant component of the adult diet, the ability to hydrolyze lactose declines between the ages of 1 and 4 years[5]. Thus lactose intolerance is common in many non-milk consuming adult populations.

Deficiencies of lysosomal α- and β-galactosidases have recently been described[6, 7]. In Fabry's disease, there is a deficiency of the α-galactosidase which normally catalyzes the hydrolysis of ceramide trihexoside[8], resulting in the accumulation of trihexosylceramide in various organs, primarily in the kidneys. Three other sphingolipidoses are attributed to deficiency of enzymes hydrolyzing β-galactosidic bonds: Krabbe's disease, ceramidelactoside lipidosis, and generalized gangliosidosis. Galactosidases obviously play an important role in the regulation of tissue glycolipid levels.

Lactose biosynthesis

From radio-isotope experiments, it was concluded[9] that UDP-galactose was the donor and glucose the acceptor for the synthesis of lactose (Figure 4.1). Extracts of mammary tissue were subsequently found to catalyze the synthesis of lactose from the predicted substrates, UDP-galactose and glucose. Lactose synthetase was resolved into two components, a mixture of galactosyl transferase protein fractionated from mammary glands, and of α-lactalbumin, a protein normally found in milk[10, 11]. In the absence of α-lactalbumin, the transferase catalyzes galactosyl transfer to either free or

UDP-Galactose + Acetyl-Glucosamine-(R) $\xrightarrow[\substack{Mn^{++} \\ Ca^{++}}]{transferase}$ Galactosyl-Acetylglucosamine-(R) + UDP

Where (R) is a Glycoside, such as Glycoprotein or Glycolipid

UDP-Galactose + Glucose $\xrightarrow[\substack{\alpha\text{-lactalbumin} \\ Mn^{++} \\ Ca^{++}}]{transferase}$ Galactosyl-Glucose + UDP
(Lactose)

Figure 4.1   Galactosyl transfer; lactose synthesis in mammary tissue extracts

bound N-acetylglucosamine[12, 13]. With the transferase alone, glucose is not a good acceptor as it has a high apparent Michaelis constant (K_m) of 1 M. In the presence of α-lactalbumin, the transferase effectively catalyzes the synthesis of lactose, decreasing the K_m for glucose about 1000-fold[14]. The net effect of the second protein, α-lactalbumin produced only in the mammary gland, is to convert a more general glycosyl transferase enzyme for biosynthesis of complex polysaccharides, to an efficient system for lactose synthesis. The principal function of galactosyl transferases present in tissues other than lactating mammary glands is the transfer of galactose to an appropriate carbohydrate side chain of glycoproteins and lipids.

Galactose metabolism

The formation of galactose (gal) is from glucose (glc) via the phosphorylated intermediates, glc-6-P, glc-1-P, UDP-glc, and UDP-gal. There are, however, data from *in vivo* experiments with carbon labelled glycerol which suggest that UDP-gal contains more carbon label and has a distinctly different pattern of labelling than UDP-glc. Glycerol carbons predominate in positions 4, 5 and 6 of galactose. The incorporation of triose by a transaldolase-like exchange into an open chain UDP-hexose is one possibility to account for the unusual isotope pattern in galactose[9]. In the conversion of galactopyranose to galactofuranose at the nucleotide level, an open chain hexose derivative has been postulated that could incorporate triose by a transaldolase-like exchange[15] (Figure 4.2).

Galactose consumed in excess of developmental needs is metabolized for energy. In humans, the liver appears to be the primary site for galactose metabolism. Other tissues, including red cells, have this capacity and can be used to evaluate the metabolic capability of an individual. The pathways of galactose metabolism in man have been inferred by analogy to that of various micro-organisms and animals, and clarified by analysis of metabolic problems in human genetic disorders. The primary metabolic reactions of galactose are illustrated in Figure 4.3.

Reduction A non-specific enzymic reduction of the aldehyde at carbon-1 leads to the product galactitol[16, 17]. This process is especially significant in the lens of the eye which forms galactitol from excess galactose. Man has a limited capacity to further metabolize galactitol; when galactitol accumulates in the eye, it gives rise to opacity and eventually to cataracts[18]. This is important in inherited disorders of galactose metabolism where galactose accumulates.

An adaptive pathway of galactitol metabolism in micro-organisms has been recently delineated. The intermediates in this pathway include

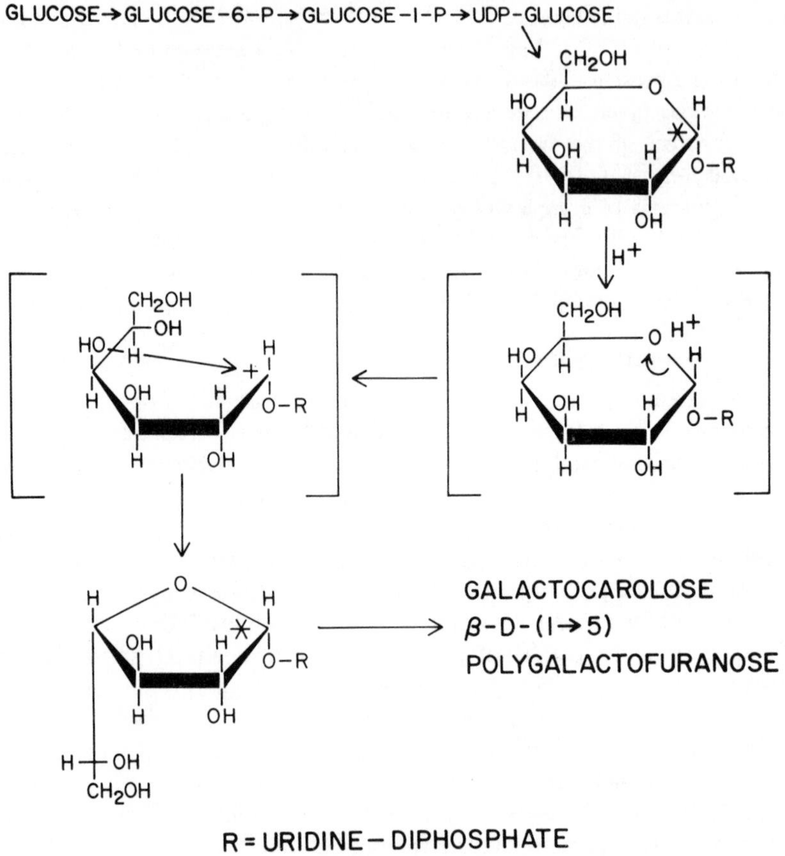

GLUCOSE→GLUCOSE−6−P→GLUCOSE−I−P→UDP−GLUCOSE

GALACTOCAROLOSE
β-D-(I→5)
POLYGALACTOFURANOSE

R = URIDINE − DIPHOSPHATE

Figure 4.2   Galactose furanose formation[53]

L-galactitol-1-phosphate (phosphoenolpyruvate being the phosphate donor), D-tagatose-6-phosphate,   D-tagatose-1,6-diphosphate,   glyceraldehyde-3-phosphate, and dihydroxyacetone-phosphate[19, 20] (Figure 4.4).

Dehydrogenation   Dehydrogenation of the aldehyde at carbon-1 results in the formation of galactonic acid in man and other animals. Galactonic acid is excreted in greater than normal amounts in cases of galactosaemia and of galactokinase deficiency when galactose is consumed[21, 22]. In man, it has not been determined whether galactonic acid arises by the action of a specific enzyme or general aldehyde dehydrogenase, or whether it is derived from some pathway as a phosphorylated intermediate. A quantitative estimation

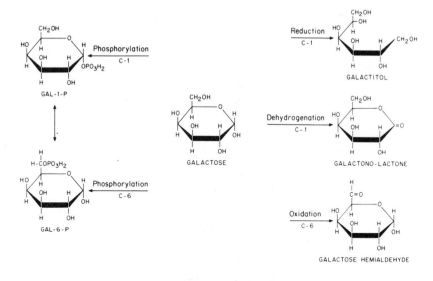

Figure 4.3 Initial steps of galactose metabolism[53]

of galactose and of galactose-1-phosphate has been based on the dehydrogenation reaction[23, 94].

Oxidation A copper-containing oxidase from moulds catalyzes oxidation of galactose at carbon-6 to galactose hemialdehyde[24]. While this reaction is of no known significance in humans, the oxidase is a useful reagent for quantitative estimates of galactose and some of its derivatives, and to differentiate between galactose in a terminal or internal position in various polysaccharides.

Phosphorylation at carbon-6: the tagatose pathway Direct phosphorylation of galactose at carbon-6 is of questionable significance in man although some evidence for the occurrence of gal-6-P has been presented[25]. Gal-6-P could arise from direct phosphorylation or from gal-1-P with a mutase type reaction[26]. In micro-organisms, gal-6-P can be metabolized by a series of reactions catalyzed by inducible enzymes analogous to glycolysis of glucose. The sequential products from gal-6-P are tagatose-6-P, tagatose-1,6-diP, then glyceraldehyde-3-P and dihydroxyacetone-P (trioses common to the glucose pathway)[27] (Figure 4.5).

Phosphorylation at carbon-1: galactokinase Phosphorylation catalyzed

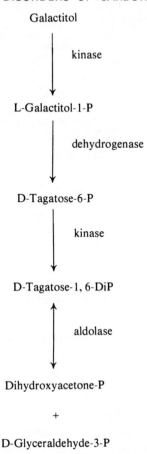

Figure 4.4   Galactitol metabolism in *Klebsiella pneumoniae*

by a kinase, appears to initiate the principal pathway of galactose metabolism in man. The resulting product (galactose-1-P) was first identified in 1943 in rabbit liver following ingestion of galactose[28]. Human liver tissue normally metabolizes most ingested galactose through the Leloir pathway, which requires two more enzymes in addition to the kinase, namely, a transferase and an epimerase[29] (Figure 4.6, reactions b and d).

Incorporation into nucleoside diphosphate hexose: transferase After phosphorylation of galactose, the next reaction in the Leloir pathway is an exchange of hexoses with UDP-glc (Figure 4.6b). The net result of the

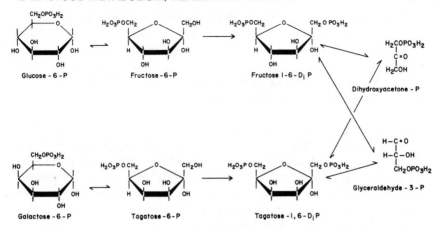

Figure 4.5 Tagatose pathway[53]

transferase reaction is: (1) the formation of glucose-1-phosphate from which energy may be derived; and (2) the formation of nucleoside diphosphate galactose which may be converted to UDP-glc, or which may be the galactosyl donor for biopolymer formation. Under normal circumstances, most

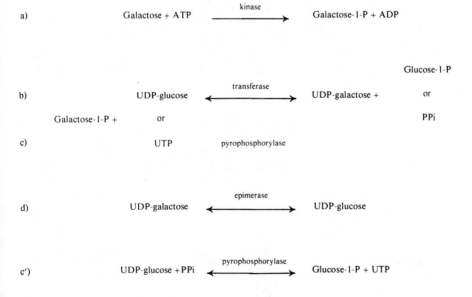

Figure 4.6 Galactose metabolism

galactose is metabolized via the transferase which is uniquely part of the Leloir pathway. Glucose-1-P, uridine mono-, di-, and tri-phosphates, and nucleoside diphosphate-glucose derivates inhibit the transferase[42]. From inhibitor constants and calculated intracellular levels of these compounds, it has been deduced that the uridine derivatives and glucose-1-phosphate could have a physiologically regulatory function.

Hexose interconversion: uridine diphosphate galactose C-4-epimerase   The epimerase and pyrophosphorylase required for galactose metabolism in man are ubiquitous and occur early in human development[37]. The epimerase-catalyzed reaction is the site of the interconversion of galactose and glucose, either when galactose is being metabolized for energy or, conversely, when galactose is needed for structural purposes. The interconversion takes place at the nucleoside-diphosphate-hexose level.

The epimerase from *E. coli* or from yeast, is a dimer containing pyridine nucleotide (NAD^+) which is inactive in reduced form. *E. coli* and yeast epimerase retain NAD^+ tenaciously but when the enzyme is from animal sources, the NAD^+ usually dissociates from the protein. The specific hydrogen atom at carbon-4, which is involved in the hexose interconversion, is removed from one hexose substrate, bound to NAD^+, and returned to the other hexose in the opposite steric mode (Figure 4.7). A keto intermediate at carbon-4 has been reported and confirmed[38, 39].

In man, ethanol oxidation generates an increase in NADH to NAD^+ ratio which apparently inhibits the UDP-galactose C-4-epimerase. This, in turn, limits the clearance of galactose from the blood[40]. Adding NAD^+ to a liver preparation has partially prevented the inhibition of epimerase by ethanol.

Biosynthesis of uridine diphosphate glucose (UDP-glc) and uridine diphosphate galactose (UDP-gal)   UDP-glc not only functions as a cofactor in the Leloir pathway for galactose utilization but also serves broader needs of the cell[30, 31]. The synthesis of glycogen requires UDP-glc. Many

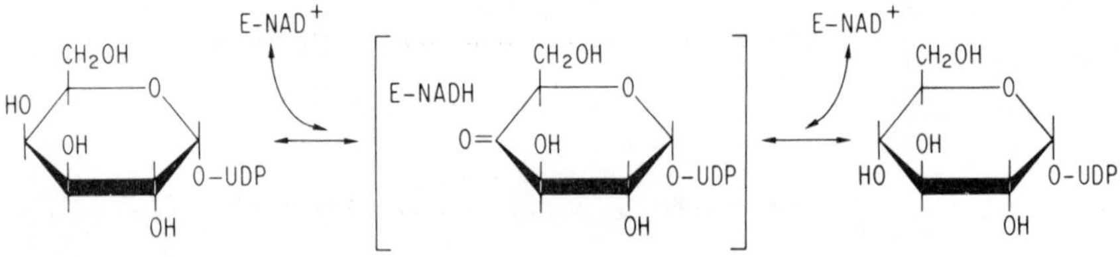

Figure 4.7   UDP-galactose 4'-epimerase: interaction with substrate

chemical compounds needed for growth and for differentiation contain a variety of saccharides. UDP-glc is the primary source of glycosyl residues for the biosynthesis of many of these saccharides. It is not surprising, therefore, that the enzyme for catalyzing the synthesis of UDP-glc is ubiquitous and abundant (Figure 4.6, reactions c and c'); in aqueous extracts of liver, more than 0.5% of the protein is this synthetase for UDP-glc[32, 33]. This reaction is reversible although the equilibrium *in vitro* favours the reactants as shown in Figure 4.6, reaction c', giving rise to the enzyme being commonly designated as a pyrophosphorylase.

In addition to being abundant, the pyrophosphorylase is not highly specific. It will catalyze the reaction with UDP-gal at about 5% of the rate of reaction with UDP-glc[34] (Figure 4.6, reaction c).

Pyrophosphorylase pathway Isselbacher has proposed a pyrophosphorylase pathway[138] of galactose utilization which is significant in humans (Figure 4.6, reactions c, d, c'). Due to its low specificity, the UDP-glc pyrophosphorylase will catalyze both reactions c and c', although claims have been made that a separate enzyme exists in human liver for each of the two reactions[35, 36].

Galactose-1-phosphate toxicity Cataracts are the only signs common to both the transferase deficiency (classical galactosaemia) and galactokinase deficiency. They are caused by osmotic swelling and disrupting of lens fibres due to accumulation of galacticol[18]. No brain, liver or kidney pathology is found in galactokinase deficiency in which galactose-1-phosphate (gal-1-P) cannot be formed. In classical galactosaemia, gal-1-P accumulates within cells and there is damage to brain, liver and kidney. It is concluded from these observations that intracellular gal-1-P is the toxic agent causing most of the changes in classical galactosaemia.

Blood glucose levels of some acutely ill infants lacking transferase are subnormal, indicating further disturbances in carbohydrate metabolism. Three key reactions involving glucose have been reported to be affected by galactose-1-phosphate; the mutase, dehydrogenase, and pyrophosphorylase reactions shown in Figure 4.8[41]. In each case the evidence has been based on kinetic studies of isolated enzymes, not always from human tissues. About a 50-fold excess of galactose-1-phosphate over glucose phosphates is required for significant inhibition of the isolated reactions.

Biosynthesis of galactose-1-phosphate from UDP-galactose The idea that the pyrophosphorylase pathway is a means of galactose metabolism in the human erythrocyte stems from the following observations. Epimerase and

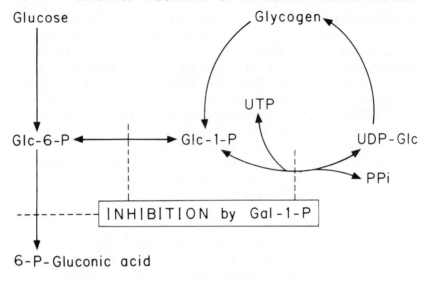

Figure 4.8   Toxicity of galactose-1-phosphate[41, 53]

UDP-glc are normal red cell constituents. Hence UDP-gal is also available as a substrate for other reactions. Incubation of haemolysates lacking transferase[43] with UDP-gal produced gal-1-P in a reaction that was absolutely dependent on inorganic pyrophosphate and was stimulated by magnesium; the production of gal-1-P was inhibited by UDP-glc, by UDP and Pi. Similar reactions may be demonstrated using the crystalline enzyme from human liver[34, 44].

UDP-glucose pyrophosphorylase of both calf and rabbit have also been purified and crystallized[32, 34, 44]. The biochemical evidence that one protein catalyzes reactions with both glucose and galactose derivatives is convincing. Throughout purification and crystallization, the ratio of activity of the enzyme towards the various substrates remains constant[34, 44, 45]. UDP-gal is bound to the purified enzyme as a function of the number of protomer subunits of pyrophosphorylase[33, 46]. This bound UDP-gal may then be stoichiometrically replaced by UDP-glc[46]. UDP-glc also limits the synthesis of gal-1-P from UDP-gal by haemolysates[43]. It is concluded, therefore, that UDP-gal competes with UDP-glc (although less effectively) for the same site on the enzyme. Immunological evidence supporting this conclusion has also been obtained[47].

The production of gal-1-P from glc-1-P by pyrophosphorylase pathway requires the enzymes pyrophosphorylase and epimerase and their substrates, the UDP-hexoses, UTP and PPi (Figure 4.9).

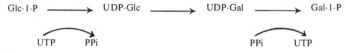

Figure 4.9 The production of galactose-1-phosphate from glucose-1-phosphate (reactions c′, d, c in Figure 4.6)

A substantial concentration of UTP is maintained intracellularly for nucleic acid synthesis and for UDP-glc formation. Besides being a precursor of UDP-gal, UDP-glc is a source of glycosyl donors for pentoses, uronic acids, and hexosamines; hence, there is a constant and vital metabolic flux through UDP-glc. Metabolic interconversions of sugars and their derivatives require epimerases, which appear to be distributed in nature. Hence, the epimerase-catalyzed formation of UDP-gal from UDP-glc is a common intracellular reaction. Under most circumstances, when nucleotides are extracted from the cell, UDP-gal and UDP-glc are present in a ratio of approximately 1:3 – 2:3, providing ample UDP-gal substrate from which gal-1-P may be enzymatically formed.

Inorganic pyrophosphate is required as the other substrate if gal-1-P is to be produced from UDP-gal (UDP-gal + PPi $\rightleftharpoons$ Gal-1-P + UTP). Pyrophosphate is a product of most biosynthetic processes, including the formation of polysaccharides, proteins and lipids. The direct hydrolysis of pyrophosphate is thought to occur in order to remove a reaction product[48, 49].

The amount of pyrophosphate produced daily by adult man may be as much as 1 kg but this amount or the turnover rate is not known with precision. Measurable quantities of pyrophosphate are present in cells and tissues, but how much is hydrolyzed, or utilized where the bond energy is consumed, or is excreted, remains to be determined[50]. Quite aside from the futile energy wastage when hydrolysis takes place, substantial evidence indicates that not only do some cells utilize the potential for productive use of the PPi, but PPi may have a regulatory function as well[51, 52]. Furthermore, PPi accumulates in man in sufficient quantity to crystallize with calcium and cause some disorders of joints[50]. The availability of PPi for gal-1-P synthesis from UDP-gal is therefore most probable.

HEREDITARY DEFECTS AND THEIR CLINICAL SIGNIFICANCE

Hereditary galactokinase deficiency

This defect was described in 1965[54] in a blind gypsy ('H.K.') who, as a 9 year old boy, had recurrent cataracts and was referred to the University

Children's Hospital in Zürich for paediatric examination. Fanconi diagnosed mellituria, and, as he was in process of evaluating the effects of 'fruit-and-vegetable diet' in diabetic children, he eliminated milk from the boy's diet, whereupon the symptoms of mellituria ceased. Mellituria reappeared only after milk or galactose ingestion, but not in response to the intake of other hexoses. With the help of a biochemist, Fanconi's curiosity led him, to identify the sugar in this boy's urine as galactose. He termed the new entity 'galactose diabetes'[55]. When we relocated this man 32 years later, he was living in a home for the blind where he still lives today at age 55 years. He is incapacitated by a polyneuritis-like condition (he has neurofibromatosis). Over the years, he has granted us permission to perform a number of metabolic studies, all conducted at the home, and through his generous cooperation and that of his clan we have obtained valuable information which I would like to summarize briefly as follows:

Galactokinase deficiency can be demonstrated in erythrocytes as well as in whole blood. The condition is inherited as an autosomal recessive[56]. Heterozygotes have approximately one half of normal activity. Galactokinase deficient adults are not mentally deficient although perhaps deprived because of blindness[56]. Blindness may be life-long as in H.K. who had several operations for recurring cataracts. However, an older affected sister[56, 57] was luckier; she retained fairly good vision after discission and was able to lead a normal life. Galactokinase deficient persons have no aversion to milk and experience no discomfort from drinking it. They are asymptomatic with the exception of nuclear cataracts, which appear in infancy. If milk intake is high, they excrete substantial amounts not only of galactose, but also of galactitol[58] (Table 4.1). After an oral galactose load, blood galactose rises excessively[57].

In H.K. galactose does not stimulate insulin release (Figure 4.10). The cause of his impaired glucose tolerance is not understood (Figure 4.11). Conversion of injected [^{14}C]galactose to $^{14}CO_2$ in expired air was minimal (Figure 4.12) which demonstrated that the enzyme defect was extensive,

TABLE 4.1   Amounts of galactose and of galactitol excreted in urine by H. K. during 5 days of high milk intake (3 l/day)[56]

	Daily range	Total of 5 days
Galactose	35.00–42.05 g	191.51 g
	192.5–231.3 mmol	1053.3 mmol
Galactitol	8.34–10.58 g	47.97 g
	45.87–58.19 mmol	400.07 mmol

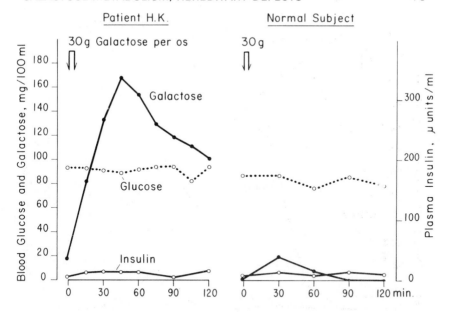

Figure 4.10 Oral galactose tolerance test in a galactokinase deficient adult and a control. (Glucose and galactose: 1 mg/100 ml = 0.055 mmol/l)[57]

probably involving all tissues[22]. Though galactonate was present in his urine, it failed to become labelled after the injection of [14C]galactose. His cultured skin fibroblasts had no galactokinase activity[22], a finding that had been reported in another kinase-deficient person[59].

Incidence and screening In 1967 we advanced two speculations, firstly, that galactokinase-deficiency could be discovered early if newborns were tested for elevated blood galactose; secondly, that heterozygosity for galactokinase deficiency could be a factor related to the formation of cataracts beyond infancy and childhood[56]. Both speculations have been shown to be correct.

The first affected newborn was detected in the Austrian mass newborn screening programme[60]. In Sweden, two newborns have been discovered[61, 62] and in Austria and Germany together 13 galactokinase-deficient babies (Table 4.2), but none in Switzerland. From population surveys[56, 63], the heterozygote frequency has been estimated to be 0.01 and hence the birth incidence at 1 in 40 000. The true incidence in Germany and Austria combined, however, was only 1 in 155 000, i.e. 3–4 times smaller. The difference is unexplained although genetic heterogeneity could be one factor.

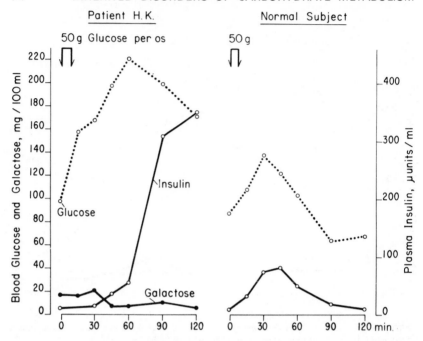

Figure 4.11 Oral glucose tolerance test in a galactokinase deficient adult and a control. (Glucose and galactose: 1 mg/100 ml = 0.055 mmol/l)[57]

Racially determined galactokinase polymorphism has been detected in North American blacks who have lower activity in red cells than whites[64, 65]. The first three families with the disorder were gypsies[56, 60, 66] but all subsequent cases were non-gypsy. There are now 19 published cases from Switzerland, Austria, Germany, Sweden, France, England, Pakistan, the USA and Italy[56, 59–61, 66–76]. One infant reported from France had transitory galactokinase deficiency[67]. Galactokinase-deficient newborns are completely asymptomatic. If fed a galactose-exclusion diet they do not develop cataracts.

Additional problems   Does untreated galactokinase deficiency cause any disorder other than cataracts? A number of authors have reported additional findings[75] such as neonatal hyperbilirubinaemia, mild hepatomegaly, and pseudotumour cerebri[76]. One 21 year old female had recurrent seizures[59] that appeared after years of milk abstinence; she had been a small-for-date baby, had required tracheotomy for acute infection at age 7 months and at age 4 years 9 months was brachycephalic and frail[77]. Two

TABLE 4.2 Detection of errors of galactose metabolism through mass newborn screening

		Tested	Detected	Incidence (1 per . . .)
Galactokinase	D	1 100 000	7	157 000
	A	920 00	6	153 000
	CH	608 000	0	?
Gal-1-P uridyl-transferase	D	1 700 000	29	59 000
	A	919 000	21	44 000
	CH	747 000	12	62 000
UDP-galactose 4'-Epimerase	D			
	A			
	CH	230 000	5	46 000

D – Germany, A – Austria, CH – Switzerland

Compiled May 1978.
Courtesy of: H. Bickel, Heidelberg; R. Bütler, Bern; O. Thalhammer, Wien

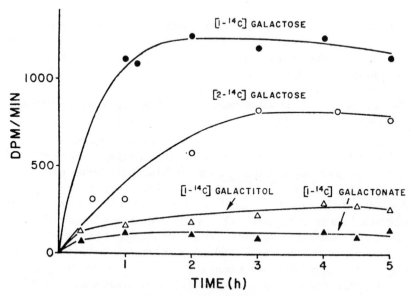

Figure 4.12 Conversion of injected ^{14}C-labelled galactose, galactitol and galactonate to $^{14}CO_2$ in a patient with galactokinase deficiency[22]

retarded galactokinase-deficient brothers, aged 11 and 7 years, with 10% residual enzyme activity have been diagnosed[78], but details have not been reported yet. At present, these additional findings are regarded as un-related[79] because a number of patients who were diagnosed after infancy and childhood[56, 70, 71, 73, 75] had neither liver pathology nor neurological disease.

Pathogenesis of cataracts   Nuclear cataracts are formed because galactitol accumulates, gets trapped and causes swelling and disruption of lens fibres[18]. The process can be imitated *in vitro*. That aldose reductase plays the key role is demonstrated by the preventive effective of inhibitors[80]. The formation of galactose cataracts is a complex sequence of events including disturbances in the balance of water, electrolytes, amino acids, proteins, energy-rich phosphates and reduced glutathione[18, 81]. Considering the multi-plicity of events in cataractogenesis, most nuclear cataracts must be multi-factorial in origin, a situation infinitely more difficult to analyse biochemically. Reduced galactokinase activity as found in heterozygotes may predispose to cataracts[56] but the number of heterozygotes *with* cataracts[66, 70, 71] is smaller than those *without*. Whether the statistically significant lowering of galactokinase activity in patients whose cataracts developed during the first year of life[73] is causally related to their cataracts remains unresolved[82].

Treatment of galactokinase deficiency with galactose exclusion diet must be continued throughout life. It can be safely assumed that minute amounts of galactose in the diet will be tolerated but this assumption *cannot* be made for transferase-deficient patients.

Hereditary deficiency of galactose-1-phosphate uridyltransferase: galactosaemia

This inborn error was recognized in 1908[83], but it took nearly 50 years to define galactose-1-phosphate as the accumulating substrate[84] and transferase deficiency as the enzyme defect[85]. Incidence figures have varied widely[86], but the pooled results from the three neighbouring countries Austria, Germany and Switzerland show that 62 galactosaemic infants were discovered among 3 366 000 newborns screened on their 5th or 6th day for high blood galactose or for absence of transferase activity (Table 4.2). This corresponds to an overall birth incidence of approximately 1: 55 000, the in-cidence in Austria being higher than in the other two countries.

Transferase deficiency is transmitted as an autosomal recessive trait[87, 88]. Absence of transferase activity is the basis for diagnosing galactosaemia. Enzyme assays are most often performed on erythrocytes and activity is usually missing or minimal. The defect can also be demonstrated in many other tissues such as cultured skin fibroblasts and in cultured amniotic fluid cells (see Chapter 9). Heterozygotes have approximately one half of normal activity in red cells.

Clinical findings and treatment Galactosaemic infants have normal weight at birth[89] but gain little as they start ingesting milk. Usually symptoms appear in the second half of the first week of life and include jaundice, vomiting, lethargy, oedema, ascites, hepatomegaly and sometimes diarrhoea[90, 91]. If milk feeding continues, the disease is usually rapidly fatal. Symptoms are milder and the course is less precipitous when milk is temporarily withdrawn and replaced by intravenous nutrition. Nuclear cataracts appear within days or weeks and become irreversible within weeks of their appearance. Diagnosis may be indicated by the presence of non-glucose reducing substance in the urine. However, galactosuria has been missed repeatedly because of the concomitant presence of glucose in urine. Glycosuria and hyperaminoaciduria are signs of proximal renal tubular damage. If milk is withdrawn and a galactose-free diet[91] is instituted, symptoms disappear promptly. Cataracts may clear, and liver cirrhosis may be prevented. Some degree of irreversible brain damage is always present resulting in delayed mental development, difficulties of visual perception, behaviour changes and sometimes epilepsy. Long term follow-up studies have been conducted in Illinois[90], in Manchester[92], and in California[91, 93].

Treatment with a galactose exclusion diet is comparatively easy. Galactose-1-phosphate in erythrocytes can be determined[94]; it decreases as galactose is excluded from the diet and then serves as an indicator of inadvertent galactose intake. However, high levels in treated infants do not always reflect poor dietary control. That galactose-1-phosphate is the toxic agent causing most of the pathology[53] was concluded from the comparison of manifestations in kinase and in transferase deficiencies (p. 69). Cataracts are caused by the deleterious effect of galactitol on the lens fibres (p. 76); although galactose-1-phosphate is also found in the lens[95] its role in cataractogenesis must be minor.

As long-term follow-up, treatment and screening are discussed in Chapters 5, 6 and 8, we would like to restrict the remainder of this Chapter to two topics: transferase polymorphism and the uncontrolled biosynthesis of galactose.

Transferase polymorphism With the advent of enzyme electrophoresis and specific staining procedures so many enzyme variants[96] have been found that enzyme diversity can no longer be regarded as an exception. In a recent

TABLE 4.3   Galactose-1-phosphate uridyltransferase polymorphism (EC 2.7.7.12)

Variant	Clinical manifestations in homozygotes (compounds)	Enzyme			Local gene frequency (Caucasians)	Refs.
		Activity*	Electrophoresis	Stability		
Galactosemia (Gal)	yes	0-few % 0 (liver, intestine)			0.005 0.0041 0.0021 0.004	114 115 97 98 Table 4.2
Negro	yes or no	0 10% (liver, intestine)				116 117 114
Duarte	no (Duarte/Gal: no?)	50%	fast 3-banded		0.040	103 118 115

Rennes	yes	7–10%	slow		0.0706	100
					0.062	101
					0.080	102
					0.0548	98
Indiana	? (Ind./Gal: yes)	0–40%	slow	unstable, P_i-sensitive		120, 121
						122
Los Angeles	no	100–140%	fast			123
Münster?	yes	30%	3-banded			124, 125
Berne	?	40%	slow		0.0009	126
Chicago fast	? (fast/Gal: mild)	25% / 25% (fibroblasts)	fast			127
Chicago labile	? (labile/fast: no)			heat-labile		

* in erythrocytes (if not specified)

survey[96] the average heterozygosity per locus was 0.063 implying that any one of us is likely to be heterozygous for alleles determining electrophoretic variants at 6% of our loci. In Caucasians, heterozygosity for the galactose-1-phosphate uridyltransferase locus may be even higher than that for other transferases[96]. For instance in a 1973 survey by Beutler[97], the average frequency of *Duarte* heterozygotes alone was 0.0678. It was even higher in Greece,[98] certain parts of Germany[99–101] and Switzerland[102] where up to approximately 16% of the population may be heterozygote for the *Duarte* allele (Table 4.3).

Duarte was the first electrophoretic variant[103] to be discovered. This was perhaps no coincidence as this variant is the most common one. The mutant enzyme is roughly 50% active. Homozygotes thus have one half normal activity; they are asymptomatic. Other electrophoretic variants are *Rennes, Indiana, Los Angeles, Berne, Chicago*. With the exception of *Los Angeles*, the activity of the variant enzyme is lower than that of the wild type. The stability of some variant enzymes is reduced. The *Negro* and *Münster* variants were recognized clinically (Table 4.3). One individual may harbour one allele coding for one variant enzyme and a second allele coding for galactosaemia; or, two alleles each coding for another variant. Partial transferase deficiency of different severity ensues in these compound heterozygotes. Symptomatic compound heterozygotes have been described with the *Indiana* and *Chicago* traits involved. Many more compounds must exist and some may be clinically important.

Owing to the high gene frequency of the *Duarte* variant, compound heterozygosity for galactosaemia/*Duarte* is relatively common. Accepting a birth incidence for galactosaemia of 1:55 000 newborns (Table 4.2) and published gene frequencies for the *Duarte* trait (0.06–0.08; Table 4.3), one must expect one compound heterozygote in approximately 3000–4000 newborns. They are discovered in mass screening programmes because of very low transferase, high blood galactose (e.g. 6 mg%, that is 0.3 mmol/l, or above), or both.

The first such case was reported in 1967[104] (Figure 4.13). D.B. had a blood galactose reading of 10 mg% (0.6 mmol/l), low transferase and excessive erythrocyte galactose-1-phosphate. His red cell transferase rose gradually to reach the level expected for his genotype, i.e. roughly 25%. Such a rise has been observed by us and by others, e.g. Dr William Murphey (personal communication) but has not been adequately explained. Eventually, a special diet was prescribed although the patient was asymptomatic. At the age of 12 years, he is a bit slow at school and poor at abstract thinking.

Levy recently reviewed his own and other published cases of compound

GALACTOSE-1-PHOSPHATE URIDYLTRANSFERASE

Genetic Compound: Galactosemia/Duarte

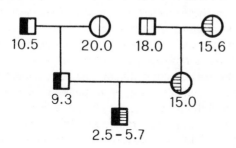

Pedigree of Newborn D.B.

Erythrocyte transferase levels (controls: 17-24 U/g Hb)

Transferase and gal-1-P in D.B., changing with age

Age	Transferase	Gal-1-P
4 w	2.5	17
5 w	2.5	5
6 w	4.2	7
3 m	4.6	1
5 m	5.0	
1 y	5.7	0
9 y	5.1	

Figure 4.13 Pedigree, erythrocyte transferase and galactose-1-phosphate levels in patient with galactosaemia/*Duarte* variant. Gal-1-P in mg/100 ml RBC ($\times$ 38.4 = μmol/l)

heterozygotes for galactosaemia/*Duarte*[105, 106] and has come to the conclusion that this common genetic variation is usually, if not always, benign. Uncertainty remains, however, even after having considered blood galactose, erythrocyte galactose-1-phosphate, transferase level, galactose tolerance curves, enzyme electrophoresis and family investigation. Careful follow-up studies[107] on these children are needed. Even with this question resolved, each newborn with partial transferase deficiency will have to be observed closely, because another genetic compound may be operative, e.g. one that involves the traits *Indiana, Rennes,* or *Chicago.*

Galactose tolerance tests do not distinguish galactosaemia heterozygotes from the normal[108, 109] but the test is noxious to the galactosaemic homozygote[90]. It is doubtful if this test has any place in evaluating the need for treatment in infants with partial transferase deficiency as the following example shows. Proband J.C.R. was discovered because he had 10 mg% (0.6 mmol/l) blood galactose on his 5th day screening. He was shown to have less than 10% of the normal level of transferase, his mother had 50%, his father unusually high activity but non-paternity was most unlikely. The exact genotype could not be established in this family. There was a rise of red cell transferase with increasing age (Figure 4.14). The rate of disappearance of blood galactose was fastest and the red cell galactose-1-phosphate 2 h after ingestion highest, at the time red cell transferase was lowest. Almost certainly, the rate of disappearance of galactose corresponded not with transferase activity but with that of galactokinase.

Uncontrolled biosynthesis of galactose-1-phosphate   Our interest in this

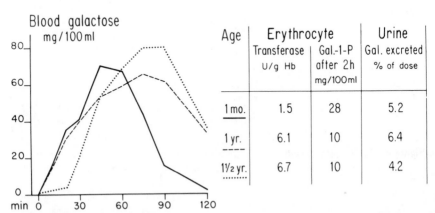

| Age | Erythrocyte | | Urine |
	Transferase U/g Hb	Gal.-1-P after 2h mg/100ml	Gal. excreted % of dose
1 mo.	1.5	28	5.2
1 yr.	6.1	10	6.4
1½ yr.	6.7	10	4.2

Figure 4.14   Oral galactose tolerance tests (1 g/kg) in patient J.C.R. with partial transferase deficiency, at various ages. Transferase activity in controls: 18–30 U/g Hb. (Galactose: 1 mg/100 ml = 0.055 mmol/l; Gal-1-P: 1 mg/100 ml = 38.4 μmol/l)

topic dates from 1966 when we treated a transferase deficient infant from birth and saw an unexplained rise of galactose-1-phosphate in her red cells[43]; the red cells accumulated the phosphate *in vitro* in the absence of galactose in the medium (Figure 4.15). Later, the same phenomenon was observed in transferase deficient fibroblasts grown in a medium devoid of

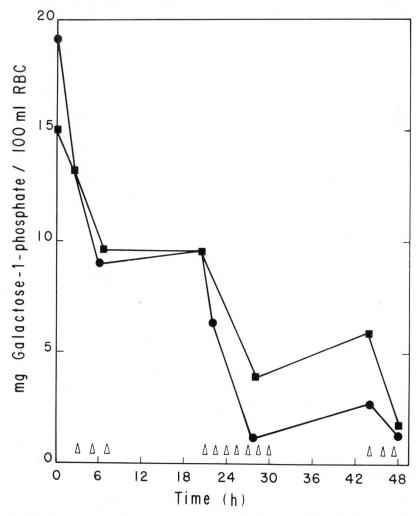

Figure 4.15 Galactose-1-phosphate content of erythrocytes of two siblings with total transferase deficiency. Red cells were incubated *in vitro* with glucose as the sole carbohydrate. Arrows indicate medium change. (Galactose-1-phosphate: 1 mg/100 ml = 38.4 μmol/l)[43]

galactose[110]. We have since demonstrated that the pyrophosphorylase pathway was implicated[47, 53, 111].

There is accumulating evidence for the biosynthesis of galactose from glucose in man[53]. The fetus of mothers who are heterozygous for galactosaemia and live without galactose during pregnancy develop normally. Galactokinase and transferase deficient children also develop normally with galactose excluded from their diet; several such infants even excreted some galactitol or small amounts of galactose[74, 112]. Transferase deficient newborns have demonstrable red cell galactose-1-phosphate in cord blood even though their mothers abstain from galactose[89].

One galactosaemic newborn was given a glucose infusion but nothing by mouth until he was 24 h old, yet his red cell galactose-1-phosphate rose (Figure 4.16)[47, 111]. Two galactosaemic infants were discovered after initial exposure to milk; both had excessive galactose-1-phosphate before we initiated a galactose free diet on day 7 and 6, respectively (Figure 4.17). Their red cell galactose-1-phosphate fell rather hesitantly and remained at potentially dangerous levels for weeks and months. Feeding isocaloric dextrimaltose for 36 h in one (R.B., indicated by arrows in Figure 4.17) did not lower his galactose-1-phosphate. The other infant (D.A.), a female, had breast swellings until her 25th day; on day 19 her breast secretions contained 2.9 mg% (0.08 mmol/l) lactose, a concentration comparable to that found in controls (Table 4.4). While she was obviously synthesizing lactose from glucose, her galactose-1-phosphate peaked again (Figure 4.17).

Such uncontrolled biosynthesis of galactose from glucose in well-treated galactosaemic infants constitutes a mechanism of potential self-intoxication[113]. It could take place not only in red cells or mammary glands but also in liver and brain. The pyrophosphorylase pathway is probably implicated but it is not known how to help these infants limit excessive synthesis of UDP-galactose and thus the formation of toxic amounts of galactose-1-phosphate. Clearly, the prognosis in some *treated* infants may depend on their ability to limit this process.

Hereditary deficiency of uridine diphosphate galactose 4′-epimerase

Epimerase is the third enzyme in the metabolic route by which man metabolizes galactose for energy. Epimerase deficiency used to be considered a defect hardly compatible with life[128]. As can be seen from this reaction sequence (Figure 4.18), mutants lacking epimerase would be true galactose auxotrophs, requiring exogenous (i.e. dietary) galactose for the

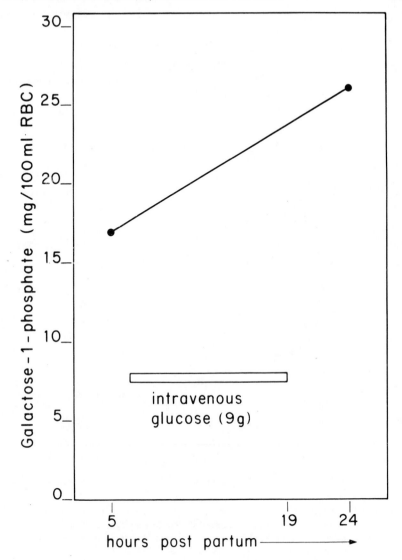

Figure 4.16 Erythrocyte galactose-1-phosphate in an unfed newborn (H.B.) with total transferase deficiency. (Galactose-1-phosphate: 1 mg/100 ml = 38.4 μmol/l)[47, 111]

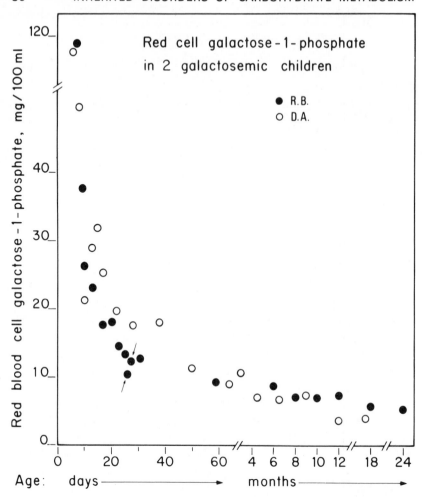

Figure 4.17 Erythrocyte galactose-1-phosphate levels in two children with total transferase deficiency. Infant R.B. received dextrimaltose by mouth but nothing else for 36 h (arrows). Infant D.A. had breast swellings until her 25th day. (Galactose-1-phosphate: 1 mg/100 ml = 38.4 μmol/l)[111]

synthesis of glycolipids and glycoproteins from UDP-galactose. The first epimerase deficient human being was discovered in our mass newborn screening programme, reported in 1971[129]. A test designed by Paigen[130] for the monitoring of galactose in blood spotted on filter paper had given a high reading. It was later discovered that the test had registered galactose-1-

TABLE 4.4   Lactose and galactose in breast secretions of newborns[111]

Patient			Lactose		Galactose	
			(g/100 ml)	(mmol/l)	(g/100 ml)	(mmol/l)
D.A.	Galactosaemia	19 days	2.9	81	0.027	1.49
	(Transferase activity:		2.5	70	0.016	0.88
	0.0 U/g Hb)					
M.J.	Compound Heterozygote	22 days	3.6	101	0.013	0.72
	(transferase activity:		2.5	70	0.013	0.72
	0.3 U/g Hb)					
E.M.	Control	11 days	5.5	154	0.005	0.28
			6.1	171	0.005	0.28
A.K.	Control	13 days	4.6	129	0.022	1.21
			5.1	143	0.016	0.88

phosphate in the red cells of the child.

To date, we have identified nine epimerase-deficient individuals in four families: five newborns, one 5 year old sibling, one grandmother and two of her sisters in their sixties. All are admirably well without the support of medicine. Since these are the only known cases, the true incidence of this peculiar defect is unknown. We have discovered our five newborns in 230 000 routine tests giving a birth incidence for epimerase deficiency of approximately 1:46 000 (Table 4.2). This preliminary estimate is of course only valid for a restricted alpine region covered by our screening programme and comprising eastern Switzerland and Liechtenstein.

The defect is easily demonstrated by assaying erythrocyte epimerase[131]. Red cells of affected individuals lack all activity and heterozygotes have intermediate activity. The defect is transmitted as an autosomal recessive trait. Two of the four families were related (Figure 4.19) and two sets of parents were consanguineous.

Nature of epimerase defect   The benign nature of hereditary epimerase deficiency was thought to be due to the defect being restricted to circulating red cells. However, one infant had some activity in her circulating lymphocytes (Table 4.5); another proband, during an upper respiratory infection at age 14 months, had considerable epimerase activity in her leukocytes[132]. The livers of two infants contained active enzyme as did cultured fibroblasts derived from the skin of four of the epimerase deficient individuals[132]. Finally, and somewhat surprisingly, a long term lymphoblast line derived from epimerase deficient lymphocytes turned out to contain active enzyme at the level comparable to that of control lines[133]. When

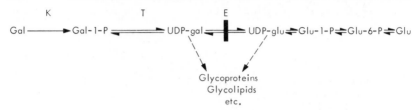

Figure 4.18   Deficiency of UDP-galactose 4'-epimerase[132]

lymphocytes were stimulated by phytohaemagglutinin, epimerase activity appeared after only 72 h of culture[133]. This mutant epimerase, partially purified from lymphoblast and fibroblast lines, had reduced heat stability and required higher concentrations of coenzyme NAD than control lines for saturation, although there was no difference in pH optimum and K_m for UDP-galactose (Table 4.6)[134]. The higher NAD requirement of mutant epimerase for stability at 40 °C *in vitro* is shown in Figure 4.20.

It is probable that there is a structural defect in the epimerase of all tissues affecting the ability of the enzyme to bind NAD and thus its stability. The unstable enzyme is active only in those tissues (or tissue cultures) where synthesis of epimerase is more rapid than degradation and/or where NAD concentrations are high enough to protect the abnormal enzyme from degradation.

An enzyme which inactivates NAD-dependent enzymes in the absence of NAD has been demonstrated in rat intestine[135] and may occur in other tissues. Such an enzyme could be responsible for the rapid proteolysis of a mutant epimerase defective in NAD binding. Therefore, tissue concentrations of NAD could be crucial for the stability of the mutant enzyme. NAD concentration in human red cells is reported to be 50–60 μmol/l in the presence of approximately 30 μmol/l NADH[136].

The detection of small amounts of epimerase in the lymphocytes of one proband during a presumed viral infection provides some evidence that *in vivo* activation of epimerase is possible, and this may explain the absence of dire metabolic consequences predicted for those with epimerase deficiency[128].

The apparent reversal of a genetically determined enzyme deficiency in human cells in culture appears to be without precedent[133]. However, the same phenomenon may be observed in other unstable enzyme mutants in the future. The demonstration of an active enzyme in human cells in culture, e.g. in skin fibroblasts or amniotic fluid cells, may not in every instance reflect the *in vivo* activity state of the enzyme. It may in fact obscure the diagnosis of an enzyme deficiency.

TABLE 4.5 UDP-galactose 4'-epimerase deficiency: epimerase activity in circulating blood cells, liver and cultivated skin fibroblasts

	RBC[1]	Leukocytes[2]	Lymphocytes[2]	Liver[3]	Fibroblasts[2]
Probands					
E.B.	0.00	0.00		1.6	3.90
B.B.	0.00				
R.B.	0.00	0.00	0.40	2.1	4.34
C.K.	0.00	0.00	0.00		5.40
T.T.	0.00	0.00			
J.P.	0.00	0.00	0.00		3.90
M.E.	0.00	0.00			
A.E.	0.00	0.00			
H.M.	0.00	0.00			
Obligate heterozygotes					
x̄	1.72	0.65			
SD	0.56	0.44			
Range	0.92–2.41	0.31–1.40			
(n)	(11)	(6)			
Controls					
x̄	4.90	2.24	6.19	3.0	6.20
SD	1.13	0.92	2.44		1.80
Range	2.72–7.91	1.02–4.64	3.10–10.90	2.1–3.6	3.6–8.9
(n)	(36)	(22)	(14)	(3)	(6)

[1]µmoles/h/ml RBC [2]U/g soluble protein [3]U/ml soluble fraction
Results of first assays are shown

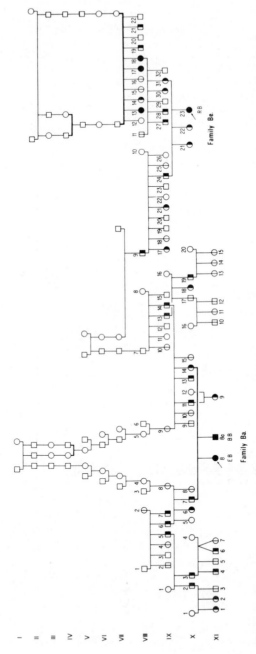

Figure 4.19 Pedigrees of families Ba. and Be. in whom newborns with epimerase deficiency were detected. Genotypes were assigned according to erythrocyte epimerase activity.[132]

□ = not tested ■ ◑ = heterozygote □ ⊕ = normal ● = homozygote

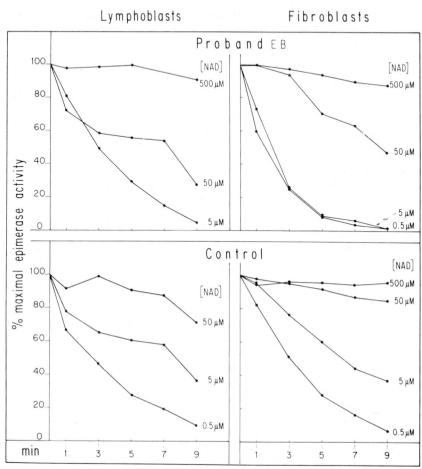

Figure 4.20 UDP-galactose 4′-epimerase: NAD requirement for stability at 40° of proband and control enzyme partially purified from lymphoblasts and fibroblasts. (Haigis E. and Gitzelmann R., in prep.)

Biochemical and haematological findings Our probands have normal or nearly normal galactose tolerance, experience no intolerance symptoms and have normal blood morphology[132]. Although galactose-1-phosphate accumulates in erythrocytes, especially after feeding in infancy (Table 4.7), red cell integrity is not affected. Up to this date, epimerase deficiency should not be considered a clinical entity although perhaps a nuisance to the newborn screening laboratory.

TABLE 4.6   UDP-galactose 4′-epimerase: Enzyme characteristics of cultured lymphoblasts and fibroblasts from probands and controls

	[NAD] required for saturation (10^{-6} mol/l)	Heat stability	Optimum pH	K_mUDP-gal (10^{-6} mol/l)
Lymphoblasts				
Proband E.B.		reduced		18–36
3 Controls				17–18
Fibroblasts				
Probands E.B. ⎫		reduced	9.0	⎫
C.K. ⎬	40–60			⎬
R.B. ⎭				⎬ 30–40
Controls R.G. ⎫	5–7			⎬
B.S. ⎭			9.0	⎭

Epimerase of lymphoblasts and fibroblasts was purified 12–30 fold and 15–40 fold respectively

TABLE 4.7   Erythrocyte galactose-1-phosphate in five infants with UDP-galactose 4′-epimerase deficiency

Initials	Age	Feeding	Galactose-1-phosphate* (mg/100 ml RC)	(μmol/l RC)
E.B.	3 months	cow's milk	19	730
B.B.	at birth	—	7	269
	5 days	breast milk	49	1882
R.B.	17 days	breast milk	70	2688
M.E.	21 days	breast milk + cow's milk	60	2304
H.M.	24 days	breast milk	41	1574

* Estimated enzymatically

Three out of nine probands had unexplained eosinophilia but otherwise unremarkable red and white blood cells. However, eight epimerase deficient persons, members of three families, had a ccdee Rhesus genotype (Table 4.8). The possibility of genetic linkage between the Rhesus locus on chromosome one[137] and the yet unassigned epimerase locus was examined[132]. With the help of Dr Margrit Metaxas and Dr Marc Metaxas, Zürich, we surveyed the distribution of the two traits in the three families. Unfortunately, red and white cell epimerase activity in a few key members

TABLE 4.8 UDP-galactose 4′-epimerase deficiency: Haematological findings in the nine known probands

	Hb (g/100 ml)	RBC indices and morphology	Reticulocyte count (%)	Osmotic fragility	Blood group	Rhesus phenotype	WBC and differential count
E.B. ○	11.0–13.0	N	0.6–2.7	N	A	ccdee	N
B.B. ○					A	ccdEe	
R.B. ♀	12.1–13.8	N	1.0–2.5	N	B	ccdee	N
C.K. ♀	15.5	N	1.0	N	O	ccdee	N
T.T. ♀	14.0	N			O	ccdee	N
J.P. ♀	12.0	N			O	ccdee	N
M.E. ○	11.2–14.1	N	1.8–2.7	N	O	ccdee	eosinophilia
A.E. ♀	12.4–14.0	N	0.6–1.1	N	O	ccdee	eosinophilia
H.M. ○	11.9	N	0.6	N	A	CcDEe	eosinophilia

proved too variable to allow the unequivocal assignment of epimerase genotype[132]. It remains to be seen whether the epimerase locus resides on chromosome one.

References

1. Lengemann, F. W., Wasserman, R. H. and Comar, C. L. (1959). Studies on the enhancement of radiocalcium and radiostrontium absorption by lactose in the rat. *J. Nutr.*, **68**, 443

2. Fournier, P., Dupins, Y. and Fournier, A. (1971). Effect of lactose on the absorption of alkaline earth metals and intestinal lactase activity. *Isr. J. Med. Sci.*, **7**, 389

3. Condon, J. R., Nassim, J. R., Millard, F. I. C., Hilbe, A. and Stainthorpe, E. M. (1970). Calcium and phosphorus metabolism in relation to lactose tolerance. *Lancet*, **1**, 1027

4. Miller, D. and Crane, R. K. (1961). The digestive function of the epithelium of the small intestine. II. Localization of disaccharide hydrolysis in the isolated brush border of intestinal epithelial cells. *Biochim. Biophys. Acta*, **52**, 293

5. Simoons, F. J. (1970). Primary adult lactose intolerance and the milking habit: a problem in biologic and cultural interrelations. II. A culture historical hypothesis. *Am. J. Dig. Dis.*, **15**, 695

6. Brady, R. O. (1973). Inborn errors of lipid metabolism. *Adv. Enzymol.*, **38**, 293

7. Brady, R. O. (1978). Sphingolipidoses. *Annu. Rev. Biochem.*, **47**, 687

8. Sweeley, C. C. and Klionsky, B. (1963). Fabry's disease: classification as a sphingolipidosis and partial characterization of a novel glycolipid. *J. Biol. Chem.*, **238**, 3148

9. Hansen, R. G., Wood, H. G., Peeters, G. J., Jacobson, B. and Wilken, J. (1962). Lactose synthesis. VI. Labeling of lactose precursors by glycerol-1, 3-C^{14} and glucose-2-C^{14}. *J. Biol. Chem.*, **237**, 1034

10. Brodbeck, U. and Ebner, K. E. (1966). Resolution of a soluble lactose synthetase into two protein components and solubilization of microsomal lactose synthetase. *J. Biol. Chem.*, **241**, 762

11. Brodbeck, U., Denton, W. L., Tanahashi, N. and Ebner, K. E. (1967). The isolation and identification of the B-protein of lactose synthetase as α-lactalbumin. *J. Biol. Chem.*, **242**, 1391

12. Brew, K., Vanaman, T. C. and Hill, R. L. (1968). The role of α-lactalbumin and the A protein in lactose synthetase: a unique mechanism for the control of biological reaction. *Proc. Natl. Acad. Sci. USA.*, **59**, 491

13. McGuire, E. J., Jourdian, G. W., Carlson, D. M. and Roseman, S. (1965). Incorporation of D-Galactose into glycoproteins. *J. Biol. Chem.*, **240**, 4112

14. Morrison, J. F. and Ebner, K. E. (1971). Kinetic effects of α-lactalbumin with N-acetylglucosamine and glucose as galactosyl group acceptors. *J. Biol. Chem.*, **246**, 3992

15. Trejo, A. G., Haddock, J. W., Chittenden, G. J. F. and Baddiley, J. (1971). The biosynthesis of galactofuranosyl residues in galactocarolose. *Biochem. J.*, **122**, 49

16. Hers, H. G. (1960). L'aldose-réductase. *Biochim. Biophys. Acta*, **37**, 120
17. Hayman, S. and Kinoshita, J. H. (1965). Isolation and properties of lens aldose reductase. *J. Biol. Chem.*, **240**, 877
18. Van Heyningen, R. (1971). Galactose cataract: a review. *Exp. Eye Res.*, **11**, 415
19. Markwell, J., Shimamoto, G. T., Bissett, D. L. and Anderson, R. L. (1976). Pathway of galactitol catabolism in *Klebsiella pneumoniae*. *Biochem. Biophys. Res. Commun.*, **71**, 221
20. Lengeler, J. (1977). Analysis of mutations affecting the dissimilation of galactitol (dulcitol) in *Escherichia coli* K12. *Mol. Gen. Genet.*, **152**, 83
21. Bergren, W. R., Ng, W. G., Donnell, G. N. and Markey, S. P. (1972). Galactonic acid in galactosemia: identification in the urine. *Science*, **176**, 683
22. Gitzelmann, R., Wells, H. J. and Segal, S. (1974). Galactose metabolism in a patient with hereditary galactokinase deficiency. *Eur. J. Clin. Invest.*, **4**, 79
23. Wallenfels, K. and Kurz, G. (1966). *Methods in Enzymology*, Vol. IX., p. 112. (New York: Academic Press)
24. Avigad, G., Amaral, D., Asensio, C. and Horecker, B. L. (1962). The D-galactose oxidase of *Polyporus circinatus*. *J. Biol. Chem.*, **237**, 2736
25. Inouye, T., Tannenbaum, M. and Hsia, D. Y.-Y. (1962). Identification of galactose-6-phosphate in galactosemic erythrocytes. *Nature*, **193**, 67
26. Posternak, T. and Rosselet, J. P. (1954). Action de la phosphoglucomutase du muscle sur des acides aldose-1-phosphoriques. Transformation de l'acide galactose-1-phosphorique. *Helv. Chim. Acta*, **37**, 246
27. Bissett, D. L. and Anderson, R. L. (1973). Lactose and D-galactose metabolism in *Staphylococcus aureus*: Pathway of D-galactose 6-phosphate degradation. *Biochem. Biophys. Res. Commun.*, **52**, 641
28. Kosterlitz, H. W. (1943). The structure of the galactose-1-phosphate present in the liver during galactose assimilation. *Biochem. J.*, **37**, 318
29. Leloir, L. F. (1951). The enzymatic transformation of uridine diphosphate glucose into a galactose derivative. *Arch. Biochem. Biophys.*, **33**, 186
30. Caputto, R., Barra, H. S. and Cumar, F. A. (1967). *Carbohydrate metabolism*. Biosynthesis of di- and tri-saccharides. *Annu. Rev. Biochem.*, **36**, 211
31. Ginsburg, V. and Neufeld, E. F. (1969). Complex heterosaccharides of animals. *Annu. Rev. Biochem.*, **38**, 371
32. Albrecht, G. J., Bass, S. T., Seifert, L. L. and Hansen, R. G. (1966). Crystallization and properties of uridine diphosphate glucose pyrophosphorylase from liver. *J. Biol. Chem.*, **241**, 2968
33. Levine, S., Gillett, T. A., Hageman, E. and Hansen, R. G. (1969). Uridine diphosphate glucose pyrophosphorylase. II. Polymeric and subunit structure. *J. Biol. Chem.*, **244**, 5729
34. Turnquist, R. L., Gillett, T. A. and Hansen, R. G. (1974). Uridine diphosphate glucose pyrophosphorylase. Crystallization and properties of the enzyme from rabbit liver and species comparisons. *J. Biol. Chem.*, **249**, 7695
35. Abraham, H. D. and Howell, R. R. (1969). Human hepatic uridine diphosphate galactose pyrophosphorylase. *J. Biol. Chem.*, **244**, 545
36. Chacko, C. M., McCrone, L. and Nadler, H. L. (1972). Uridine diphosphoglucose pyrophosphorylase and uridine diphosphogalactose pyrophosphorylase in human skin fibroblasts derived from normal and galac-

tosemic individuals. *Biochim. Biophys. Acta*, **268**, 113
37. Gitzelmann, R. and Steinmann, B. (1973). Uridine diphosphate galactose 4-epimerase deficiency. II. Clinical follow-up, biochemical studies and family investigation. *Helv. Paediatr. Acta*, **28**, 497
38. Nelsetuen, G. L. and Kirkwood, S. (1971). The mechanism of action of the enzyme uridine diphosphoglucose 4-epimerase. *J. Biol. Chem.*, **246**, 7533
39. Gabriel, O., Van Linten, L. (1978). Biochemistry of carbohydrates. II. In D. J. Manners (ed.). *International Review of Biochemistry.*, p. 1. (Baltimore: University Park Press)
40. Isselbacher, K. J. and Krane, S. M. (1961). Studies on the mechanism of the inhibition of galactose oxidation by ethanol. *J. Biol. Chem.*, **236**, 2394
41. Kalckar, H. M., Kinoshita, J. H. and Donnell, G. N. (1973). *Biology of Brain Disfunction*. p. 31. (New York: Plenum Press)
42. Segal, S. and Rogers, S. (1971). Nucleotide inhibition of mammalian liver galactose-1-phosphate uridyltransferase. *Biochim. Biophys. Acta*, **250**, 351
43. Gitzelmann, R. (1969). Formation of galactose-1-phosphate from uridine diphosphate galactose in erythrocytes from patients with galactosemia. *Pediatr. Res.*, **3**, 279
44. Knop, J. K. and Hansen, R. G. (1970). Uridine diphosphate glucose pyrophosphorylase. IV. Crystallization and properties of the enzyme from human liver. *J. Biol. Chem.*, **245**, 2499
45. Ting, W. K. and Hansen, R. G. (1968). Uridine diphosphate galactose pyrophosphorylase from calf liver. *Proc. Soc. Exp. Biol. Med.*, **127**, 960
46. Turnquist, R. L., Turnquist, M. M., Bachmann, R. C. and Hansen, R. G. (1974). Uridine diphosphate glucose pyrophosphorylase: Differential heat inactivation and further characterization of human liver enzyme. *Biochim. Biophys. Acta*, **364**, 59
47. Gitzelmann, R. and Hansen, R. G. (1974). Galactose biogenesis and disposal in galactosemics. *Biochim. Biophys. Acta*, **372**, 374
48. Kornberg, A. (1957). Pyrophosphorylases and phosphorylases in biosynthetic reactions. *Adv. Enzymol.*, **18**, 191
49. Wood, H. G., O'Brien, W. E. and Michaels, G. (1977). Properties of carboxytransphosphorylase; pyruvate, phosphate dikinase; pyrophosphate-phosphofructokinase and pyrophosphate-acetate kinase and their roles in the metabolism of inorganic pyrophosphate. *Adv. Enzymol.*, **45**, 85
50. Russel, R. G. G. (1976). Metabolism of inorganic pyrophosphate (PPi). *Arthritis Rheum.*, **19**, 465
51. Schwenn, J. D., Lilley, R. M. and Walker, D. A. (1973). Inorganic pyrophosphatase and photosynthesis by isolated chloroplasts. I. Characterization of chloroplast pyrophosphatase and its relation to the response to exogenous pyrophosphate. *Biochim. Biophys. Acta*, **325**, 586
52. Levine, G. and Bassham, J. A. (1974). Inhibition of photosynthesis in isolated spinach chloroplasts by inorganic phosphate or inorganic pyrophosphatase in the presence of pyrophosphate and magnesium ions. *Biochim. Biophys. Acta*, **333**, 136
53. Hansen, R. G. and Gitzelmann, R. (1975). The metabolism of lactose and galactose. In A. Jeanes and J. Hodge (eds.). *Physiological Effects of Food Carbohydrates*, Vol. 15, pp. 100–122. (Am. Chem. Soc. Symposium Series)
54. Gitzelmann, R. (1965). Deficiency of erythrocyte galactokinase in a patient

with galactose diabetes. *Lancet*, **2**, 670

55. Fanconi, G. (1933). Hochgradige Galaktose-Intoleranz (Galaktose-Diabetes) bei einem Kinde mit Neurofibromatosis Recklinghausen. *Jb. Kinderheilk.*, **138**, 1

56. Gitzelmann, R. (1967). Hereditary galactokinase deficiency, a newly recognized cause of juvenile cataracts. *Pediatr. Res.*, **1**, 14

57. Gitzelmann, R. and Illig, R. (1969). Inability of galactose to mobilize insulin in galactokinase-deficient individuals. *Diabetologia*, **5**, 143

58. Gitzelmann, R., Curtius, H. C. and Müller, M. (1966). Galactitol excretion in the urine of a galactokinase-deficient man. *Biochem. Biophys. Res. Commun.*, **22**, 437

59. Pickering, W. R. and Howell, R. R. (1972). Galactokinase deficiency: clinical and biochemical findings in a new kindred. *J. Pediatr.*, **81**, 50

60. Thalhammer, O., Gitzelmann, R. and Pantlitschko, M. (1968). Hypergalactosemia and galactosuria due to galactokinase deficiency in a newborn. *Pediatrics*, **42**, 441

61. Dahlqvist, A., Gamstorp, I. and Madsen, H. (1970). A patient with hereditary galactokinase deficiency. *Acta Paediatr. Scand.*, **59**, 669

62. Dahlqvist, A. (Personal communication)

63. Mayes, J. S. and Guthrie, R. (1968). Detection of heterozygotes for galactokinase deficiency in a human population. *Biochem. Genet.*, **2**, 219

64. Tedesco, T. A., Nonow, R., Miller, K. and Mellman, W. J. (1972). Galactokinase: evidence for a new racial polymorphism. *Science*, **178**, 176

65. Tedesco, T. A., Miller, K. L., Rawnsley, B. E., Adams, M. C., Markus, H. B., Orkwiszewski, K. G. and Mellman, W. J. (1977). The Philadelphia variant of galactokinase. *Am. J. Hum. Genet.*, **29**, 240

66. Linneweh, F., Schaumlöffel, E. and Vetrella, M. (1970). Galaktokinase-Defekt bei einem Neugeborenen. *Klin. Wochenschr.*, **48**, 31

67. Vigneron, C., Marchal, C., Deifts, C., Vidailhet, M., Pierson, M. et Neimann, N. (1970). Déficit partiel et transitoire en galactokinase érythrocytaire chez un nouveau-né. *Arch. Fr. Pédiatr.*, **27**, 523

68. Cook, J. G. H., Don, N. A. and Mann, T. P. (1971). Hereditary galactokinase deficiency. *Arch. Dis. Child.*, **46**, 465

69. Kerr, M. M., Logan, R. W., Cant, J. S. and Hutchison, J. H. (1971). Galactokinase deficiency in a newborn infant. *Arch. Dis. Child.*, **46**, 864

70. Monteleone, J. A., Beutler, E., Monteleone, P. L., Utz, C. L. and Casey, E. C. (1971). Cataracts, galactosuria and hypergalactosemia due to galactokinase deficiency in a child. *Am. J. Med.*, **50**, 403

71. Levy, N. S., Krill, A. E. and Beutler, E. (1972). Galactokinase deficiency and cataracts. *Am. J. Ophthalmol.*, **74**, 41

72. Kaloud, H., Sitzmann, F. C., Mayer, R. und Paltauf, F. (1973). Klinische und biochemische Befunde bei einem Kleinkind mit hereditärem Galaktokinase-Defekt. *Clin. Paediatr.*, **185**, 18

73. Beutler, E., Matsumoto, F., Kuhl, W., Krill, A., Levy, N., Sparkes, R. and Degnan, M. (1973). Galactokinase deficiency as a cause of cataracts. *N. Engl. J. Med.*, **288**, 1203

74. Olambiwonnu, N. O., McVie, R., Ng, W. G., Frasier, S. D. and Donnell, G. N. (1974). Galactokinase deficiency in twins: clinical and biochemical studies. *Pediatrics*, **53**, 314

75. Vecchio, F., Carnevale, F. and Di Bitonto, G. (1976). Galactokinase deficiency in an Italian infant. In H. Bickel and J. Stern (eds.). *Inborn Errors of Calcium and Bone Metabolism*, pp. 317–324. (Lancaster: MTP Press)

76. Litman, N., Kanter, A. I. and Finberg, L. (1975). Galactokinase deficiency presenting as pseudotumor cerebri. *J. Pediatr.*, **86**, 410

77. Ritter, J. A. and Cannon, E. J. (1955). Galactosemia with cataracts. *N. Engl. J. Med.*, **252**, 747

78. Segal, S. (Personal communication)

79. Gitzelmann, R. (1975). Additional findings in galactokinase deficiency. *J. Pediatr.*, **87**, 1007

80. Kinoshita, J. H., Dvornik, D., Kraml, M. and Gabbay, K. (1968). The effect of an aldose reductase inhibitor on the galactose-exposed rabbit lens. *Biochim. Biophys, Acta*, **158**, 472

81. Kinoshita, J. H. (1965). Cataracts in galactosemia. *Invest. Ophthalmol.*, **4**, 786

82. Prchal, J. T., Conrad, M. E. and Skalka, H. W. (1978). Association of presenile cataracts with heterozygosity for galactosaemic states and with riboflavin deficiency. *Lancet*, **1**, 12

83. Von Reuss, A. (1908). Zuckerausscheidung im Säuglingsalter. *Wien. Med. Wochenschr.*, **58**, 800

84. Schwarz, V., Golberg, L., Komrower, G. M. and Holzel, A. (1956). Some disturbances of erythrocyte metabolism in galactosaemia. *Biochem. J.*, **62**, 34

85. Kalckar, H. M., Anderson, E. P. and Isselbacher, K. J. (1956). Galactosemia, a congenital defect in a nucleotide transferase. *Biochim. Biophys. Acta*, **20**, 262

86. Komrower, G. M. (1973). Treatment of galactosaemia. In J. W. T. Seakins, R. A. Saunders and C. Toothill (eds.). *Treatment of Inborn Errors of Metabolism*, pp. 113–120. (Edinburgh: Churchill Livingstone)

87. Segal, S. (1978). Disorders of galactose metabolism. In J. B. Stanbury, J. B. Wyngaarden and D. S. Fredrickson (eds.). *The Metabolic Basis of Inherited Disease*, pp. 160–181. (New York: McGraw-Hill)

88. Tedesco, T. A., Wu, J. W., Boches, F. S. and Mellman, W. J. (1975). The genetic defect in galactosemia. *N. Engl. J. Med.*, **292**, 737

89. Donnell, G. N., Koch, R. and Bergren, W. R. (1969). Observations on results of management of galactosemic patients. In D. Y.-Y. Hsia (ed.). *Galactosemia*, pp. 247–268. (Springfield: Charles C. Thomas)

90. Nadler, H. L., Inouye, T. and Hsia, D. Y.-Y. (1969). Classical galactosemia: a study of fifty-five cases. In D. Y.-Y. Hsia (ed.). *Galactosemia*, pp. 127–139. (Springfield: Charles C. Thomas)

91. Donnell, G. N. and Bergren, W. R. (1975). The galactosaemias. In D. N. Raine (ed.). *The Treatment of Inherited Metabolic Disease*, pp. 91–114. (Lancaster: MTP Press)

92. Komrower, G. M. and Lee, D. H. (1970). Long-term follow-up of galactosaemia. *Arch. Dis. Child.*, **45**, 367

93. Fishler, K., Donnell, G. N., Bergren, W. R. and Koch, R. (1972). Intellectual and personality development in children with galactosemia. *Pediatrics*, **50**, 412

94. Gitzelmann, R. (1974). α-D-galactose-1-phosphate determination as galactose after hydrolysis of phosphate. In H. U. Bergmeyer and K. Gawehn (eds.).

Methods of Enzymatic Analysis, pp. 1291–1295. (New York: Weinheim Academic Press)

95. Gitzelmann, R., Curtius, H. C. and Schneller, I. (1967). Galactitol and galactose-1-phosphate in the lens of a galactosemic infant. *Exp. Eye Res.*, **6**, 1

96. Harris, H. (1976). Enzyme variants in human populations. *Johns Hopkins Med. J.*, **138**, 245

97. Beutler, E. (1973). Screening for galactosemia. Studies of the gene frequencies for galactosemia and the Duarte variant. *Isr. J. Med. Sci.*, **9**, 1323

98. Thomakos, A., Beutler, E. and Stamatoyannopoulos, G. (1977). Variants of galactose-1-phosphate uridyl transferase in the Greek populations. *Hum. Genet.*, **36**, 335

99. Bissbort, S. and Kömpf, J. (1972). Population genetics of red cell galactose-1-phosphate-uridyl-transferase (EC: 2.7.7.12). *Humangenetik*, **17**, 79

100. Kühnl, P., Nowicki, L. und Spielmann, W. (1974). Untersuchungen zum Polymorphismus der Galaktose-1-Phosphat-Uridyltransferase (EC: 2.7.7.12) mittels Agarosegelelektrophorese. *Humangenetik*, **24**, 227

101. Martin, W. und Kienzler, G. (1975). Polymorphismus der menschlichen Erythrozyten-Uridyltransferase (E.C. 2.7.7.12). Untersuchung an einer Stichprobe aus der Berliner Bevölkerung. *Blut*, **30**, 59

102. Pflugshaupt, R., Scherz, R. and Bütler, R. (1976). Polymorphism of human red cell adenosine deaminase, esterase D, glutamate pyruvate transaminase and galactose-1-phosphate-uridyltransferase in the Swiss population. *Hum. Hered.*, **26**, 161

103. Mathai, C. K. and Beutler, E. (1966). Electrophoretic variation of galactose-1-phosphate uridyltransferase. *Science*, **154**, 1179

104. Gitzelmann, R., Poley, J. R. and Prader, A. (1967). Partial galactose-1-phosphate uridyltransferase deficiency due to a variant enzyme. *Helv. Paediatr. Acta*, **22**, 252

105. Levy, H. L., Sepe, S. J., Walton, D. S., Shih, V. E., Hammersen, G., Houghton, S. and Beutler, E. (1978). Galactose-1-phosphate uridyltransferase deficiency due to Duarte/galactosemia combined variation: clinical and biochemical studies. *J. Pediatr.*, **92**, 390

106. Wharton, C. H., Berry, H. K. and Bofinger, M. K. (1978). Galactose-1-phosphate accumulation by a Duarte-transferase deficiency double heterozygote. *Clin. Genet.*, **13**, 171

107. Schwarz, H. P., Zuppinger, K., Zimmerman, A., Dauwalder, H. and Scherz, R. (1978). Doppeltheterozygotie für Duarte-Variante und Galaktosämie – genetische Variation oder Krankheit? (Abstr.). *Helv. Paediatr. Acta*, **40**, 14

108. Holzel, A. and Komrower, G. M. (1955). A study of the genetics of galactosemia. *Arch. Dis. Child.*, **30**, 155

109. Donnell, G. N., Bergren, W. R. and Roldan, M. (1959). Genetic studies in galactosemia. I: The oral galactose tolerance test and the heterozygous state. *Pediatrics*, **24**, 418

110. Mayes, J. S. and Miller, L. R. (1973). The metabolism of galactose by galactosemic fibroblasts in vitro. *Biochim. Biophys. Acta*, **313**, 9

111. Gitzelmann, R., Hansen, R. G. and Steinmann, B. (1975). Biogenesis of galactose, a possible mechanism of self-intoxication in galactosemia. In F. A. Hommes and C. J. Van den Berg (eds.). *Normal and Pathological Develop-*

ment of Energy Metabolism, pp. 25–37. (London: Academic Press)

112. Roe, T. F., Ng, W. G., Bergren, W. R. and Donnell, G. N. (1973). Urinary galactitol in galactosemic patients. *Biochem. Med.*, **7**, 266

113. Gitzelmann, R. and Hansen, R. G. (1974). Biogenesis of galactose: evidence in galactosemic infants. (Abstr.) *Pediatr. Res.*, **8**, 137

114. Rogers, S., Holtzapple, P. G., Mellman, W. J. and Segal, S. (1970). Characteristics of galactose-1-phosphate uridyl transferase in intestinal mucosa of normal and galactosemic humans. *Metabolism*, **19**, 701

115. Mellman, W. J., Tedesco, T. A. and Feigl, P. (1968). Estimation of the gene frequency of the Duarte variant of galactose-1-phosphate uridyl transferase. *Ann. Hum. Genet.*, **32**, 1

116. Segal, S., Blair, A. and Roth, H. (1965). The metabolism of galactose by patients with congenital galactosemia. *Am. J. Med.*, **38**, 62

117. Baker, L., Mellman, W. J., Tedesco, T. A. and Segal, S. (1966). Galactosemia: symptomatic and asymptomatic homozygotes in one Negro sibship. *J. Pediatr.*, **68**, 551

118. Ng, W. G., Bergren, W. R., Fields, M. and Donnell, G. N. (1969). An improved electrophoretic procedure for galactose-1-phosphate uridyl transferase: demonstration of multiple activity bands with the Duarte variant. *Biochem. Biophys. Res. Commun.*, **37**, 354

119. Beutler, E. and Mathai, C. K. (1968). Genetic variation in red cell galactose-1-phosphate uridyl transferase. In *Hereditary Disorders of Erythrocyte Metabolism*, pp. 66–86. (USA: Grune Stratton)

120. Schapira, F. and Kaplan, J.-C. (1969). Electrophoretic abnormality of galactose-1-phosphate uridyl transferase in galactosemia. *Biochem. Biophys. Res. Commun.* **35**, 451

121. Hammersen, G., Houghton, S. and Levy, H. L. (1975). Rennes-like variant of galactosemia: clinical and biochemical studies. *J. Pediatr.*, **87**, 50

122. Chacko, C. M., Christian, J. C. and Nadler, H. L. (1971). Unstable galactose-1-phosphate uridyl transferase: a new variant of galactosemia. *J. Pediatr.*, **78**, 454

123. Ng, W. G., Bergren, W. R. and Donnell, G. N. (1973). A new variant of galactose-1-phosphate uridyltransferase in man: the Los Angeles variant. *Ann. Hum. Genet.*, **37**, 1

124. Matz, D., Enzenauer, J. and Menne, F. (1975). Ueber einen Fall von atypischer Galaktosämie. *Humangenetik*, **27**, 309

125. v. Figura, K., Lang, A. and Gröbe, H. (1979). Eine neue Galaktosämievariante: Hemmung der Uridyltransferaseaktivität durch Glucose 1-Phosphat. (In preparation).

126. Scherz, R., Pflugshaupt, R. and Bütler, R. (1976). A new genetic variant of galactose-1-phosphate uridyl transferase. *Hum. Genet.*, **35**, 51

127. Chacko, C. M., Wappner, R. S., Brandt, I. K. and Nadler, H. L. (1977). The Chicago variant of clinical galactosemia. *Hum. Genet.*, **37**, 261

128. Kalckar, H. M. (1965). Galactose metabolism and cell 'sociology'. *Science*, **150**, 305

129. Gitzelmann, R. (1972). Deficiency of uridine diphosphate galactose 4-epimerase in blood cells of an apparently healthy infant. Preliminary communication. *Helv. Paediatr. Acta*, **27**, 125

130. Paigen, K. and Pacholec, F. (1979). A new method of screening neonates for

galactosemia. *J. Lab. Clin. Med.* (In press).
131. Gitzelmann, R. and Steinmann, B. (1973). Uridine diphosphate galactose 4-epimerase deficiency. II. Clinical follow-up, biochemical studies and family investigation. *Helv. Paediatr. Acta*, **28,** 497
132. Gitzelmann, R., Steinmann, B., Mitchell, B. and Haigis, E. (1976). Uridine diphosphate galactose 4'-epimerase deficiency. IV. Report of eight cases in three families. *Helv. Paediatr. Acta*, **31,** 441
133. Mitchell, B., Haigis, E., Steinmann, B. and Gitzelmann, R. (1975). Reversal of UDP-galactose 4-epimerase deficiency of human leukocytes in culture. (Gene expression/enzyme deficiency/lymphocyte transformation). *Proc. Natl. Acad. Sci. USA*, **72,** 5026
134. Gitzelmann, R. and Haigis, E. (1978). Appearance of active UDP-galactose 4'-epimerase in cells cultured from epimerase-deficient persons. *J. Inher. Metab. Dis.*, **1,** 41
135. Katunuma, N., Kito, K. and Kominami, E. (1971). A new enzyme that specifically inactivates apoprotein of NAD-dependent dehydrogenases. *Biochem. Biophys. Res. Commun.*, **45,** 76
136. Marshall, W. E. and Omachi, A. (1974). Measured and calculated NAD$^+$/NADH ratios in human erythrocytes. *Biochim. Biophys. Acta*, **354,** 1
137. McKusick, V. A. (1975). *Mendelian Inheritance in Man*, 4th ed., entry No. 11170, p. 39. (Baltimore: Johns Hopkins University Press)
138. Isselbacher, K. J. (1957). Evidence for an accessory pathway of galactose metabolism in mammalian liver. *Science*, **126,** 652

5

Clinical aspects of galactosaemia

G. N. Donnell, R. Koch, K. Fishler and
W. G. Ng

INTRODUCTION

Classical galactosaemia (transferase deficiency) is a relatively rare metabolic disorder, which is important to the paediatrician as a model for the interdisciplinary approach to the treatment of children with inborn errors of metabolism. Early diagnosis and prompt treatment with a galactose-free diet can lead to excellent immediate results and a favourable long term prognosis. Mass neonatal screening constitutes an essential first step in reducing mortality and morbidity among galactosaemic children.

Galactosaemia has been an area of intensive research involving close collaboration of the paediatrician, biochemist, psychologist and nutritionist. Our preliminary results from treatment of galactosaemic infants and children were reported in 1967[1]. The present communication outlines new findings collected from 59 patients during the succeeding decade, including observations on some older patients during adolescence and early adult life.

PATIENTS IN THE STUDY

Fifty-nine children with galactosaemia from 47 families have been followed at the Children's Hospital of Los Angeles from 1949–1978. Based upon the

103

clinical findings and conventional biochemical studies it has been assumed that the same defect in galactose metabolism exists throughout the whole sample but it is likely that variants of the transferase defect will be found as newer biochemical methods are applied to the evaluation of patients with galactosaemia.

The age distribution of our patients is shown in Table 5.1. Approximately half of the individuals are of school age, and one third has progressed beyond that stage. Twenty-seven are male and thirty-two female; they range

TABLE 5.1   Present age distribution

Status	Age	Number
Pre-school	0–6	13
School	6–17	25
Post-school	17+	21

in age from 1 to 29 years. Forty-three (73%) are Caucasian, nine (15%) are Mexican–American and seven (12%) are Black. None is of Oriental or of American Indian origin. Seventeen of 59 were diagnosed at birth or within the first week of life; of these, fifteen were born to families known to be at risk and two were identified by newborn screening. Of the remaining 42, 18 were diagnosed between 8 and 30 days of age and an additional 17 between 1 and 3 months. Seven were not diagnosed until after 4 months of age.

Three of the 59 have been lost to follow-up. Information concerning these individuals will be included until the time they were last seen at the Children's Hospital of Los Angeles.

FACTORS IN MANAGEMENT

The clinical manifestations of galactosaemia are well known[2, 3]. The findings in this series were typical (Table 5.2). With the exception of the seventeen infants diagnosed at birth, all children were moderately to severely ill. Recurrent vomiting, weight loss, jaundice, and hepatomegaly occurred in the majority. The occurrence of other features of the disorder was variable.

As soon as the diagnosis was suspected, each patient was given a lactose free diet[4]. Milk, milk products and all foods containing milk were eliminated; a casein hydrolysate formula (Nutramigen: Mead Johnson) or soya bean preparations were substituted. Dietary restriction was rigid until school age was reached and then minor relaxation was allowed. Milk and foods obviously containing milk, such as ice cream, were still excluded, but small

TABLE 5.2   Clinical data among 43 symptomatic galactosaemic subjects

Major organ systems	Signs and symptoms	Number of subjects
General	Anorexia and weight loss (failure to thrive)	23
	Lethargy	7
	Pallor and/or cyanosis	6
Hepatic	Hepatomegaly	39
	Jaundice	34
	Ascites and/or oedema	7
Gastrointestinal	Vomiting	17
	Abdominal distention	9
	Diarrhoea	3
	Light stool	1
Ophthalmological	Cataracts	19
Spleen	Splenomegaly	6
Blood	Haemorrhagic phenomenon	3
Genito-urinary	Dark urine	6
	Dysuria and frequency	1
Central Nervous System*	Bulging anterior fontanel	4
	Neonatal anoxia suspected	1
	Mental retardation	2
	Cerebral palsy	1
	Speech delay	1
Infection	Sepsis	5
	Meningitis	1
	Septic joint	1
	Osteomyelitis	1
	Ethmoiditis	1
	Genito-urinary	1

* 1. Includes one individual diagnosed at 11 years of age who remained untreated (and not included in study except as noted in Table 5.6)
  2. The 17 individuals diagnosed and treated at birth remained symptom free

amounts of bread and other foods containing milk products were permitted. In some instances dietary indiscretions became evident, especially during adolescence.

Discontinuation of the restricted diet was never recommended because adaptation to galactose was never documented. Galactose tolerance tests remained abnormal in all the subjects selected for study. Concern about the development of cataracts was an important factor in the decision against discontinuation.

Progress of patients was assessed at regular visits for clinical evaluation, nutritional assessment and psychological testing. Determination of erythrocyte galactose-1-phosphate was carried out routinely.

OUTCOME

Dietary treatment may be life saving for individuals affected with galactosaemia. Without removal of galactose, many of the 59 patients would have died in infancy and many of those that survived might have become severely mentally retarded. With treatment, at least half of the 59 individuals have developed very well; some have normal IQs ranging up to 125.

General health

Most of the clinical evidence of the disorder was reversed a few weeks after treatment was initiated. Usually jaundice disappeared in a few days and weight gain was restored within a week or two.

Twenty-one children exhibited cataracts, two strabismus and two severe hyperopia. Seventeen of 21 patients have minimal cataracts and do not require surgery; in one child the cataracts completely resolved.

Three children required surgery for cataracts; one an iridectomy (bilateral), one capsulotomy and one lysis of cataracts by laser beam. Eye changes in the latter two progressed while on a well controlled galactose restricted diet. The individual with bilateral iridectomy has dense cataracts, but surgery has been refused because she is afraid of losing financial aid for the blind. Strabismus was corrected by surgery in two children with this problem and hyperopia corrected by refraction in another two.

One patient had seizures but their relationship to galactosaemia remains uncertain. During the follow-up there was no evidence of liver involvement in any of the children but gallstones were discovered and removed in one of them. One child developed osteogenic sarcoma; no relationship to galactosaemia was proven. This patient underwent surgical amputation. She has not had a recurrence in over five years. Ovarian insufficiency was diagnosed in a seventeen year old girl when she did not develop secondary sexual characteristics at the appropriate time. She was of normal height and had no stigmata of Turner's syndrome. Her karyotype was normal.

Growth

The birthweights of the galactosaemic patients were within normal limits.

Sufficient data on 8 males and on 8 females have been collected for growth curves from birth to 18 years of age for comparison with normal standards of the National Center of Health Statistics (Figures 5.1 and 5.2). The growth velocity for male and female patients was similar. In terms of height; all patients lagged behind normal standards until 18 years of age when they finally approached normal. The weight throughout the 18 year span was slightly below that of the normals.

Intellectual development

All patients were periodically assessed with the same developmental and psychological testing procedures. These studies were coordinated with medical, social, nutritional and laboratory evaluations. The Gesell Developmental Scales were used for infants and children up to 3 years of age. Because estimates of early infant abilities are based on sensory and

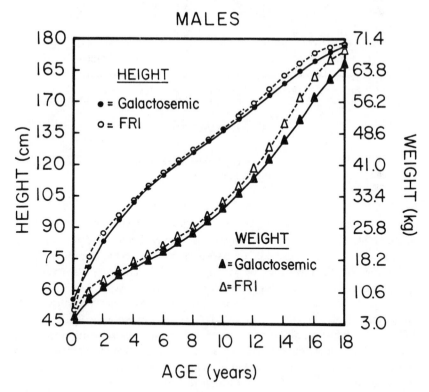

Figure 5.1 Mean growth curve of eight galactosaemic males compared to normal mean of the Fels Research Institute (FRI)

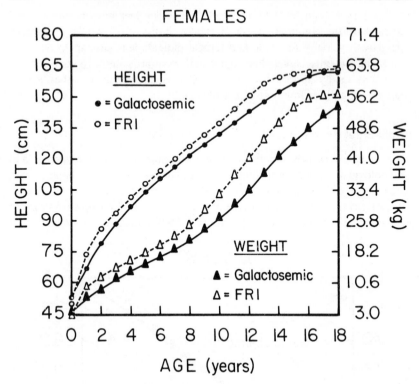

Figure 5.2   Mean growth curve of eight galactosaemic females compared to normal mean of the Fels Research Institute (FRI)

neuromuscular functions, they are reported as developmental quotient (DQ), rather than intellectual quotient (IQ). Intelligence, as determined by various mental functions, can be assessed only if verbal communication exists. The Stanford–Binet Scale was used for children from 3 to 7 years of age, and the Wechsler Intelligence Scale for Children (WISC) over 8 years. After age 16 years, the adult extension of the WISC, the Wechsler Adult Intelligence Scale (WAIS), was utilized. Comparisons between age groups is difficult due to known differences amongst the testing instruments employed.

Each child under the age of 5 years was given the Seguin formboard test and a drawing test which included copying simple geometric forms (circle, cross, square, etc.). The Bender–Gestalt test, Raven's Matrices and Draw-A-Person were administered routinely to older children. These techniques facilitated early identification of possible visual perceptual limitations.

Earlier studies had suggested that such disabilities might be frequent among school-age galactosaemic patients.

The overall findings are summarized in Table 5.3. For purposes of discussion, the sample has been divided into three groups, corresponding to the grouping in Table 5.1.

Group I This group is composed of 13 children from 5 months of age to 5.5 years. The range of DQ/IQ is from 70 to 125, with a mean of 102. In general, dietary control has been good to excellent. Visual–perceptual performance is normal for the four children old enough to be tested. Significant behavioural problems were not identified. For the most part, they can be described as happy, sociable children.

TABLE 5.3   Distribution of intelligence in galactosaemic patients

Group number	Number cases	Age range (years)	DQ/IQ range	Mean DQ/IQ	SD
I	13	0–6	70–125	102	12.8
II	25	6–17	50–117	91	17.5
III	21	17–29	72–119	94	18.2
			Total sample:	95	16

Group II Group II consists of 25 individuals from 6 to 17 years of age. Intelligence quotients vary from 50 to 117, with a mean of 91. All children attend school. Of the 25 children, 12 are in the proper grade for their age. The educational needs of the remaining 13 are shown in Table 5.4. Eighteen of the 25 show mild to moderate degrees of visual-perceptual difficulties which may have had a bearing upon their academic progress. The school problems most frequently encountered were difficulties in writing, reading and arithmetic. Some require special tutoring and other help with their school work.

Some of the older children are rather shy and restrained in interpersonal contacts even though basically they are friendly and cooperative. None of the children above the age of 12 years is described by school personnel as 'hyperactive'.

Group III This group includes the 21 individuals ranging from 17 to 29.5 years. Two in this group have been lost to follow-up. The mean IQ is 94 with a range of 72–119.

The six youngest attend high school, three in regular classes and three in

TABLE 5.4   School status in galactosaemic children

Elementary school (Grades K–6):	7
Regular class:	5
1 Grade below normal	1
2 Grades below normal	0
Special class:	
Educable mentally retarded	1
Secondary School (Grades 7–12):	18
Regular class:	7
1 Grade below normal	2
2 Grades below normal	1
Special class:	
Educationally handicapped (IQ 70+)	2
Educable mentally retarded (IQ 50–70)	3
Trainable mentally retarded (IQ 30–50)	2
Aphasic:	1

special classes (two are educable and one trainable). Of the children in regular class placement, one is an Alpha student who will enter college after graduation, another plans to enter college and the other is considering this possibility.

Two of the 15 individuals beyond high school age are in college. Five are gainfully employed, including one in the Air Force and one who is a programme director for a radio station. The oldest, a male, has joined a religious order. The two oldest females have married and have had four normal heterozygous children. One of these two has succeeded as a housewife and mother of her one child in spite of borderline intelligence. The other is alcoholic and separated from her husband. She lives in a sociologically unfavourable environment and has emotional problems. Her three heterozygous children, all developmentally normal, have been placed in a foster home by court order.

One other patient, a male, also has an unstable home background and a history of alcoholism. Two other adults, a brother and sister, have had difficulty establishing independence; they are working, but living at home. In addition to participating in household tasks they have established a home industry for selling canaries.

DISCUSSION

Galactosaemia, if untreated, usually results in early death for many affected children and creates the prospect of severe mental retardation for those who survive. Among the families included in the present study, there was a history of 13 neonatal deaths prior to initial diagnosis of a galactosaemic homozygote. The deaths occurred at an average age of 6 weeks and were usually attributed to liver disease or infection. The history and autopsy findings were found to be consistent with a diagnosis of galactosaemia. Only one death from galactosaemia occurred in a family known to have a child with the disease. Early testing and treatment could not be provided because the mother failed to inform the staff of her pregnancy. The high rate of early death emphasizes the need to consider galactosaemia in the differential diagnosis of the sick neonate.

One other individual, not included in the present study, was identified at age 11 years as a galactosaemia homozygote at the time a much younger sibling was diagnosed. This older child was in an institution for the retarded. He had bilateral cataracts, cerebral palsy and severe mental retardation. He remained in the institution until his death at age 24 years.

Galactosaemia is a devastating disease. Treatment results in survival and reversal of the acute symptoms, but the long term outcome (intellectual development) is not entirely certain. Experience gained in the present study has shown that many have developed very well, but others have had more or less severe problems; the causes of this variability in response to treatment need exploration.

Family differences related to genetic or sociological factors may account for some of these findings. Table 5.5 presents a comparison of the IQ results for homozygote galactosaemics with those for fathers and mothers, normal brothers and sisters and heterozygote siblings. These data are for a group and are not a comparison family by family. The spread of values within an individual group is broad, and drawing conclusions from the means is difficult. In considering individual patients in relation to their parents, there is a tendency, not apparent in the grouped data, for patients with higher IQ scores to come from parents with higher than average IQ.

Another determinant for outcome is the age at which diagnosis was made. The relationship between intellectual development and the time of initiation of dietary treatment is shown in Table 5.6. The data in this table tend to support the impression that a more favourable outcome results if the patients are treated at an earlier age. The mean IQs for the children in the first three groups are about the same. However, one of the patients included in the 0–7 day group was improperly treated elsewhere and was taken off

TABLE 5.5   Intellectual status of the parents and unaffected siblings of galactosaemic patients

Subjects	Number	IQ range	Mean	S.D.
Fathers	33	87–138	110	12.7
Mothers	33	70–127	106	14.2
Normal siblings				
Brothers	5	92–114	103	8.9
Sisters	9	82–116	101	12.5
Heterozygote siblings				
Brothers	13	91–123	105	11.3
Sisters	13	86–125	105	11.1
Homozygote	59	50–125	95	16.0

diet at age 6 months. He has the lowest IQ of the group (56) and was not seen by us until 3–4 years of age. If this case were eliminated, the mean IQ for the remaining 16 would be 99.5. In patients treated after 4 months, there is a precipitous drop in mean IQ as compared to the first three groups, although the numbers are small. Five individuals diagnosed at 4–11 months were all treated adequately after diagnosis, but two of three in the last group never received adequate therapy. The mean IQ value for the three individuals in this group (after 1 year of age) is biased by the inclusion of the patient (mentioned earlier) who was not diagnosed until age 11 years and who is not otherwise a part of this study. Another of the three patients, who was diagnosed at 17 months, received inadequate treatment due to poor compliance and subsequently was lost to the study.

Assessment of the relationship of late diagnosis to intellectual ability requires more data but it is reasonable to consider that symptoms should be avoided and that diagnosis should be made and treatment instituted at the earliest possible age. Neonatal screening is an important step in this direction.

Electroencephalographic findings were non-specific and variable; 73% of those diagnosed before 7 days of age exhibited normal tracing whereas 50% of those diagnosed after the age of 4 months were abnormal. In view of the small sample size in the latter group, reliable interpretation of this data is not feasible. Our oldest patient was diagnosed at 14 months of age and his most recent electroencephalogram, at age 23, was normal.

While diagnosis and treatment from birth are desirable objectives, the possibility exists that galactosaemic homozygotes may have experienced un-

TABLE 5.6 **Relationship between the age of diagnosis, intelligence, visual-perceptual status and EEG results**

	Age of Diagnosis				
	Birth (0–7 days)	*Days* (8–30)	*Months* (1–3)	*Months* (4–11)	*Years* (over 1)
Number of cases	17	18	17	5	3 *
Mean IQ	97	94	91	62	57
Visual-perceptual status	7 N	6 N	8 N	0 N	1 N
	7 A	6 A	7 A	5 A	0 A
	3 NA	6 NA	2 NA	0 NA	2 NA
EEG results	11 N	7 N	9 N	2 N	2 N
	4 A	4 A	6 A	2 A	0 A
	2 NA	7 NA	2 NA	1 NA	1 NA

N – Normal; A – Abnormal; NA – Not available

* Includes one individual diagnosed at 11 years of age who remained untreated (and not included in study except as noted in Table 5.2)

favourable intrauterine exposure to galactose or its metabolites. This concept is supported by comparisons between homozygotes diagnosed at birth, who had no post-natal exposure to galactose, and older siblings who were diagnosed and treated at varying intervals from 2 weeks to 11 months after birth (Table 5.7). Comparison of the mean IQ scores reveals that the mean values for the two groups are similar. Moreover, the mean IQ for the 17 galactosaemic children treated at birth is 97; this is close to that for all 59 patients (94). These results do not support the conclusions of our earlier studies, summarized in 1967, that patients treated from birth appeared to have a better outcome than those exposed to milk for varying short periods of time.

Cord blood erythrocyte galactose-1-phosphate determination was obtained for 12 homozygotes (Table 5.8). All values demonstrated an accumulation of galactose-1-phosphate which occurred during intra-uterine life even though the mothers had been on a restricted lactose intake throughout pregnancy. The obvious inference is that the intra-uterine environment is unfavourable for the homozygous fetus. That this is most likely the result of the metabolic processes of the fetus is suggested by the fact that the two treated galactosaemic homozygous mothers have had clinically normal heterozygous children. This is in contrast to the problems experienced in untreated maternal phenylketonuria.

TABLE 5.7   Comparison of ten pairs of galactosaemic siblings

Age diagnosed and treated (months)		Latest IQ		Visual-perceptual		EEG	
Index case	Younger sib	Index case	Younger sib	Index case	Younger sib	Index case	Younger sib
3	Birth	119	118	N	N	N	N
3	0.5	106	79	N	A	N	N
1.5	Birth	79	94	A	N	A	N
1.5	Birth	92	80	N	A	N	N
1.5	Birth	121	117	N	N	N	N
Birth	Birth	110	90	N	A	N	N
0.5	Birth	95	84	A	A	N	A
11	Birth	83	115	A	N	A	N
3	Birth	67	92	A	N	A	N
1	Birth	100	93	A	A	N	A
	Mean IQ:	97	96				
	S.D.:	17.6	15.1				

N – Normal
A – Abnormal

TABLE 5.8   Relationship of cord blood erythrocyte galactose-1-PO_4 content and subsequent IQs

Case	Cord blood erythrocyte galactose-1-PO_4 content		Latest IQ
	(μg/ml)	(μmol/l)	
1	246	945	103
2	177	680	97
3	164	630	103
4	127	488	110
5	127	488	115
6	116	445	100
7	91	349	97
8	90	346	107
9	87	334	93
10	47	180	81
11	47	180	100
12	39	150	128
	Average 113	434	Mean 102

CONCLUSIONS

The outcome of dietary treatment of 59 individuals with galactosaemia cared for at the Children's Hospital of Los Angeles during the past 30 years suggests that dietary management is effective. All patients survived and general health and growth approximate to normal. Most have attained satisfactory intellectual development. For the remainder the outcome has been less favourable for reasons that are ill understood.

Data from this study suggest that the intrauterine environment may be one factor in variability. Other variables may include age of diagnosis and treatment, family background and genetic factors unrelated to the disease. The necessity for prolonged adherence to diet also poses problems in compliance and in the maintenance of nutritional adequacy. Finally, the affected individuals are the offspring of families of varying economic status which may influence the development independently of galactosaemia and its treatment.

The principles of dietary management of galactosaemia remain simple but their application is more complex. There is no doubt that as we gain experience we will gain greater insight enabling us to improve the approach to management.

Acknowledgements

The authors wish to express their appreciation to W. R. Bergren, Elizabeth Wenz and Malcolm Williamson for their assistance in the preparation of this manuscript. Special thanks to Lee Mollison for her patience in typing and retyping this manuscript.

This work was supported by Grants Nos. 911 and 422 of the Maternal and Child Health Service, D.H.E.W. (USA) and the Michael J. Connell Foundation.

References

1. Donnell, G. N., Koch, R. and Bergren, W. R. (1967). Observations on results of management of galactosemic patients. In D.Y.-Y. Hsia (ed.). *Galactosemia*, pp. 247–268. (Springfield, Illinois: Charles C. Thomas)
2. Komrower, G. M., Schwarz, V., Holzel, A. and Goldberg, L. (1956). A clinical and biochemical study of galactosaemia. A possible explanation of the nature of the biochemical lesion. *Arch. Dis. Child.*, **31**, 254
3. Nadler, H. L., Inouye, T. and Hsia, D. Y.-Y. (1969). Classical Galactosemia: A study of fifty-five cases. In D. Y.-Y. Hsia (ed.). *Galactosaemia*, pp. 127–139. (Springfield, Illinois: Charles C. Thomas)
4. Koch, R. Donnell, G. N., Wenz, E., Fishler, K., Graliker, B. and Bergren, W. R. (1973). Galactosaemia. In V. C. Kelly (ed.). *Brennemann's Practice of Pediatrics*. (New York: Harper and Row)

6

How long should galacto-saemia be treated?

N. J. Brandt

INTRODUCTION

Numerous recent publications on hereditary galactosaemia indicate that many problems still remain: too many late diagnosed patients; the question of whether population screening is necessary; the atypical cases of galactosaemia; and finally, another major dilemma, should treatment be lifelong or not?

There are many excellent reviews on galactosaemia in the literature, including detailed instructions on the composition of the diet and management in the neonatal period and early childhood. Everyone agrees with the proposals put forward by the Manchester group[1] that the diet should be very restricted in the first few years of life; but generally no one mentions the older child nor the adult patient. The American Academy of Pediatrics summarised their recommendations in 1967[2] but even here it is not stated how long treatment should be continued. There are notable exceptions however, namely Komrower's review in 1973[3] and Donnell's in 1975[4]. They both accept a relaxed attitude towards dietary treatment when the patients are a few years old.

Classical galactosaemia

Features of classical galactosaemia which form a basis for discussion include:

117

(1) Galactose-1-phosphate-uridyltransferase is absent in all tissues and the enzyme deficiency persists throughout life.
(2) Galactose-1-phosphate is very toxic as we know from late diagnosed patients and also from groups of patients in bad dietary control.
(3) In the normal liver as well as in the galactosaemic liver, there are abundant amounts of galactokinase and, as the formation of galactose-1-phosphate by this enzyme is almost irreversible, most ingested galactose will quickly be transformed to galactose-1-phosphate. The inhibition of galactokinase by galactose-1-phosphate is not of an order of magnitude to be self limiting, at least not when we are dealing with smaller amounts of galactose.
(4) Galactose-free diet is not harmful and is relatively simple to compose.
(5) Although the patients are able to metabolize small amounts of galactose, this ability does not improve with age[5].

ΜG GAL-1-P/ML ERYTHROCYTES

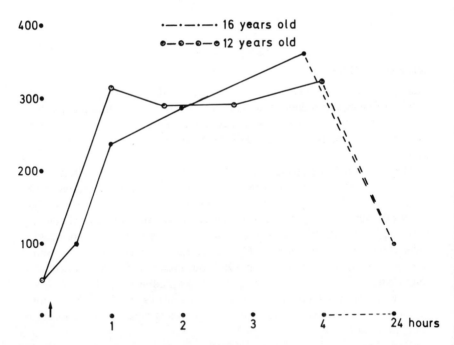

Figure 6.1a Galactose-load (100 mg/kg body weight) in a patient at different ages. Galactose-1-phosphate accumulation in the erythrocytes (1 μg/ml = 3.84 μmol/l) is remarkably constant. The galactose load corresponds to one small glass of milk. Return to initial levels of galactose-1-phosphate has not occurred after 24 h

µG GAL-1-P/ML ERYTHROCYTES

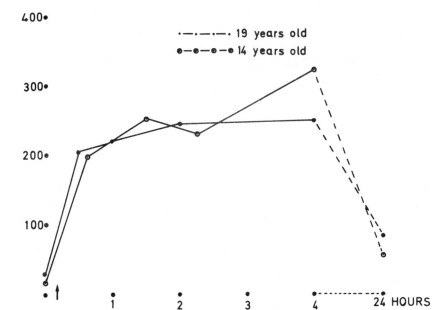

Figure 6.1b   Galactose load in a further patient at different ages. For details see Figure 6.1a

Galactose loading test

We have studied the effect of oral galactose loads on erythrocyte galactose-1-phosphate in a few patients followed over many years. Various amounts of galactose have been tried but now our usual procedure is to give 100 mg/kg body weight. For the 12–14 year old child with a bodyweight of 40 kg, the galactose load is equivalent to one glass of milk. Looking at the galactose-1-phosphate accumulation the same pattern is found irrespective of age (Figures 6.1a and 6.1b); we have done this yearly in three patients and the results are identical. Galactose-1-phosphate reaches a level of 300 µg/ml (1152 µmol/l) erythrocytes for several hours. Even at 24 h, the galactose-1-phosphate level has not fallen to the pretest figure. Donnell's group has obtained similar results[6]. Using this low dose of galactose only a few percent is excreted in the urine. If 50 mg/kg bodyweight is given a lower level of galactose-1-phosphate is found and the patients excrete only minimal amounts of galactose. With larger doses the excretion in the urine will be raised relatively more than the erythrocyte galactose-1-phosphate. Red blood cells are easy to obtain for analysis but their specialised nature may prevent them reflecting accurately changes in other cells, particularly brain and liver.

A few patients have been studied with a battery of psychological tests before and during a galactose load of 100 mg/kg body weight. Although the interpretation of the data is complex, there is a poor performance in most tests during the load. To illustrate this the results of Bender tests performed before and after a galactose load are shown in Figure 6.2 and 6.3. In some tests, for instance the Goldstein–Scheerer block pattern test, there is some

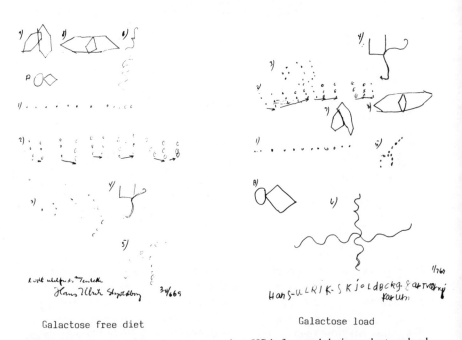

Galactose free diet   Galactose load

Figure 6.2 Results of Bender-test on patient HS before and during galactose load (100 mg/kg body weight). Erythrocytic galactose-1-phosphate around 250 μg/ml (960 μmol/l) erythrocytes

improvement on high galactose. Also, there is a relaxation of inhibitory traits similar to that observed during alcohol intoxication.

Relaxing the diet

For several reasons it seems logical that classical hereditary galactosaemia should be treated throughout life. How could this assumption ever be

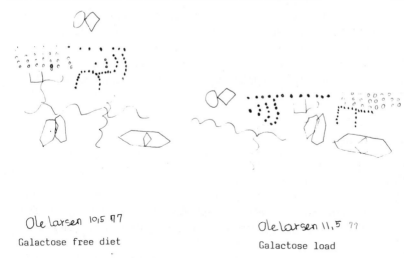

Ole Larsen 10,5 77

Galactose free diet

Ole Larsen 11,5 77

Galactose load

Figure 6.3   Results of Bender test on patient OL before and during galactose load (100 mg/kg body weight). Erythrocytic galactose-1-phosphate around 250 μg/ml (960 μmol/l) erythrocytes

questioned? No one would stop treating patients suffering from diabetes mellitus or congenital hypothyroidism. We know much more about the pathogenesis of galactosaemia. The more relaxed attitude towards treatment is due to several false assumptions. For instance, it has been said that around 2 years of age brain growth is finished, but physically, intellectually and psychosocially many years, perhaps more than 20 years, of growth remain. School performance should be optimal but it is even more important to adapt to society as an adult.

The relaxed attitude towards treatment of galactosaemia in older children may have been influenced by the policy of termination of dietary treatment in phenylketonuria when the patients are around 5 years old. Most centres involved in the treatment of phenylketonuria and galactosaemia have probably had the same experience as we have. When patients with either of these two disorders are taken off diet, poor performance at school and behaviour problems follow. There is a difficult period when the diet is reinstituted, but subsequently normal behaviour and better school performance returns. Centres treating phenylketonuria are gradually changing their policy[7]. It would not be surprising if it is finally concluded that phenylketonuria should be treated throughout life.

Another factor is that it is usually the paediatrician who takes care of patients with inborn errors of metabolism and traditionally he does not take care of adult patients. This attitude should be changed because internists are not ready to take over the specialised treatment required for phenylketonuria, galactosaemia and cystic fibrosis. The paediatrician must face the fact that he must take care of an increasing proportion of adult patients.

Conclusion

We do not know if patients with classical galactosaemia should be treated lifelong, but in our clinic we certainly recommend it. Ethanol inhibits hepatic galactose elimination[8] and in pig liver experiments, this inhibitory effect is associated with elevated galactose-1-phosphate[9]. It is probably justified to recommend that the youngster and adult with galactosaemia should avoid not only lactose but also alcohol.

The only way to give a clear, scientifically based answer to the question of how long galactosaemia should be treated is a prospective, controlled, double blind trial. To be of any value, such a study should include a large group of patients followed over many years. The data collected should include physical, cognitive and psychosocial variables. The sampling procedure and stratification of the material should be well defined, including proper control groups, altogether so cumbersome a study that probably it will never be carried out.

Meanwhile we must not let down our youngster and adult patient with classical galactosaemia. We must recommend them lifelong lactose free diet and proper control.

ATYPICAL GALACTOSAEMIA

In the atypical cases of galactosaemia, with a residual activity of galactose-1-phosphate-uridyl transferase, there can be little doubt that the patients should be on a galactose free diet in the first months of life. Without diet these patients would in fact be under a constant galactose load. With the atypical cases the combined *Duarte*/galactosaemia heterozygotes should be included. In Figure 6.4 the result of galactose loading (1 g/kg body weight) in two such individuals is shown. Although the galactose-1-phosphate level is not of the same magnitude as seen in classical galactosaemia, the test is clearly abnormal and galactose-1-phosphate has not disappeared from the blood even after 4 hours. After the first 2 years of life the diet could probably be less restricted.

JJG GAL-1-P/ML ERYTHROCYTES

400•

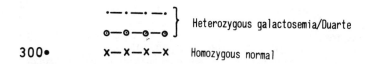

300• Homozygous normal

200•

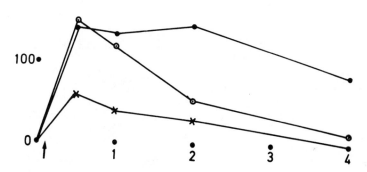

100•

0

Figure 6.4 Erythrocyte galactose-1-phosphate levels (1 μg/ml = 3.84 μmol/l) present in double heterozygotes for galactosaemia/*Duarte*. Galactose load; 1 g/kg body weight

References

1. Holzel, A., Komrower, G. M. and Schwarz, V. (1957). Galactosaemia. *Mod. Probl. Paediatr.*, **3**, 359
2. American Academy of Pediatrics. (Committee on Nutrition) (1967). Nutritional management in hereditary metabolic disease. *Pediatrics*, **40**, 289
3. Komrower, G. M. (1973). Treatment of galactosaemia. In J. W. T. Seakins, R. A. Saunders and C. Toothill (eds.). *Treatment of Inborn Errors of Metabolism*, pp. 113–120. (Edinburgh: Churchill Livingstone)
4. Donnell, G. N. and Bergren, W. R. (1975). The Galactosaemias. In D. N. Raine (ed.). *The Treatment of Inherited Metabolic Disease*, pp. 91–114. (Lancaster: MTP Press)

5. Segal, S., Blair, A. and Roth, H. (1965). The metabolism of galactose by patients with congenital galactosaemia. *Am. J. Med.*, **38,** 62
6. Donnell, G. N., Koch, R. and Bergren, W. R. (1969). Observations on results of management of galactosaemic patients. In D. Y.-Y. Hsia (ed.). *Galactosemia*, pp. 247–268. (Springfield, Illinois: Charles C. Thomas)
7. Cabalska, V., Duczynska, N., Borzymowska, J., Zorska, K., Koslacz-Folga, A. and Bozkowa, K. (1977). Termination of dietary treatment in phenylketonuria. *Eur. J. Pediatr.*, **126,** 253
8. Tygstrup, N. and Lundquist, F. (1962). The effect of ethanol on galactose elimination in man. *J. Lab. Clin. Med.*, **59,** 102
9. Keiding, S. (1973). Galactose elimination capacity in the rat. *Scand. J. Clin. Lab. Invest.*, **31,** 319

7

Pregnancy in classical galactosaemia

I. B. Sardharwalla, G. M. Komrower and V. Schwarz

Much has been written about the diagnosis and treatment of galactosaemia in childhood but so far there are only three reports describing the outcome of pregnancies in galactosaemic mothers[1-3]. The purpose of this paper is to report on two sisters with galactosaemia whom we have followed from the neonatal period, to comment on biochemical observations made during their recent pregnancies and to describe the early progress of their babies.

CASE HISTORIES

Patient A. J.   This patient presented in 1953, (aged 2 weeks) with clinical features of classical galactosaemia (galactose-1-phosphate uridyl transferase deficiency), namely vomiting, failure to thrive, obstructive jaundice and hepatomegaly. Investigations revealed raised blood galactose, increased galactose excretion in the urine and abnormal generalized aminoaciduria. Deficiency of the transferase was not unequivocally demonstrated until 3 years later when the assay became available. The introduction of a galactose free diet led to the resolution of all her symptoms. The values of galactose-1-phosphate, recorded from 1956 onwards, ranged between

30–45 μg/ml (115–172 μmol/l) of packed red cells. Her physical development gave no cause for concern but her mental development was disappointing. At the age of 25 years she attained an IQ score of 65.

In October 1976, this girl informed us that she was 10 weeks pregnant. She was advised to remain on a strict galactose free diet and we were assured that she did so throughout her pregnancy which proceeded normally. The father's genotype for the transferase enzyme was homozygous normal. The mother's levels of red cell galactose-1-phosphate were measured at 4–8 weekly intervals. An amniocentesis was done a week before delivery and the fluid was examined for sugars by thin layer chromatography. At delivery cord blood and maternal venous blood were checked for red cell galactose-1-phosphate. At the same time, the cord blood was assayed for the transferase enzyme. The mother did not wish to breast feed the infant who was put on an artificial milk preparation from birth.

Patient B. J.   This patient's galactosaemia was diagnosed *at birth* in 1957. The concentration of galactose-1-phosphate in the cord blood was 51 μg/ml (196 μmol/l) packed red cells. With the early introduction of dietary treatment, biochemical control was satisfactory from birth, the values of galactose-1-phosphate ranging between 40–50 μg/ml (154–192 μmol/l) packed red cells. The pattern of physical and mental development was very similar to that of her sister and her IQ at the age of 21 was also 65.

In June 1977, she reported that she was 16 weeks pregnant. Advice was given about the importance of keeping to a strict galactose free diet, as in her sister's case; similarly, B. J.'s blood was checked for galactose-1-phosphate levels at 1–3 weekly intervals. The father's genotype was found to be homozygous normal. Her pregnancy was complicated by a mil i rise in blood pressure and slight proteinuria which required a short admission to hospital prior to delivery. At the time of delivery, amniotic fluid was obtained for investigation of galactose and samples of cord blood and maternal venous blood were taken for the estimation of levels of galactose-1-phosphate. This mother decided to breast feed her baby.

Methods

Erythrocyte galactose-1-phosphate levels were determined by the method of Schwarz[4]. Erythrocyte galactose-1-phosphate uridyl transferase activity was assayed by the procedure of Beutler[5]. Galactose and lactose in amniotic fluid and colostrum respectively were demonstrated by thin layer chromatography (microcrystalline cellulose) using ethyl acetate, pyridine and water 6 : 3 : 2 as solvent. The sugars were located by staining the chromatrograms with phenylenediamine–stannous chloride. Cord blood specimens were centrifuged as soon as possible after collection; the erythrocytes were washed twice with N saline and then stored at −20 °C until they were analysed for galactose-1-phosphate.

Biochemical results

Patient A. J.   The results of red cell galactose-1-phosphate measurements are shown in Figure 7.1; concentration remained steady throughout pregnancy but there was a slight rise to 50 μg/ml (192 μmol/l) packed red cells at the time of delivery. The galactose-1-phosphate in cord blood was 5 μg/ml (19μmol/l) packed red cells and a trace of galactose was demonstrated in the amniotic fluid (Table 7.1).

Patient B. J.   The levels of red cell galactose-1-phosphate are shown in Figure 7.2. They remained steady while the patient was at home but rose slightly during her admission to hospital prior to delivery; sharp rises to 111 μg (426 μmol/l) and 139 μg/ml (534 μmol/l) of packed red cells were recorded 3 and 6 days respectively after delivery. The galactose-1-phosphate in cord blood was 3 μg/ml (12 μmol/l) and trace amounts of galactose and lactose were found in the amniotic fluid (Table 7.1).

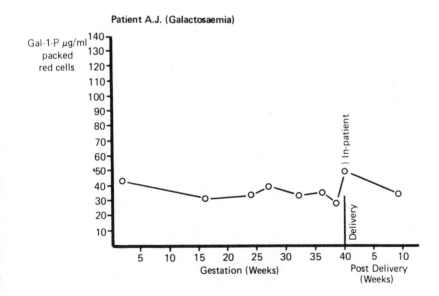

Figure 7.1   Red cell galactose-1-phosphate (Gal-1-P) concentrations during pregnancy, delivery and post-partum in patient A. J. (1 μg/ml = 3.84 μmol/l)

TABLE 7.1   Results of biochemical investigations on cord blood, maternal blood at delivery, amniotic fluid and colostrum

	A.J.	B.J.
Gal-1-P in red cells (cord blood)	5 μg/ml (19 μmol/l)	3 μg/ml (12 μmol/l)
Gal-1-P in red cells (maternal at delivery)	50 μg/ml (192 μmol/l)	60 μg/ml (230 μmol/l)
Amniotic fluid (TLC)	Trace of galactose	Trace of galactose and lactose
Colostrum (TLC)	Large amounts of lactose present	Large amounts of lactose present

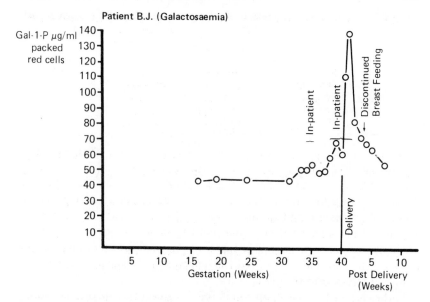

Figure 7.2 Red cell galactose-1-phosphate (Gal-1-P) concentrations during pregnancy, delivery and post-partum in patient B. J. (1 μg/ml = 3.84 μmol/l)

Colostrum obtained from both mothers was checked for lactose by thin layer chromatography and large amounts of the sugar were demonstrated.

Progress of infants

The physical measurements at birth of the infants born to the two mothers are shown in Table 7.2; they were normal.

Both children are developing normally, mentally and physically. The child of the first mother is 14 months old and the Development Quotient at the age of one year was 104. A similar test on the child born to the second mother gave a Development Quotient of 117 at the same age.

DISCUSSION

Red cell galactose-1-phosphate during the two pregnancies

The steady levels of red cell galactose-1-phosphate during A.J.'s pregnancy were considered to be a reflection of good dietary control at home and the small rise at the time of delivery to be due to a possible dietary indiscretion

TABLE 7.2   Physical measurements of infants born to A.J. and B.J. taken at birth

	Infant of A.J.	Infant of B.J.
Sex	Female	Male
Gestation	40 weeks	40 weeks
Weight	2.35 kg	3.6 kg
Length	45.07 cm	48.3 cm
Head circ.	32.00 cm	36.0 cm

in the hospital or to endogenous synthesis of galactose-1-phosphate from glucose via UDP galactose using the pyrophosphorylase pathway[6]. The formation of UDP galactose which is the donor of galactose moiety in the synthesis of lactose for breast milk[7], is likely to be increased during the late stages of pregnancy and during lactation. However, the rise of red cell galactose-1-phosphate was not significant and as the mother decided to feed her baby with an artificial milk preparation, lactation was immediately suppressed. The concentration of red cell galactose-1-phosphate 9 weeks after birth had returned to the prenatal levels.

In the case of B.J. the sharp rise in red cell galactose-1-phosphate during the first week after delivery was largely due to a dietary indiscretion (the Senior Nursing Officer saw the patient eating chocolate). However, there was the real possibility that a lesser but significantly high level would be maintained by the endogenous synthesis of galactose-1-phosphate, thus creating a harmful situation for the mother; for this reason lactation was suppressed. On reflection, we now feel that endogenous synthesis of galactose-1-phosphate would have made a smaller contribution because of the rapid rate of fall of the galactose-1-phosphate immediately after delivery and the subsequent slower change after stopping lactation.

Red cell galactose-1-phosphate in cord blood

The low levels of galactose-1-phosphate in the cord blood of the two heterozygous infants compared with the relatively high levels found in their mothers' blood at the time of delivery is due to the fact that galactose-1-phosphate is an intracellular compound which cannot cross the cell membrane or the placenta. In addition, the heterozygous fetus who has about 50% of the normal transferase activity is well able to metabolise any galactose that might cross the placenta.

Galactose in the amniotic fluid

There is evidence that endogenous synthesis of galactose occurs in man[6]. Roe et al.[1,8] observed that their patients with classical galactosaemia excreted small amounts of galactitol in the urine even when on galactose restricted diets. Olambiwonnu et al.[9] reported that galactose remained detectable in plasma and urine in galactokinase deficient twins who were maintained on strict diets. It would seem therefore that galactose formed endogenously in the mother was the source of galactose found in the amniotic fluid. After crossing the placenta, only a small proportion of the galactose in the blood entering the fetus via the umbilical vein would pass through the hepatic sinusoids[10] where galactose would be metabolized. Some of the galactose carried to the systemic circulation, would be metabolised by other fetal tissues and the remainder be excreted unchanged in the fetal urine and consequently appear in the amniotic fluid. The small amounts of galactose in the amniotic fluid of our well controlled mothers means that the formation of galactitol will be insignificant and therefore the risk of damage to the fetal lens minimal. The eyes of both infants were examined by ophthalmoscopy and there was no evidence of lenticular opacities.

CONCLUSION

The toxic effect of galactose-1-phosphate on the homozygous galactosaemic fetus of the heterozygous mother has been suggested as a cause of brain damage during the intrauterine period[11]. In support of this view is the fact that the red cell galactose-1-phosphate in the cord blood of a galactosaemic infant is always elevated. It has been shown that the heterozygous fetus of a homozygous galactosaemic mother is not exposed to raised galactose-1-phosphate tissue concentrations. It appears that the infant born to a galactosaemic mother has a much better chance of ultimate intellectual achievement than had his well treated but homozygous mother.

Acknowledgements

We would like to thank Mr J. Firth, Consultant Obstetrician, and all staff of the Maternity Unit at Bolton District General Hospital for assisting with the collection of amniotic fluids, maternal blood and cord blood from each of the patients and their infants. We also wish to express our appreciation to Dr A. H. Fensom, Guy's Hospital, London, for assaying the red cell galactose-1-phosphate uridyl transferase activity to determine the genotype of the fathers.

References

1.   Roe, T., Hallatt, J., Donnell, G. and Ng, W. (1971). Childbearing by galactosemic women. J. Pediatr., **78**, 1026

2. Tedesco, T. A., Marrow, G. and Mellman, W. J. (1972). Normal pregnancy and childbirth in a galactosemic woman. *J. Pediatr.*, **81,** 1158

3. Samuels, S., Sun, S. C. and Verasestakul, S. (1976). Normal infant birth in white galactosemic women. *J. Med. Soc. N. J.*, **73,** 309

4. Schwarz, V. (1969). Galactose oxidation methods. In Hsia, D. Y. (ed.). *Galactosemia*, pp. 37–41. (Springfield, Illinois: Charles C. Thomas)

5. Beutler, E. (1971). *Red Cell Metabolism: A Manual of Biochemical Methods*, p. 83. (New York and London: Grune and Stratton)

6. Gitzelmann, R., Hansen, R. G. and Steinmann, B. (1975). Biogenesis of galactose, a possible mechanism of self-intoxication in galactosemia. In Hommes, F. A. and Van den Berg, C. J. (eds.). *Normal and Pathological Development of Energy Metabolism.*, pp. 25–36. (London: Academic Press)

7. Leloir, L. F. and Cardini, C. E. (1961). The biosynthesis of lactose. In Kon S. K. and Cowie A. T. (eds.). *Milk: The Mammary Gland and Its Secretion.* Vol. I, pp. 421–440. (New York: Academic Press)

8. Roe, T. F., Ng, W. G., Bergren, W. R. and Donnell, G. N. (1973). Urinary galactitol in galactosemic patients. *Biochem. Med.*, **7,** 266

9. Olambiwonnu, N. O., McVie, R., Ng, W. G., Frasier, S. D. and Donnell, G. N. (1974). Galactokinase deficiency in twins: clinical and biochemical studies. *Pediatrics*, **53,** 314

10. Rudolph, A. M. (1970). The fetal circulation and its adjustments after birth in congenital heart disease. In F. H. Adams, H. J. C. Swan and V. E. Hall (eds.). *Pathophysiology of Congenital Heart Disease.* pp. 105–107. (Berkeley, Los Angeles and London: University of California Press)

11. Komrower, G. M. and Lee D. H. (1970). Long-term follow-up of galactosaemia. *Arch. Dis. Child.*, **45,** 372

8

Screening for galactosaemia

H. L. Levy

Newborn screening for galactosaemia has not been as widely accepted as screening for phenylketonuria (PKU) nor as excitedly embraced as the recently introduced screening for hypothyroidism. Experience of over ten years, however, indicates that galactosaemia screening should be included in all programmes of newborn screening for metabolic disorders.

JUSTIFICATION

Of those metabolic disorders for which there is both therapy and an available screening test, galactosaemia is perhaps unique in being opposed for routine newborn screening on grounds that such screening is unnecessary. Screening for PKU, for instance, though now widely accepted, was once opposed on the basis of treatment being ineffective[1]. Maple syrup urine disease and homocystinuria have been thought not only to lack effective treatment but also to be too rare to justify newborn screening. Galactosaemia is believed to be a different sort of disease; it is acknowledged as one that occurs sufficiently often to constitute a recognizable paediatric problem. Widely accepted also is the concept that early treatment is effective in preventing the chronic complications of cataracts, cirrhosis, and mental retardation[2]. Why then is routine screening for galactosaemia believed by some to be unnecessary? Simply because most physicians, particularly paediatricians, make two incorrect assumptions: (1) that galactosaemia always presents in the neonatal period with at least jaundice and vomiting of milk; and (2) that this clinical presentation will lead to a proper urine test and thus to the correct diagnosis and treatment.

The facts are quite contrary to these views. First, a number of galactosaemic individuals never have clinical abnormalities in the early neonatal period. Among the ten galactosaemic infants that we have detected by routine newborn screening, four were entirely normal as late as 5–10 days of age and had never been detectably jaundiced, much less ill. Second, in only one of these ten galactosaemic infants detected did the clinical signs lead to a suspicion of galactosaemia; this includes three infants who were markedly jaundiced and three others who died after having clinical courses that included jaundice, hepatomegaly, failure to thrive, diarrhoea, and *Escherichia coli* sepsis[3]. The reason for lack of diagnosis in this latter group of infants is either that galactosaemia was never considered or that an insufficient test was performed on the urine and was then misinterpreted.

This last point warrants illustration. In my hospital office, I saw a galactosaemic neonate who had just been detected by routine newborn screening. This infant had been brought over from another hospital where he had been found to have jaundice and hepatomegaly of undetermined aetiology. I obtained a urine specimen and performed a test for reducing substance (Clinitest, Ames Company, Elkhart, Indiana) which gave a strongly positive result. The infant was admitted to the hospital nursery where a urine specimen was obtained for analysis. Shortly thereafter I checked the hospital chart and discovered that the second urine test was recorded on the laboratory report slip and in the chart as 'negative for sugar'. Upon investigation it was found that the urine test that had been performed and that was routine in the nursery utilized a popular dipstick (Clinistix, Ames Company, Elkhart, Indiana). This responds only to glucose and in no manner constitutes an adequate test for urinary reducing substances. I am certain that this story could be repeated many times in many different hospitals over the world.

In my opinion, therefore, it is important to include galactosaemia among those disorders screened in the neonate. This can readily be accomplished using the same filter paper blood specimen that is submitted for PKU testing.

SCREENING TESTS

The first test that was developed for this purpose was a direct *Escherichia coli* inhibition assay[4]. Professor Paigen of Buffalo suggested this test and Professor Guthrie and his coworkers in Buffalo refined the assay and made it available to many newborn screening laboratories in 1964. The principle is one of growth inhibition produced by galactose toxicity to a mutant *Escherichia coli* that lacks galactose-1-phosphate uridyl transferase (transferase) activity (Figure 8.1). This test has resulted in the detection of several galactosaemic neonates and is still in use by Professor Thalhammer in Vienna[5]. However, this mutant bacterium is unstable and most screening laboratories have neither the expertise nor the time to maintain it.

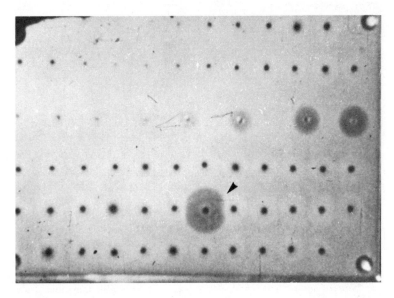

Figure 8.1 The *Escherichia coli* bacterial inhibition assay for galactose. Control discs containing galactose are in the third row from the top. The arrow indicates the large zone of inhibition surrounding a blood specimen from a galactosaemic neonate.

Because of problems with this galactose assay the 'Beutler test' was welcomed. This ingenious test is really a spot enzyme assay for transferase activity[6]. A small disc from the newborn blood specimen is incubated with the appropriate reagents and, if transferase activity is present, reduced nucleotide is formed. This indirect reaction product can be detected by fluorescence of the filter paper discs (Figure 8.2). While the 'Beutler test' has resulted in the detection of many infants with galactosaemia, the problem of many false positive results has greatly complicated its use. These 'positive' results seem to be due mainly to inactivation of enzyme in the heat and humidity of summer months[7] and to benign enzyme variations[8].

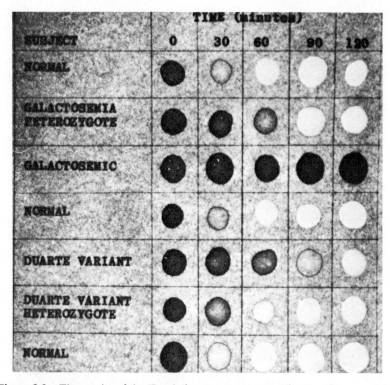

Figure 8.2 The results of the 'Beutler' spot enzyme assay for transferase activity. The amount of fluorescence under long-wave ultraviolet illumination is shown following incubation periods of the reaction varying from 0 to 120 minutes. The tests were conducted on blood from three normal subjects, one who was heterozygous for galactosaemia, one homozygous for the Duarte variant and one heterozygous for the Duarte variant. (Reproduced from the *J. Lab. Clin. Med.* (1966), **68,** 137 with permission of the authors and publishers).

Fortunately for galactosaemia screening, Professor Paigen has now produced an assay that is stable, reliable and associated with few false positive results. This is a bacterial assay that responds to galactose[9] and, when modified by the addition of alkaline phosphatase to the assay media, also responds to galactose-1-phosphate[10]. The principle of this assay is growth of a mutant *Escherichia coli* that lacks UDP-Galactose-4-epimerase and is resistant to bacteriophage lysing when exposed to galactose (Figure 8.3). We have used this assay for six years in testing over 500 000 filter paper specimens of umbilical cord blood and newborn blood and continue to be pleased with it.

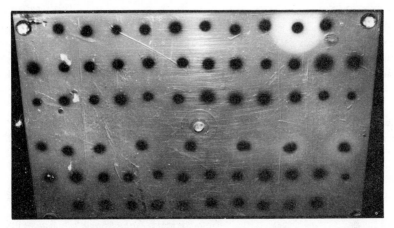

Figure 8.3 The 'Paigen' *Escherichia coli* bacteriophage assay for galactose and galactose-1-phosphate. Control discs are in the fourth row from the top. The large bacterial growth surrounding a blood specimen from a galactosaemic neonate in the top row indicates increased galactose and galactose-1-phosphate in this disc.

In our estimation the Paigen assay, when constituted to detect elevations of galactose and galactose-1-phosphate in blood, is preferable to the Beutler enzyme spot assay. First, there are many fewer false positive reactions with the Paigen assay and, as a consequence, many less 'false alarms' and requests for repeat specimens. Second, the Paigen test allows for the identification of galactose metabolic defects other than classical galactosaemia, such as galactokinase deficiency or UDP-Galactose-4-epimerase (epimerase) deficiency. Finally, the Paigen assay obviates the problem of transferase activity in the blood of a galactosaemic newborn as a result of exchange transfusion[11] and thus passed as normal in the Beutler assay. On the basis of data that we recently compiled it would appear that assaying newborn blood for galactose elevations has probably been more effective in the detection of galactosaemia than has been the use of the Beutler test[12]. In Massachusetts, for instance, we detected one galactosaemic infant among almost 200 000 infants screened by the Beutler test[7] but by routine screening using the Paigen test, we have detected eight galactosaemic infants among 400 000 screened newborns giving a frequency of one per 50 000.

RESULTS OF SCREENING

Throughout the world about six million newborn infants have now been screened for galactosaemia and/or other galactose metabolic defects[12]. A summary of this screening is given in Table 8.1. The 97 galactosaemic infants detected yield a frequency of one per 62 000. Whether this represents the true frequency is debatable. I suspect that many galactosaemic infants have been overlooked, either missed by screening or because a newborn blood specimen was never obtained when the infant became ill and died soon after with *Escherichia coli* sepsis[3].

In addition, infants with galactokinase deficiency and with epimerase deficiency have been detected among the 2.5 million infants screened by a galactose assay. Some of these may have been overlooked also if their galactose elevations were only moderate.

TABLE 8.1   Results of routine newborn screening for galactosaemia

	Newborns tested	*Newborns with disorder*		
		Galactokinase deficiency	*Galactosaemia*	*Epimerase deficiency*
North America	3 099 462	1	40	0
Europe	2 317 083	5	47	2
Asia	550 544	0	10	0
Total	5 967 089	6	97 (1:62 000)	2

SUMMARY

Routine newborn screening for galactosaemia can be effectively performed on filter paper blood specimens obtained on the second or third day of life and mailed promptly to the testing laboratory. This effectiveness is reduced when the blood specimen is obtained later in the neonatal period (e.g. on the fifth day) but is still of value in that most galactosaemic infants can still be treated at 2 weeks of age, or even later. This type of screening should be combined with screening for PKU and hypothyroidism. It is best performed with the Paigen assay modified to respond to both galactose and galactose-1-phosphate. Screening of umbilical cord blood for galactosaemia using the Paigen assay to detect galactose-1-phosphate, as performed in Massachusetts, may be effective in very early diagnosis and treatment, but needs further study.

Acknowledgements

Newborn screening for metabolic disorders, including galactosaemia, has received continuous support in Massachusetts from the Department of

Public Health and from the federal government through a project grant (01-H-000111-08-0). Study of this type of screening has also been made possible by grant NS 05096 from the National Institutes of Health.

References

1. Bessman, S. P. (1966). Legislation and advances in medical knowledge – acceleration or inhibition? *J. Pediatr.*, **69**, 334
2. Donnell, G. N., Koch, R. and Bergren, W. R. (1969). Observations on results of management of galactosemia patients. In D. Y.-Y. Hsia (ed.). *Galactosemia*, pp. 247–275. (Springfield, Illinois: Charles C. Thomas)
3. Levy, H. L., Sepe, S. J., Shih, V. E., Vawter, G. F. and Klein, J. O. (1977). Sepsis due to *Escherichia coli* in neonates with galactosemia. *N. Engl. J. Med.*, **297**, 825
4. Guthrie, R. (1964). Routine screening for inborn errors in the newborn: 'inhibition assays', instant bacteria and multiple tests. In *Proceedings of the International Copenhagen Congress on the Scientific Study of Mental Retardation.* Vol. II, p. 495. (Copenhagen)
5. Thalhammer, O. (1975). Frequency of inborn errors of metabolism, especially PKU, in some representative newborn screening centers around the world. A collaborative study. *Humangenetik*, **30**, 273
6. Beutler, E. and Baluda, M. C. (1966). A single spot screening test for galactosemia, *J. Lab. Clin. Med.*, **68**, 137
7. Shih, V. E., Levy, H. L., Karolkewicz, V., Houghton, S., Efron, M. L., Isselbacher, K. J., Beutler, E. and MacCready, R. A. (1971). Galactosemia screening in Massachusetts. *N. Engl. J. Med.*, **284**, 753
8. Levy, H. L., Sepe, S. J., Walton, D. S., Shih, V. E., Hammersen, G., Houghton, S. and Beutler, E. (1978). Duarte/galactosemia genetic compound variant of galactose-1-phosphate uridyl transferase deficiency: clinical and biochemical studies. *J. Pediatr.*, **92**, 390
9. Paigen, K. and Pacholec, F. (1979). A new method of screening neonates for galactosemia. *J. Lab. Clin. Med.* (In press)
10. Gitzelman, R. (1976). Früherfassung von Anomalien im Galaktosestoffwechsel Methoden und Resultate. *Monatsschr. Kinderheilkd.*, **124**, 654
11. Schwartz, R. P., Roesel, R. A., Blankenship, P. R. and Hall, W. K. (1975). Loss of transferase enzyme activity of transfused erythrocytes in galactosemia. *South Med. J.*, **68**, 301
12. Levy, H. L. and Hammersen, G. (1978). Newborn screening for galactosemia and other galactose metabolic defects. *J. Pediatr.*, **92**, 871

9

Prenatal diagnosis of classical galactosaemia

J. B. Holton and C. M. Raymont

The successful prenatal detection of classical galactosaemia by the assay of galactose-1-phosphate uridyl transferase (GalPUT) in amniotic fluid cells, has been reported by several groups of workers[1-3]. In fact, it is accurate, precise and one of the more satisfactory prenatal diagnostic tests presently available. Doubts are likely to arise, however, over the place of *in utero* detection and pregnancy termination in the management of this particular disorder. Opinion on this issue will vary, largely depending on one's view about the alternative, of neonatal diagnosis and long term dietary treatment. It is apparent that there are different opinions on the success of this[4, 5].

Because of the choice of management available to parents, careful genetic counselling is of paramount importance. The data in Table 9.1 shows that, in our series, the cases (nos. 2–5) in which prenatal detection and termination were considered seriously, each had an affected child dying in the neonatal period, prior to diagnosis. It seems likely that the possibility of dietary treatment was not fully appreciated by all of these parents. The experience of the parents of case 4, who had three sequential affected pregnancies and no live child, makes termination seem relatively less attractive.

METHODOLOGICAL CONSIDERATIONS
The widely used UDPGlc consumption test for red cell GalPUT[6] is not sen-

TABLE 9.1 Details of prenatal diagnoses performed in Bristol

Case number	History of previous pregnancies	Record of prenatal diagnoses	
		Prediction*	Outcome of pregnancy/ Confirmation of result
1	1. Girl with severe jaundice on 4th day. Reducing substances found in urine and GalPUT deficiency confirmed. Satisfactory progress on treatment	Gt+/Gt^G heterozygote	Live child. Genotype supported by GalPUT assay on erythrocytes
2	1. Normal boy		
	2. Boy, died on 16th day. Symptoms suggested galactosaemia, but no confirmation of diagnosis. Erythrocyte and skin fibroblast studies indicated that parents were heterozygous for galactosaemia	2. Gt+/Gt+ homozygote	No follow-up available
3	1. Child died with symptoms suggesting galactosaemia but no confirmatory data available on child or parents	Gt+/Gt^G or Gt+/Gt^D heterozygote	Live, healthy child No enzyme follow-up
4	1. Child died with jaundice and septicaemia. No positive diagnosis, but parents were in heterozygote range in erythrocyte and skin fibroblast GalPUT assays	1. Gt^G/Gt^G homozygote	Pregnancy terminated. Genotype confirmed on skin fibroblast cells from fetus
		2. Gt^G/Gt^G homozygote	Pregnancy terminated and genotype confirmed as above
5	1. Child died		
	2. Child died at 2 weeks and diagnosis of galactosaemia was made by erythrocyte GalPUT assay. Erythrocyte and skin fibroblast assay suggested mother was Gt+/Gt^G heterozygote and father Gt+/Gt variant heterozygote	2. Gt+/Gt^G heterozygote	Pregnancy continued; outcome unknown

* Genotype shown as follows: Gt+ – normal, wild type; Gt – galactosaemia; Gt^G – galactosaemia; Gt^D – Duarte; Gt variant – variant enzyme (described in text)

sitive enough for routine prenatal diagnosis and recent techniques are all modifications of Ng's erythrocyte assay[7]. This uses [^{14}C]galactose-1-phosphate and UDPGlc as substrates and measures the transfer of label to UDPGal. The method has been scaled down and optimised for cultured skin fibroblasts or amniotic fluid cells, so that a reliable result may be obtained using about 150 000 cells[2]. A firm diagnosis should be available in less than 3 weeks from the time of the amniocentesis.

One problem that has been reported is a variation of specific enzyme activity depending on the time of harvesting the cells after sub-culture[8, 9]. Cells harvested in a rapid growth phase displayed significantly higher enzyme levels than those which were approaching confluency. Even cell strains from galactosaemic patients may have considerable activity, which could lead to some difficulty in interpreting a prenatal diagnosis. Our assay has not demonstrated this phenomenon (Figure 9.1), which appears to be a methodological variation rather than a characteristic of certain cell strains, because the galactosaemic cells we used had displayed high enzyme activity early in the growth cycle in the hands of others.

DIAGNOSTIC PROBLEMS

The results of assaying GalPUT in skin fibroblasts and amniotic fluid cells are shown in Figure 9.2. For a successful diagnostic test it is necessary to distinguish clearly between cells with the low enzyme activity associated with classical galactosaemia (up to 5% of normal) and those found in clinically normal subjects possessing other enzyme variants with reduced activity. The gene combination in which this difficulty will occur most commonly is heterozygous for the *Duarte* and galactosaemia variants. Such individuals have 20–25% of mean normal activity. Recently some *Duarte*/galactosaemia infants have been reported with galactosaemic symptoms and were treated[10, 11]. It is very doubtful, however, whether this should constitute a valid reason for pregnancy termination.

There is a potential danger in all prenatal diagnoses that the enzyme activity of cultured skin and amniotic fluid cells may not be typical of other tissue cells in the body, particularly those actually concerned *in vivo* with the metabolic pathway being studied. An example of this sort of problem occurred on investigating the mother and father of case 5, prior to performing a prenatal diagnosis. Both parents had red cell GalPUT activities in the expected range for galactosaemia/normal heterozygotes. However, on assaying their skin fibroblasts only the mother fell in the expected heterozygote range. The father had a significantly higher enzyme level, about 70% of normal. Skin fibroblast enzymes were then followed up on the

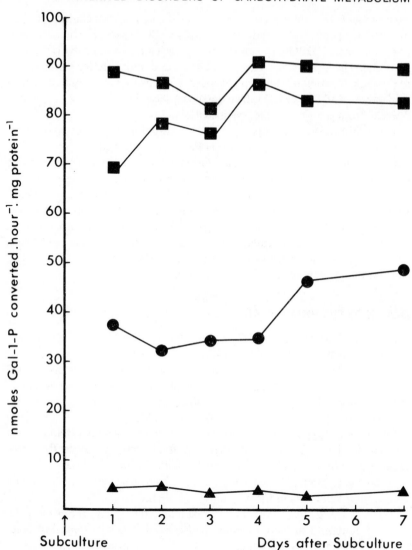

Figure 9.1   Specific activity of GalPUT in amniotic fluid cell cultures on the 7 days after subculture ■ – two normal amniotic fluid cell strains (Gt+/Gt+); ● – an amniotic fluid from a pregnancy at risk for galactosaemia (fetus predicted to be Gt+/Gt^G); ▲ – an amniotic fluid from a pregnancy in which the fetus was shown to be affected with classical galactosaemia

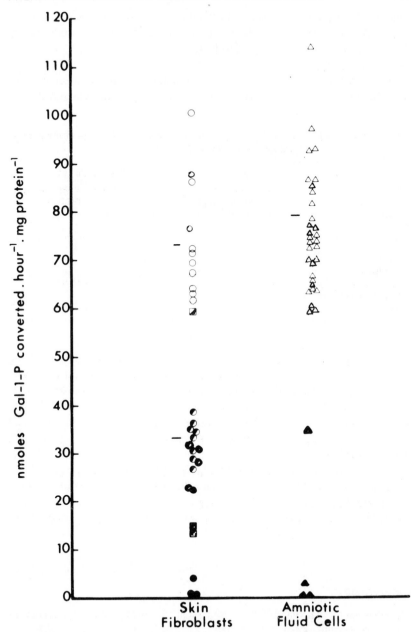

Figure 9.2 Activity of GalPUT in cultured cells with various genotypes. Skin fibroblasts: $\circ$ – Gt$^+$/Gt$^+$; $\mathbf{0}$ – Gt$^+$/Gt^G; $\bullet$ – Gt^G/Gt^G; $\blacksquare$ – Gt$^+$/Gt^D; $\blacksquare$ – Gt^D/Gt^G; Amniotic fluid cells: $\triangle$ – Gt$^+$/Gt$^+$; $\blacktriangle$ – Gt^G/Gt^G; $\blacktriangle$ – Gt$^+$/Gt^D

father's parents, when the paternal grandfather had the same atypical levels as his son, and the grandmother was in the homozygous normal range. Table 9.2 shows the enzyme levels obtained in this family, which we reproduced on many occasions.

The most logical explanation of these findings is that the affected child, his father and grandfather, were all heterozygous for a gene which codes for

TABLE 9.2   GalPUT activities in erythrocytes and skin fibroblasts of the parents and paternal grandparents of case 5

	Erythrocytes μmol Gal-1-P converted/ h/g haemoglobin	*Skin fibroblasts* nmol Gal-1-P converted/ h/mg protein
Mother	8.5	36
Father	9.1	46
Paternal grandmother	19.4	69
Paternal grandfather	8.1	47
Homozygous normals	18–24	62–101
Normal/galactosaemic heterozygotes	8–12	23–39

a variant enzyme that produces about 40% of the enzyme activity of the normal gene in cultured cells but no measurable activity in red cells. The father and grandfather possess the variant gene in combination with a normal gene, but the affected child was heterozygous for the galactosaemic gene. From the severe clinical manifestations of the child it must be assumed that galactose was not metabolised *in vivo*. However, it would be anticipated that cultured cells from a fetus or infant with the genotype would show 15–20% of normal enzyme level. This level would not usually be considered to be associated with severe abnormality. In fact, the first prenatal diagnosis performed has indicated a fetus heterozygous for galactosaemia/normal genes. It has not yet been established whether the atypical enzyme is the same as one of the reported variants[12].

References

1. Fensom, A. H., Benson, P. F. and Blunt, S. (1974). Prenatal diagnosis of galactosaemia. *Br. Med. J.*, **4**, 386
2. Monk, A. and Holton, J. B. (1976). Galactose-1-phosphate uridyl transferase in cultured cells. *Clin. Chim. Acta*, **73**, 537

3. Ng, W. G., Donnell, G. N., Bergren, W. R., Alfi, O. and Golbus, M. S. (1977). Prenatal diagnosis of galactosaemia. *Clin. Chim. Acta*, **74,** 227
4. Donnell, G. N., Koch, R., Fishler, K. and Ng, W. G. (1979). Clinical aspects of galactosaemia. This volume, p. 103
5. Sardharwalla, I. (1979). Discussion. This volume p. 151
6. Anderson, E. P., Kalckar, H. M., Kurahaski, K. and Isselbacher, K. J. (1957). A specific enzymatic assay for the diagnosis of congenital galactosemia. *J. Lab. Clin. Med.*, **50,** 469
7. Ng, W. G., Bergren, W. R. and Donnell, G. N. (1967). An improved procedure for the assay of haemolysate galactose-1-phosphate uridyl transferase by the use of C^{14} labelled galactose-1-phosphate. *Clin. Chim. Acta*, **15,** 489
8. Russell, J. D. and De Mars, R. (1967). UDPglucose: αD-galactose-1-phosphate uridyl transferase activity in cultured human fibroblasts. *Biochem. Genet.*, **1,** 11
9. Fensom, A. H. and Benson, P. F. (1975). Assay of Galactose-1-phosphate uridyl transferase in cultured amniotic cells for prenatal diagnosis of galactosaemia. *Clin. Chim. Acta.*, **62,** 189
10. Wharton, C. H., Berry, H. K. and Bofinger, M. K. (1978). Galactose-1-phosphate accumulation by a Duarte-transferase deficiency double heterozygote. *Clin. Genet.*, **13,** 171
11. Christensen, E. and Brandt, N. J. (1979). Prenatal and postnatal diagnostic difficulties in a family with rare alleles of the galactose-1-phosphate uridyl transferase locus. *J. Inher. Metab. Dis.* (In press)
12. Gitzelmann, R. and Hansen, R. G. (1979). Galactose metabolism, hereditary defects and their clinical significance. This volume p. 61

Discussion

Hereditary defects of galactose metabolism

BRANDT (Copenhagen): Prof. Gitzelmann mentioned the presence of cataract in individuals who are heterozygous carriers for galactokinase deficiency. Can he describe the morphologic appearance of the cataract in these cases and does he know the age of the individuals when the examination was made? Cataract is a rather common finding, especially in elderly people. Did he have the opportunity to measure galactokinase in the lens of such individuals?

GITZELMANN (Zurich): Some heterozygotes for galactokinase deficiency were discovered from among a group of patients who developed nuclear cataracts during the first year of life. Others have been found from many centres where patients with presenile cataracts are screened for galactokinase activity. In the latter group cataract appeared later, so it appears that the development of cataracts due to galactokinase deficiency can occur at any time of life.

I have not seen a very good description of cataracts in heterozygotes yet, but I think they are nuclear cataracts. The part of the lens that is damaged shortly before birth, or immediately after birth, remains in the centre and is the most susceptible to cataractogenic factors.

Estimation of galactokinase in the lens has not been done and such an enterprise would not make much sense because all, or most, enzyme activity would be lost because of denaturation of the protein.

NG (Los Angeles): Prof. Gitzelmann presented data which shows that Duarte-galactosaemia compound heterozygotes had much lower transferase activity in the newborn period than at a later age. Could this be due to the use of the UDPG consumption assay, since UDP-Galactose-4-epimerase is very active? We have measured the enzyme activity using radioactive galactose-1-phosphate in several Duarte variants and have found no change in activity with age.

GITZELMANN: No, we see the same when we use radioactive galactose-1-phosphate as the substrate.

RAINE (Birmingham): Can we accept the concept that an enzyme may be nearly totally deficient in one tissue but present in another tissue; or are you suggesting that, if it is absent in one and appears to be present in another, we should look more closely at the enzyme kinetics of the tissue in which it is present?

GITZELMANN: The latter is correct.

HUG (Cincinnati): Has anybody measured galactokinase in a liver biopsy in galactokinase deficient children?

GITZELMANN: I do not think it is necessary to biopsy infant livers in order to measure galactokinase. Red-cell galactokinase has so far been shown to be representative of liver activity and for the moment we do not need such assays. I have never had a galactokinase deficient infant in my care, although I have adults with the disease.

FERNANDES (Groningen, Netherlands): Would Prof. Gitzelmann comment on the galactose tolerance test? In some circumstances it is justifiable to perform the test and under other circumstances it is not.

GITZELMANN: The test should not be done in the homozygote where enzyme activity is completely missing. It was done in compound heterozygotes in order to find out if it had any value and I think it had not.

KOMROWER (Manchester): Most of us would agree that this is a very dangerous procedure that we shouldn't undertake in classical galactosaemia. Could I ask you about your observations on the slow diminution of galactose-1-phosphate in the first year of life and your interpretation of this. I have seen this on several occasions where the dietary regime was good. Even in hospital galactose-1-phosphate levels did not come down to levels which were considered to be reasonable and we never got them to normal levels. In the second year of life, in the same children continuing the same dietary regime, the levels do come down much further. Is there an explanation? Is galactokinase more active in the first year of life or is pyrophosphorylase more active in the first year than in the second year? Is there some other regulating mechanism that comes into operation?

GITZELMANN: Galactokinase cannot play a role because if you restrict your galactose intake very severely it has no substrate. There could be some hidden galactose in the diet as is known to all those concerned in administering such diets. I think the pyrophosphorylase reaction is the one that is the real culprit and it can easily be demonstrated in red cells of these transferase deficient individuals, be they infants or not.

KOCH (Los Angeles): A compound heterozygote was identified on our newborn screening programme but was not treated and was subsequently mentally retarded. Do you think there is a cause and effect relationship?

GITZELMANN: I do not believe there is but it is a view held by others. The answer will come from careful observations on older double heterozygotes that are found in family investigations. The literature so far indicates that most compound heterozygotes (galactosaemia/Duarte) are perfectly healthy, but we would need some careful follow-up on these later.

Treatment of galactosaemia

KOMROWER: Dr Brandt is not quite right to say that we recommended some relaxation of diet since there was a very significant qualification; that the diet should be relaxed only to make it a socially sensible and satisfactory diet. Patients were not expected to be obsessional about whether or not a sandwich had some margarine that contained a small amount of butter, but we never suggested that they should have milk or any of the milk products in quantity. I do not think that anyone would disagree with what you have said about the basic premise of continued dietary treatment. It is my strong impression that any galactosaemic adult or adolescent who takes milk or milk products will feel very ill with abdominal pain and cramps, so I do not think they will want to drink milk.

SARDHARWALLA (Manchester): We have 14 patients under review, of whom seven are over the age of 15 years. Their ages range between 15 and 27 years with a mean of 19 years. These patients were born in five families and, with the exception of one who was diagnosed at the age of 13 months, they were all diagnosed either at birth or within the first two weeks of life. A review of their physical development showed that their growth was slightly retarded in early childhood but continued after puberty, and they are now all of average height and weight. Their IQ scores are not as good as those of the group that Dr Koch has just reported, since, with the exception of two patients with IQ scores of 107 and 80 respectively, they have IQs in the lower 60 range. This is in spite of what would be regarded as satisfactory control on the basis of the red blood cell galactose-1-phosphate levels which have always been 40 μg (154 μmol)/ml of packed red cells, or less. In fact two patients with IQ scores of 62 and 61 have generally had red blood cell galactose-1-phosphate levels of less than 25 μg (96 μmol)/ml.

Three patients were initially found to have cataracts but these have all resolved following treatment. Electroencephalograms have been carried out on four patients and two of them have shown no specific changes. None of these patients have shown any aggressive or antisocial behaviour, but as a group they tend to be passive and lack initiative. One has no real occupation, two are in a special school and two of the girls are able to cope with simple factory work and have made good mothers. One patient is working under sheltered conditions and the man who has an IQ of 107 has open employment. He enjoys his work and his wife is currently expecting a baby. On the whole our results have been somewhat disappointing.

KOMROWER: Dr Koch, I interpreted your data relating visual perceptual status to the time of treatment as meaning that there was no indication that early treatment was beneficial in respect of these visual perceptual difficulties.

KOCH: I think the data relating to visual perceptual status at the time of treatment suggests that treatment at birth is beneficial; from 0–7 days there were equal numbers of normal and abnormal patients. However, over the age of 4–11 months after diagnosis there were no normals and five abnormals in terms of visual perceptual status.

RAINE: It is important to have controls when assessing psychosocial deficiencies. I would very much like to hear Dr Koch's thoughts about the difficulty of choosing a suitable control group.

KOCH: I think it would be difficult, but there have been school studies in our part of the country which show that 10–20% of children have perceptual problems on entry to kindergarten. I look upon perceptual defects as a delay in maturation, not as indicators of organic brain damage, because if you follow these individuals into adulthood their perceptual difficulties cease to be demonstrable.

CLAYTON (Southampton): I should be interested to know the Panel's views on whether or not galactosides should be allowed in the diet. In the United Kingdom soya flour is added to a wide variety of foodstuffs and also masquerades as 'meat'. Whereas a galactose-free diet is relatively easy to attain, it would not be all that easy to be certain of excluding galactosides once mixed feeding is introduced.

GITZELMANN: To release galactose from raffinose and stachyose in our intestine we would need an α-galactosidase which we do not have in the intestinal mucosa. These saccharides will reach the colon and will be fermented by bacteria and a small part of their galactose moiety will probably be taken up. We have studied the feeding of saccharides to patients with galactosaemia and have shown that only small amounts of galactose is absorbed, except when the patient has diarrhoea. We do not know why the latter occurs.

My best dietary preparation is a soya milk prepared by dialysis of soya flour and therefore stachyose and raffinose and a trypsin inhibitor are removed; in the process, oligosaccharides are also removed, so that galactose from these sources will be minimal.

BRANDT: For practical purposes you should avoid milk and everything made of milk, that is enough.

KOCH: I would agree with Dr Brandt. We do not restrict soya beans in our preparations.

LEVY (Boston, USA): Dr Komrower is worried that red-cell galactose-1-phosphate during the first year of life indicates possible accumulation of galactose-1-phosphate in other body cells, particularly the brain, and that this could be causing harm. Professor Clayton worries about the soya bean based preparations and their containing polysaccharides that may be a source of galactose in a galactosaemic patient. Dr Brandt has said that we should exclude all milk and milk products. What does one substitute for the milk? In the United States we generally use either Nutramigen which contains some lactose, or a soya bean based formula which, as Professor Gitzelmann points out, may contain some available galactose. Should we be worried about even the small amounts of lactose or galactose in the presently used formulas; and if so, should we be preparing synthetic diets that totally exclude lactose for the treatment of galactosaemia?

KOMROWER: Yes, I am worried about galactose-1-phosphate. I think it is an indicator of what goes on in other cells of the body. The limited autopsy material that we have comparing galactose-1-phosphate levels in red cells with those in the brain, heart and other organs would indicate that a raised level of red-cell galactose-1-phosphate is indicative of an accumulation in other organs. The reverse is probably true during treatment, since there appears to be good reversibility of liver damage and cataract formation. I would be careful to ensure that lactose and galactose were eliminated from the diet in the first few years of life, as far as humanly possible. I agree that we should aim to produce totally lactose and galactose free diets.

GITZELMANN: I am convinced that one should not administer Nutramigen in the first year of life. We do give soya bean protein, but this soya bean protein has been shown to contain minimal amounts of galactose. I would not advocate the use of *any* soya bean extract, only a *good* soya bean extract. I do not think there is any one single nutrient or nutrient mixture, except for a totally synthetic preparation, that would not contain a small amount of galactose.

Pregnancy in galactosaemia

KOCH: We have two galactosaemic women who have had four normal heterozygous children. The first galactosaemic mother comes from a socially inept family in which her mother is an alcoholic, as well as she herself. In each of her four pregnancies erythrocyte galactose-1-phosphate levels were maintained within the normal range but we were unsuccessful in obtaining cord blood studies due to the patient's unreliability. Her three children resulting from these pregnancies are apparently normal and are now 5 years, 4 years and 6 months old. Our second mother was seen in our clinic on a routine visit and on physical examination an abdominal mass was paipated. Since the mass was midline and compatible with a pregnant uterus a pregnancy test was arranged and was found to be positive. She was kept on a galactose free diet and gave birth to a normal infant. Unfortunately she failed to notify us of her delivery and the opportunity to obtain a cord blood specimen was missed. Both of these mothers are markedly mentally retarded.

THURSBY-PELHAM (Stoke-on-Trent): We have one patient with galactosaemia who was diagnosed in 1951 and has been on a lactose free diet since the age of 6 weeks. She has had an uneventful pregnancy; the baby appears so far to be quite normal and has normal galactose-1-phosphate transferase activity. The child's development is being followed, but at present has not been fully assessed.

BRENTON (London): I can understand the need to keep the homozygous galactosaemic mother on her strict diet during pregnancy, but do you place the heterozygous galactosaemic mothers on a lactose free diet and is there any evidence that it is advantageous to do so?

SARDHARWALLA: I cannot say from my own experience.

KOCH: We must assume that the last statement is correct, as our data is insufficient to prove a relationship between cord blood galactose-1-phosphate levels and dietary management of the pregnancy and its subsequent outcome, but there may be a relationship, so that your question is quite pertinent.

Prenatal diagnosis of galactosaemia

NG: We now have experience of nine prenatal diagnoses of galactosaemia of which two were affected. One of the affected cases resulted in abortion. I would like to draw your attention to one of our cases which was referred to us as fetal galactosaemia, based on assays done in another laboratory using the UDP glucose consumption test. Transferase activity could not be demonstrated using this method. However, by application of the radioactive procedure we were able to demonstrate activity in cultured amniotic fluid cells. Postnatal analysis of blood from the newborn revealed that this baby is a carrier for galactosaemia.

Prenatal diagnosis with carbon labelled galactose-1-phosphate is accurate and relatively simple. The UDP glucose test is unreliable as there is an unidentified enzyme reaction, possibly a pyrophosphorylase or hydrolase, which is very active and interferes with the UDP glucose consumption test.

KOMROWER: John Holton posed the question 'Is prenatal diagnosis a right and proper thing to do in galactosaemia'? If I interpret the question rightly it would go on '. . . Because you can treat if they are diagnosed at birth'. Is this right, or why did you ask us that question?

HOLTON (Bristol): Yes, I think that the prospects for treatment may be acceptable for some parents. The peculiar thing about our series of prenatal diagnoses is that only one case had a previous child which had been treated and the other four had children who died neonatally.

BRENTON: Prenatal diagnosis is only indicated in a woman who has already had a child with the disease. Cord blood can be collected at birth and the child placed on a lactose-free diet until we have the results of the red-cell enzyme assay. Prenatal diagnosis would not alter that policy. The justification for prenatal diagnosis must therefore rest on the prognosis for the affected child treated from birth. If you think that the outcome of treatment is so poor that the risk of having a damaged child is high and that you would terminate the pregnancy because of the risk of severe mental retardation, then prenatal diagnosis would be justified. If the prognosis is good, abortion would not seem justified.

BRANDT: Although there has been some discussion on the safety of prenatal diagnosis in hereditary galactosaemia, I think we can agree that prenatal diagnosis is possible.

Whether or not the prenatal diagnosis should be offered to parents who have already had one child with galactosaemia is a matter of good genetic counselling. Many will probably find prenatal diagnosis unjustified when you are dealing with a rather easily treatable disorder such as hereditary galactosaemia. However, the long term prognosis is not as good as many of us anticipated. We must also remember that in most societies where we are wealthy enough to deal with inborn errors of metabolism the law allows free abortion, and the next logical step is free selective abortion. It is totally up to the parents to decide.

Good genetic counselling includes intimate knowledge not only of the disorder in question, but also of the intellectual and psychosocial status of the family involved. Furthermore, one must know quite a lot on the safety of the biochemical system used and the efficiency of the tools on which judgement is to be based. Most often the paediatrician who has been involved in diagnosis and treatment of the index case will be the most appropriate person to give confident genetic counselling, calling for the specialized paediatrician to be the clinical geneticist.

HARPER (Cardiff, Wales): I think it is essential that a laboratory undertaking prenatal tests should take the responsibility of checking carefully that the couple concerned have received correct clinical information about the prognosis and the genetic risks, especially when samples are being sent from other centres. If this is not done there is a serious danger that investigations will be undertaken because they are feasible rather than because they represent the most desirable way of managing the problem. Before the laboratory gets involved in a test they have to be as sure as they possibly can that the physician at the other end has gone into all the options; otherwise, it would be very easy for one option only, that of prenatal diagnosis, to be considered without a full explanation of the question of treatment being given.

HOLTON: I consider that the principal responsibilities of a laboratory undertaking prenatal diagnosis are to provide tests for which there is a justifiable demand and to give a reliable service. I cannot agree that you must ensure the parents have had all the management options put to them in every case. The tests are frequently arranged over very great distances and if they come from a clinical genetics centre or clinical geneticist we accept them in good faith.

HARPER: I strongly disagree with that. The laboratory must take some responsibility even though that does not absolve the clinician at the other end.

NG: In our laboratory I, as a biochemist, work closely with clinicians in answering patients' queries. We never recommend abortion; firstly because we have always thought that galactosaemia can be treated and secondly because it is the mother's decision.

LEVY: I would like to emphasise the need for proper genetic counselling to be given in conjunction with prenatal diagnosis testing. The case of false positive prenatal diagnosis of galactosaemia that Dr Ng mentioned was complicated by the fact that incorrect genetic counselling was given to the parents. Following the neonatal death of their first offspring who had galactosaemia and *E. coli* sepsis, they were told that galactosaemia is a fatal and untreatable disease. On this basis they adopted a child, but four years later a pregnancy occurred for which they sought prenatal diagnosis. Following our diagnosis of an affected fetus I asked the obstetrician what made the family desire this prenatal diagnosis, and was told of the genetic counselling information given to them. I then gave the parents the information that galactosaemia is a treatable disorder. They elected to continue the pregnancy, whereupon a clinically normal heterozygous infant was born. Our previous problem was lack of proper information being given, and every prenatal diagnosis laboratory has the responsibility of being certain that such information is given to the families involved.

KOMROWER: Should there be some mechanism of variant identification as well as classical identification? Is there enough cooperation or is there a network of collaboration between units working in these particular fields whereby you can double check certain of your more doubtful cases if you wish to do so, and if not should there be some mechanism of laboratory double check?

HOLTON: There is an organisation in this country (UK) called 'The Prenatal Diagnosis Group' which exists to catalogue the laboratories which are doing certain prenatal diagnoses. The members of this group are committed to share samples when a prenatal diagnosis is requested. At the present time we have had insufficient experience to see how this is working.

SARDHARWALLA: Samples we receive are shared with another laboratory so that we have two independent answers on the same sample and that in some way provides some measure of safety. It is also a question of speed. I think if two laboratories get a certain result simultaneously, then they are more confident about it. If only one laboratory does the test and gets a result which indicates that the fetus is affected it may wish to repeat the test, which takes longer.

Screening for galactosaemia

CAHALANE (Dublin): Our newborn screening programme over a period of several years has given an incidence of 1 in 33 000. Six of the eleven cases detected died in the neonatal period and, therefore, we must conclude that although screening is worthwhile, it must be done on cord blood.

KOCH: The *average* age of death in our 13 patients was 6 weeks. Six neonatal deaths out of eleven in Ireland is an unfortunate occurrence.

CLAYTON: Screening for galactosaemia raises problems in the UK. Our Guthrie collections are made between the 6th and 14th days of life. Blood collected on the 6th day would have to be sent to a laboratory and tested, and this would mean the result would be too late to save some of those infants who have the acute form presenting as an overwhelming fulminant infection. These infants are the problem, the more classical presentation appears to be recognised by the paediatricians. To be useful therefore, it would be necessary to screen cord blood. To perform this on a national scale would put an extra burden on hard pressed nursing staff who would have to collect cord blood, fill up yet another form and send it to the laboratory. The problem does not lie in the laboratory, but rather in the administrative arrangements.

GITZELMANN: Whether newborn screening or screening of samples taken on the 5th day works for galactosaemia is a matter of organisation. The assay does not take long and if provided efficiently, including telephone contact in the event of a positive result, you can have the result back by the 6th to 7th day. You may find the child is already in hospital, but in my experience it helps the hospital if they can be informed early of the diagnosis.

KOMROWER: I think that information about a suspected diagnosis is slightly different from population screening, because if you give a laboratory an index of suspicion, they have responsibility to deal with the sample promptly. Professor Clayton is talking about collection of specimens throughout the whole of the country, which varies in efficiency in terms of delivery of the samples. I can see the arguments in favour of cord blood analysis and in the best of all possible worlds that is what I would want for the diagnosis of galactosaemia.

CLAYTON: I too would go for cord blood.

WORTHY (Sheffield): In view of the difficulty in delays with neonatal screening, ought we not to consider taking the screening one stage earlier and screening mothers for heterozygosity in the antenatal clinic?

BRADLEY (Cardiff): Whilst the benefit of early treatment of galactosaemia is recognised there is some reluctance to institute cord blood screening programmes in the UK. In Wales both blood and urine filter paper specimens are collected at 6–10 days for newborn screening. The urine specimen is tested for reducing substances using Benedict's reagent. Should an infant's urine give a positive test, the blood filter is immediately assayed for galactose-1-phosphate uridyl transferase activity. Whilst we would not claim this procedure is ideal since galactosaemic infants may not excrete galactose, it has nevertheless proved useful in detecting 4 cases over a 7 year period, an incidence of 1 in 6700 births. This figure is comparable with that provided by cord blood screening. As a biproduct of this screening programme, the use of Benedict's reagent has also led to the finding of 6 infants with alcaptanuria, giving an incidence of 1 in 4500 which would indicate that this condition may be more common than has previously been suggested. The fact that we have not missed any cases of galactosaemia would seem to obviate the necessity to have a separate cord blood screening system.

CAHALANE: One of our patients did not have reducing substances and did not have galactosuria by urine chromatography. Our patients in common with those of Dr Levy sometimes die in the first 6—11 days of life which overlaps the point in time at which screening would be instituted.

HOLTON: There is another factor which comes into this problem and that is cost. Whether we should introduce hypothyroid screening, or galactosaemia screening, or screening for neural tube defects, one has to look at the frequency and one has to look at the relative cost of these things.

SECTION FOUR

Disorders of Fructose Metabolism

10

Clinical and genetic studies of disorders in fructose metabolism

K. Baerlocher, R. Gitzelmann and
B. Steinmann

Fructose is a major food constituent in human nutrition. In the form of refined sugar its consumption has steadily increased during recent decades. It has been used widely for clinical purposes as it has been claimed to be of advantage for diabetics, and for parenteral nutrition in adults and children. The latter use has remained controversial as many studies have indicated that for infusion therapy glucose is safest and cheapest[1, 2]. The clinical and metabolic aspects of fructose have been discussed at several symposia[3-6].

Fructose is metabolized in two different ways in the mammalian body (Figure 10.1). If ingested, it is in part assimilated to glucose in the intestine by phosphorylation by fructokinase to fructose-1-phosphate. The greater part reaches the liver, where it is mostly extracted and rapidly phosphorylated to fructose-1-phosphate. Fructaldolase will then split fructose-1-phosphate into two trioses which may be used for energy by entering the Krebs cycle, or they may be condensed to fructose-1,6-diphosphate and used for glucose or glycogen formation. A small part of fructose passes through the liver and is transported to other organs like adipose or muscle tissue, where it is metabolised to fructose-6-phosphate by the enzyme

Clinical and biochemical aspects

The carriers of this defect are clinically healthy. The diagnosis is suspected when a urine test for reducing substances is positive. Diabetes mellitus may be erroneously diagnosed if urinary sugar is not identified by specific methods (paper chromatography, enzymatic methods). Diagnosis of EF can be confirmed by the determination of fructose in blood and urine after intake of fructose (e.g. 1 g/kg up to 50 gm). Figure 10.3 demonstrates the results of a peroral fructose or sorbitol tolerance test (1 g/kg) in two siblings with EF: fructose is absorbed unchanged in a normal fashion from the gut and rises to very high levels in blood (up to 60 mg/100 ml; 3.3 mmol/l) after 30–60 minutes. It declines thereafter only slowly. Glucose, lactic acid and uric acid are unchanged[11]. In healthy adults insulin increased by about 20 μU/ml when 50 g of fructose were given orally[12], whereas in our patients with EF, insulin remained below 5 μU/ml during the loading test. Thus at these concentrations, fructose alone does not influence insulin release in patients with EF. Since the renal threshold for fructose lies between 20 and 30 mg/100 ml (1.1–1.7 mmol/l)[13], 5–10% of the fructose ingested during the tolerance test was excreted in the urine of our patients within the first 2 h compared to approximately 1% in controls. A considerable portion of fructose is metabolised by muscle and adipose tissue; this can be seen from the fall in levels of free fatty acids in serum during the fructose tolerance test[14].

Sorbitol is absorbed from the intestine at a slower rate than fructose and is oxidized to fructose by liver sorbitol dehydrogenase[15]. After sorbitol, fructosaemia also appears although to a lesser degree (Figure 10.3). 3% of the ingested sorbitol (1 g/kg) was found in the urine of our patients as fructose.

Since fructose administration does not lead to any symptoms in patients with EF, dietary restrictions are unnecessary.

Genetic aspects

The incidence of fructosuria is usually given as 1:130 000 of the general population[9]. Four patients with EF were seen among 29 000 individuals with mellituria at the Joslin Clinic[16]. Of 57 persons with EF reported by Sachs *et al.*[17], 12 were Jewish.

EF is inherited as an autosomal recessive[9]. In heterozygotes fructose tolerance tests are normal[18] but enzyme studies have not been done.

HEREDITARY FRUCTOSE INTOLERANCE (HFI)

HFI is the most important inherited disorder of fructose metabolism. It was first described in 1956 as idiosyncratic to fructose by Chambers and Pratt[19].

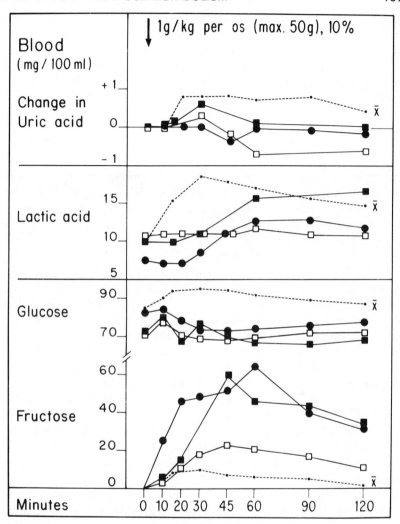

Figure 10.3 Oral fructose (sorbitol) tolerance test in two children with essential fructosuria ■ R.K., 19 years old; ● A.K., 16 years old; controls (adults) (·····); □ R.K. after sorbitol. Reproduced with permission from J. Nutr. Metab. (Karger)[11]. (Uric acid, 1 mg/100 ml = 0.06 mmol/l; lactic acid, 1 mg/100 ml = 0.11 mmol/l; glucose and fructose, 1 mg/100 ml = 0.055 mmol/l)

In 1957, Froesch et al.[20] reported hereditary fructose intolerance in two siblings and two relatives. They recognized that the disorder is inherited and that it differs from EF. In 1961 Hers and Joassin[21] demonstrated reduced activity of fructaldolase B in a liver biopsy from a patient with HFI. A deficiency or reduction of fructaldolase B has also been shown in kidney[22] and intestine[23].

Clinical aspects

Symptoms and signs   In patients with HFI, appearance and severity of symptoms depend upon the intake of fructose. In the absence of fructose (e.g. breast milk feeding) no metabolic derangement occurs. With the intake of sucrose in form of fruits and vegetables at weaning, the first symptoms are observed. The younger the child the more severe its reaction to dietary fructose; this may even be life threatening.

Older infants and children develop an aversion against sweets and protect themselves from most or all exposure to the noxious sugar. If they consume fructose repeatedly in small amounts, a milder but chronic form of HFI is observed. The clinical manifestations following a single (acute) or repeated (chronic) exposure to fructose are summarized in Table 10.1.

We have recently compiled the histories, clinical and laboratory findings of 20 symptomatic children with HFI from 17 families[23]. They were selected because of early onset of the disease and the availability of a detailed history. Fructose was first ingested and produced symptoms during the first 2 weeks of life in 5 of them, within the first 6 weeks in 11, and within the first 6 months in 17. Four patients were diagnosed during the first 2 months of life, and 11 within the first 7 months. In a further four patients diagnosis was made between 10 months and 2 years. Three patients with symptoms during infancy protected themselves later on by strong aversion against sweets and were only diagnosed because a younger sibling was also affected by HFI.

Prevailing symptoms (Figure 10.4) were poor feeding (20/20), vomiting (18/20) and failure to thrive (16/20). Drowsiness, crying, jaundice, abdominal distension, haemorrhages, irritability and diarrhoea were present in 5–8 patients out of 20.

On clinical examination (Figure 10.5), hepatomegaly was most often present (18/20). Paleness, partly due to anaemia, partly due to shock, was seen in 13 patients. Haemorrhages which occurred spontaneously or after venipuncture or finger pricks were observed in 12 patients. Trembling and jerks did not occur with low blood glucose and are therefore considered to be related to shock. They were present in 12 patients. Jaundice was

TABLE 10.1 **Symptoms, signs and laboratory findings in hereditary fructose intolerance**

Acute exposure	Chronic exposure
Sweating	Failure to thrive
Trembling	Vomiting, poor feeding
Dizziness	Jaundice
Nausea	Hepatomegaly
Vomiting	Oedema
Apathy, lethargy, coma	Ascites
Convulsions	Haemorrhages

Signs	Aversion to sweets
	Lack of dental caries
Laboratory	Fructosaemia, fructosuria
findings	Hypoglycaemia
	Hypophosphataemia
	Hyperbilirubinaemia
	Hyperuricaemia, hypermagnesaemia
	Increased serum amino acids (tyrosine, methionine)
	Increased serum levels of hepatic enzymes
	Decreased coagulation factors
	Renal tubular syndrome

observed in more than one half of patients and ascites, oliguria and splenomegaly in a quarter.

Laboratory findings

Findings in the 20 symptomatic patients are listed in Figure 10.6 in order of the frequency with which examinations were done. One or more chemical signs of liver dysfunction were always found. Abnormal results were most frequent for serum transaminases, prothrombin time, serum protein, plasma methionine and/or tyrosine. Remarkably, two HFI infants were discovered by finding a high blood methionine at routine newborn screening.

A second group of chemical tests was indicative of disturbed renal function: mellituria, proteinuria, hyperaminoaciduria and acidosis. In 14 of 20 children, mellituria and proteinuria were present. Screening for hyperaminoaciduria while in hospital led to the diagnosis of HFI in four patients.

Derangements of intermediate metabolism were mirrored by the lowering of serum phosphorus and potassium, by fructosuria, organic aciduria and

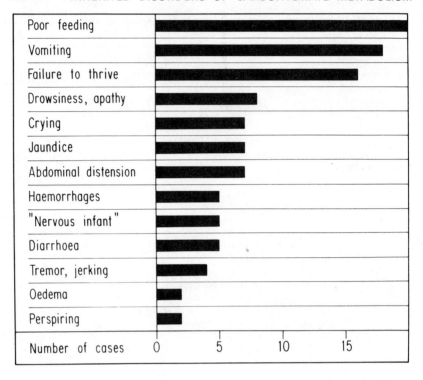

Figure 10.4 Symptoms (anamnestic data) in 20 children with hereditary fructose intolerance[23]. With permission from *Helv. Paediatr. Acta*

also by metabolic acidosis. Not mentioned in this figure are determinations of serum uric acid, magnesium and lactate. Uric acid was abnormally high in 4 of 9 children, magnesium in 3 of 5 and lactate in 1 of 2. Acanthocytes or fragmentocytes, thrombocytopenia and hypoglycaemia were seen infrequently.

Morphology of liver tissue in patients with HFI revealed fatty changes with vacuolization, fibrosis and formation of bile ductules. Two children died of acute liver failure.

Diagnosis and differential diagnosis

Diagnosis of HFI can be suspected from a detailed nutritional history and the clinical picture. Since the spectrum of symptoms and signs may be non-specific, other metabolic disorders (tyrosinosis, glycogenosis), hepatitis, liver

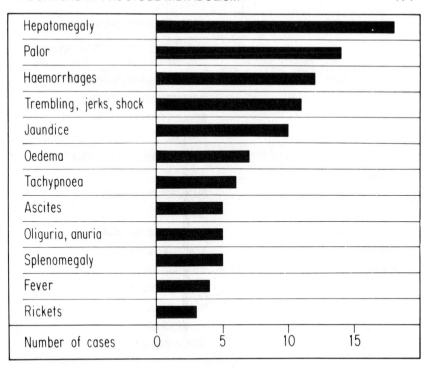

Figure 10.5 Clinical findings in 20 children with hereditary fructose intolerance[23].
With permission from *Helv. Paediatra. Acta*

cirrhosis or liver tumour may be considered. Pyloric stenosis or hiatus hernia
are often suggested if vomiting is the leading symptom. Septicaemia or intrauterine infection may present clinically in the same way as HFI, especially if clotting disturbances and haematological changes are obvious.
Haemolytic-uraemic syndrome may be considered[23].

Diagnosis is confirmed by a fructose tolerance test and/or the enzyme
assay in liver tissue or intestinal mucosa. The fructose tolerance test (FTT)
using a single intravenous dose of 0.2–0.3 g/kg body weight is more conclusive than the oral FTT. The oral FTT should be abandoned as it causes
severe gastrointestinal symptoms. The effect of an *i.v.* fructose load on
different chemical parameters in five children with HFI is summarized in
Figure 10.7. Fructose decreased rapidly with a mean half-disappearance
rate of 11 ± 2 minutes, which is normal. Blood glucose fell immediately and
was lowest after 40 minutes. Decrease of phosphate and increase of lactic

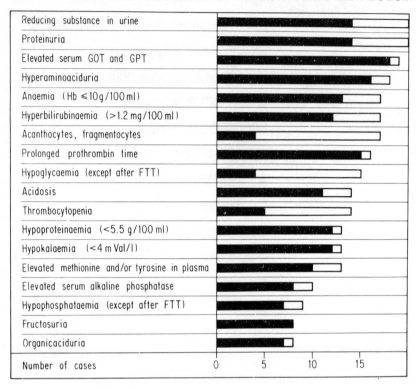

Figure 10.6 Laboratory findings in 20 symptomatic children with hereditary fructose intolerance. Open bars represent numbers of examinations performed, closed bars numbers of positive results[23]. With permission from *Helv. Paediatr. Acta*

acid and magnesium preceded the lowest glucose level. The response to the same amount of sorbitol was almost identical (1 patient shown in Figure 10.7) except that fructose could not be detected in serum.

Details for the estimation of liver or intestinal fructaldolase B activity are given by Gitzelmann[24]. Normal liver fructaldolase is almost equally active with both fructose-1,6-diphosphate and fructose-1-phosphate as substrate; the ratio of the activities is close to 1. In patients with HFI, enzyme activity is reduced with both substrates but more so with the 1-phosphate; the activity ratio is higher than normal (Table 10.2).

Therapy and prognosis

Once the diagnosis is established treatment must be started immediately

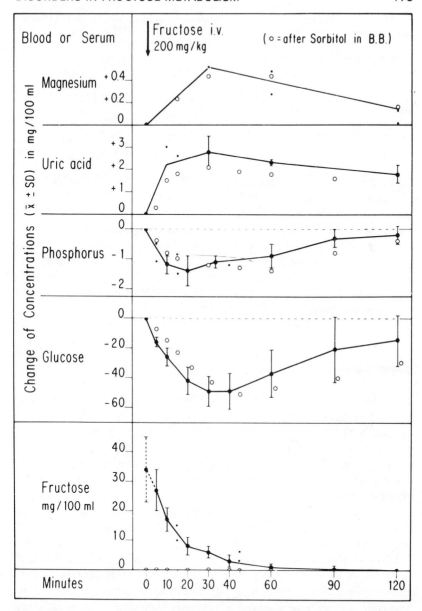

Figure 10.7 Intravenous fructose tolerance test (200 mg/kg body wt) in 5 children with hereditary fructose intolerance (HFI). I – mean ± 1 standard deviation; – values after sorbitol (1 g/kg per os) in patient B.B. with HFI[11] (Magnesium, 1 mg/100 ml = 0.41 mmol/l; uric acid, 1 mg/100 ml = 0.06 mmol/l; phosphorus, 1 mg/100 ml = 0.32 mmol/l; glucose and fructose, 1 mg/100 ml = 0.055 mmol/l)

TABLE 10.2   Activity ($\bar{X} \pm$ S.D.) of fructaldolase in liver extracts of HFI patients and controls (U/g of liver tissue) measured with fructose-1,6-diphosphatase (F-d-P) or fructose-1-phosphate (F-1-P)[11]

	(a) F-d-P	(b) F-1-P	a/b
Controls ($n = 7$)	2.64 ± 0.58	2.48 ± 0.57	1.07 ± 0.07
HFI ($n = 13$)	0.43 ± 0.19	0.08 ± 0.11	$>4(n = 12)$
			$1.7 (n = 1)$

with a fructose free diet. This regimen results in almost immediate clearance of symptoms and signs with the exception of hepatomegaly, which may persist for many months although the liver size decreases slowly[25]. Fatty changes of hepatocytes were occasionally seen many months after the diet was started[23, 25]. In young infants with severe liver damage, immediate withdrawal of fructose from the diet and/or infusions does not guarantee survival. One of our patients died in liver failure a full week after diagnosis had been made. Haemorrhages as a consequence of severe liver dysfunction may lead to complications[23].

Genetic aspects

In recent years it has become evident that HFI is more common than previously thought. Gitzelmann and Baerlocher[26] have estimated an incidence in Switzerland of about 1:20 000. About 100 cases were reported until 1972 in the literature[27]. A survey of 55 patients has been published recently[28]. In different countries many more cases have been diagnosed but not published[29], and still many will remain undiagnosed because of self imposed low fructose diet.

The defect is inherited as an autosomal recessive. Reports of apparent dominant inheritance[30–32, 56] could well indicate homozygosity in one and heterozygosity in the other parent.

Fructose-1-phosphate aldolase activity in heterozygotes does not differ from that of controls[33]. Beyreiss et al.[34] reported that parents of HFI patients receiving a constant fructose infusion have a higher plateau of fructose concentration than controls. This could not be confirmed by our group in seven parents when compared to six controls (Figure 10.8). Although in the parents the standard deviations were greater for some parameters, the differences were not significant.

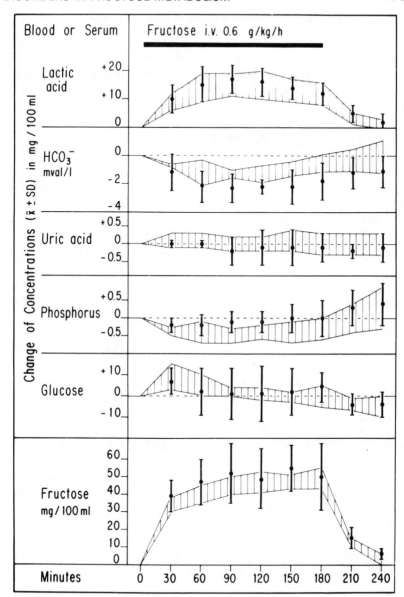

Figure 10.8 Infusion of fructose during 3 h (0.6 g/kg/h) in 6 adult controls and 7 parents of children with hereditary fructose intolerance. Changes of concentrations are given in mean ± 1 SD for parents (⚡) and controls (‖‖‖)[11] (Lactic acid, 1 mg/100 ml = 0.11 mmol/l; uric acid, 1 mg/100 ml = 0.06 mmol/l; phosphorus, 1 mg/100 ml = 0.32 mmol/1; glucose and fructose, 1 mg/100 ml = 0.055 mmol/l)

FRUCTOSE-1,6-DIPHOSPHATASE DEFICIENCY

Infantile lactic acidosis is commonly associated with different biochemical defects of gluconeogenesis[35]. In 1970, Baker and Winegrad[36] succeeded in defining fructose-1,6-diphosphatase deficiency in a patient with episodes of hypoglycaemia and severe metabolic acidosis. Since then a total of 16 patients with this defect have been reported to our knowledge[36–48] and at least 7 siblings with symptoms suggestive of the disorder were mentioned. Some patients have been diagnosed but not yet published[49].

Clinical aspects

Fructose-1,6-diphosphatase (FDPase) is a key enzyme of gluconeogenesis; its deficiency hinders endogenous formation of glucose from lactate, alanine and glycerol. Administration of these substrates and of fructose does not cause a rise of blood glucose but immediate hypoglycaemia and lactic acidosis occur. Since newborns depend upon gluconeogenesis in the first few days[35], symptoms tend to appear during this period in patients with FDPase deficiency. This has been demonstrated in 8 of 16 patients. The main findings in 16 symptomatic children with this defect reported in the literature are summarized in Table 10.3.

Acute episodes are often triggered by infections. They present with the symptoms of metabolic acidosis and acute hypoglycaemia: hyperventilation, shock, apnoea, trembling, lethargy, loss of consciousness and convulsions. Acute episodes although dramatic and life threatening may be promptly overcome by infusion of glucose and bicarbonate. During the intervals between acute episodes, mild hyperventilation and lactic acidosis persist but their severity depends on the frequency of food intake.

Hepatomegaly, slight muscular hypotonia and hyporeflexia are common findings throughout childhood. Some patients tend to be obese. In the surviving patients intellectual development seems unimpaired. Our patient, now aged 8.5 years, is slightly retarded and attending special school. EEG tracings were normal in the patient under dietary management but during the acute episode peculiar spindle-shaped bursts of fast activity (13 cps) together with severe diffuse slowing of background activity were recorded in both the patient and his affected sister[38].

Laboratory findings

Abnormal findings include hypoglycaemia, severe acidosis (pH 7.1 or lower), excessive lactic acid in serum (up to 200 mg/100 ml; 22 mmol/l)[37]

TABLE 10.3 Synopsis of 16 symptomatic patients with fructose-1,6-diphosphatase deficiency[36-48]

Consanguinity	4/12
Sex	5 m, 10 f
Deceased siblings with similar symptoms	7
Appearance of symptoms	
Perinatal period (1–4 days)	8/16
1–6 months	4/16
> 6 months	4/16
First symptoms	
Hyperventilation	11/16
Hepatomegaly	5/16
Muscular hypotonia	4/16
Lethargy	4/16
Vomiting	4/16
Failure to thrive	4/16
Convulsions (hypoglycaemic)	3/16
Further course	
Hepatomegaly	11/12
Laboratory findings	
Acidosis	15/15
Ketosis	13/15
Fasting hypoglycaemia	15/15
Fasting lactacidaemia	13/13
Special investigations	
Normal reaction to glucagon after 8–12 h fasting	6/6
No reaction to glucagon after 14–25 h fasting	8/8
Hypoglycaemic response to	
Fructose	12/15
Glycerol	8/10
Alanine	5/8
Dihydroxyacetone	1/1
Histology of liver	
Fatty infiltration	12/12
Fibrosis	4/12
Activity of fructose-1,6-diphosphatase in liver	
No activity	9/14
1–6% of normal activity	1/14
15–30%	4/14
Effect of folate administration	3/6

and urine, pyruvic acidaemia, high values of free fatty acids in serum, increased alanine and ketone bodies in serum and urine.

In contrast to HFI, disturbances of liver function were rarely observed[41]. Only one patient showed severe liver dysfunction suggestive of tyrosinosis[37, 50]. On a diet containing sucrose, severe abnormalities of aminoacid metabolism and renal reabsorption were present in this patient[50]. In other patients with this disorder such abnormalities, renal tubular dysfunction, haematological changes or coagulation defects have not been observed.

Functional studies

Prolonged fasting induces the typical biochemical derangements, hypoglycaemia and lactic acidosis. This is demonstrated in Figure 10.9. The patient remained normoglycaemic during the first 18 h although glucose dropped slowly. After 18 h a sharp decrease of glucose and an increase of lactic acid occurred. The patient was somewhat floppy at this time and respiration rose from 24 to 40 per minute. Glucagon given *i.m.* had no effect but *i.v.* glucose produced normoglycaemia.

Loading tests with fructose, glycerol, dihydroxyacetone, alanine or lactate may have a similar effect but to a lesser degree. The results of an *i.v.* fructose tolerance test (0.5 g/kg body weight) are presented in Figure 10.10[51]. Fructose induced hypoglycaemia and compensated metabolic acidosis. Lactic acid rose and phosphate dropped, as is observed in patients with HFI. No gastrointestinal symptoms occurred. The biochemical response seemed less severe and more easily overcome than in patients with HFI.

Glycerol (Figure 10.11) and dihydroxyacetone (DHA) (Figure 10.12), both metabolites which enter the gluconeogenetic pathway induced hypoglycaemia as well as compensated metabolic acidosis. A DHA tolerance test provoked similar changes to fructose, a rise of lactic acid and a fall of phosphorus. They were not seen in a patient with HFI (Figure 10.12), nor in normal individuals (Figure 10.13); in both these situations gluconeogenesis is normal.

Diagnosis and differential diagnosis

Diagnosis must be considered in patients with lactic acidosis and hypoglycaemia. It can be difficult to distinguish FDPase deficiency from other inherited disorders of gluconeogenesis (e.g. deficiencies of glucose-6-phosphatase[44], pyruvate carboxylase or pyruvate dehydrogenase) or ketotic hypoglycaemia[40].

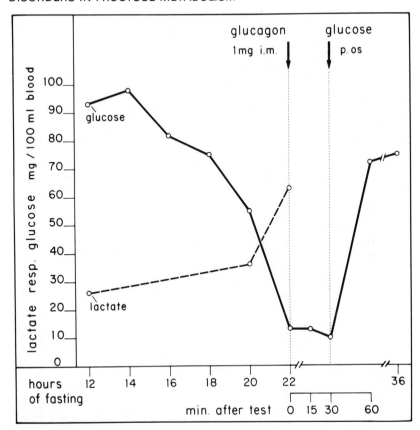

Figure 10.9 Effect of prolonged fasting on blood glucose and lactate concentrations in a 17-months-old boy with FDPase-deficiency[38]. With permission from *Helv. Paediatr. Acta*[38]. (Glucose, 1 mg/100 ml = 0.55 mmol/l; lactate, 1 mg/100 ml = 0.11 mmol/l)

Tolerance tests with fructose, alanine or DHA may prove helpful for clinical evaluation (see above and Table 10.3). Oral fructose loading should not be performed until HFI is excluded, because dangerous hypoglycaemia and gastrointestinal side effects may ensue in such patients. Final proof of the defect is obtained by the *in vitro* demonstration of enzyme deficiency in a liver biopsy. In 9 of 14 patients no enzyme activity was detected. In 4 patients activity of 15–30% of normal was measured. Patients with partial enzyme defect reacted differently to various tolerance tests but fasting hypoglycaemia was present in all (Table 10.3).

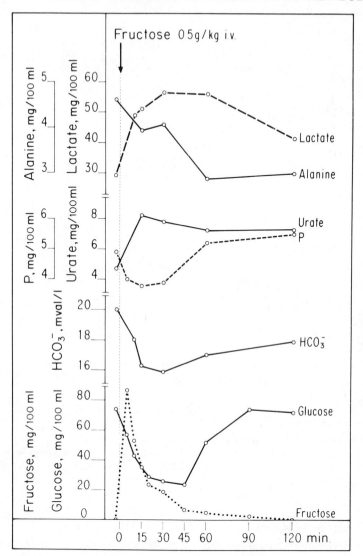

Figure 10.10　Intravenous fructose tolerance test (0.5 g/kg) in a boy with FDPase-deficiency at age 19 months[51]. With permission from *J. Vit. Nutr. Res.* (Lactate, 1 mg/100 ml = 0.11 mmol/1; alanine, 1 mg/100 ml = 0.11 mmol/1; urate, 1 mg/100 ml = 0.06 mmol/1; phosphorus, 1 mg/100 ml = 0.32 mmol/1; glucose and fructose, 1 mg/100 ml = 0.055 mmol/l).

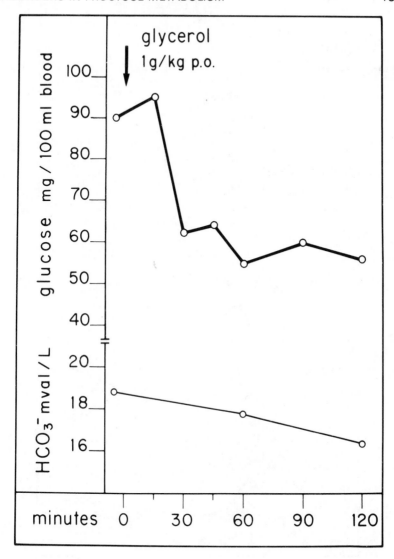

Figure 10.11   Oral glycerol tolerance test (1 g/kg) in a boy with FDPase-deficiency at 17 months of age. With permission from *Helv. Paediatr. Acta*[38]. (Glucose, 1 mg/100 ml = 0.055 mmol/l)

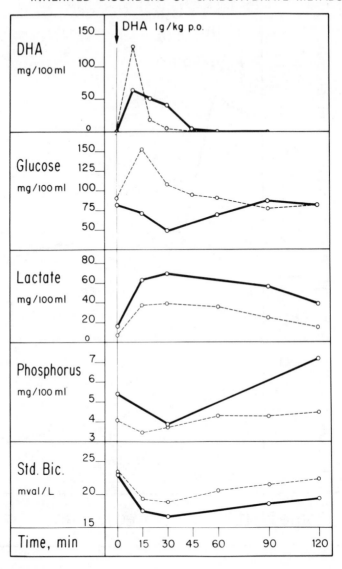

Figure 10.12 Oral dihydroxyacetone (DHA) tolerance test (1 g/kg) in a child with FDPase deficiency ——————— and in a child with hereditary fructose intolerance (--------)[38]. With permission from *Helv. Paediatr. Acta* (DHA, 1 mg/100 ml = 0.11 mmol/l; glucose, 1 mg/100 ml = 0.055 mmol/l; lactate, 1 mg/100 ml = 0.11 mmol/l; phosphorus, 1 mg/100 ml = 0.32 mmol/l)

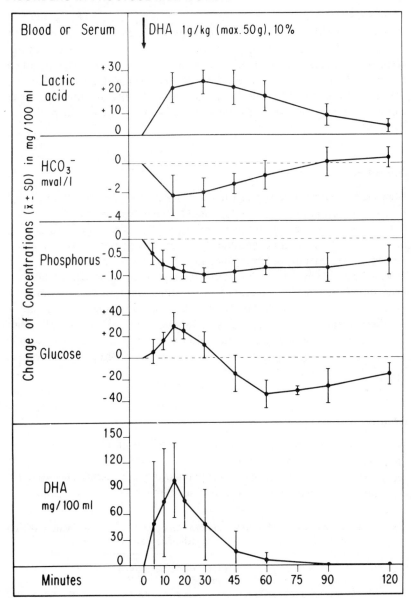

Figure 10.13   Oral dihydroxyacetone (DHA) tolerance test (1 g/kg, max. 50 g) in 6 normal adults. With permission from *J. Nutr. Metab.* (Karger)[11]. (Lactic acid, 1 mg/100 ml = 0.11 mmol/l; phosphorus, 1 mg/100 ml = 0.32 mmol/l; glucose, 1 mg/100 ml = 0.055 mmol/l; DHA, 1 mg/100 ml = 0.11 mmol/l)

Diagnosis can also be made from a biopsy specimen of intestine[40] or kidney[37]. It is still controversial whether the defect can be recognised by the estimation of fructose-1,6-diphosphatase in leukocytes. Melançon et al.[42] and also Schrijvers and Hommes[52] have found very low but significant enzyme activity in leucocytes of normal controls, whereas Cahill and Kirtley[53] did not. Gitzelmann could not reproduce these results (unpublished observation). The enzyme does not seem to be active in cultured skin fibroblasts.

Treatment

Long-term treatment consists of frequent meals and the restriction of fructose or sorbitol intake. Dietary fat should be partly restricted[39].

One child has been treated with a fructose free diet since birth and has never had hypoglycaemic episodes or liver enlargement[45]. Avoidance of fasting, especially during febrile infections, is probably more important than fructose restriction for the long-term management. Folic acid, which has been shown to increase the activity of intestinal and liver enzymes involved in gluconeogenesis had a beneficial effect in two patients[40] but not in another[45]. Patients with no enzyme activity did not respond[41]. Once diagnosis is established and acute episodes have been overcome without handicap, prognosis is good. Ten patients were recorded in good condition in 1973[41].

Genetic aspects

We can only speculate about the incidence of the disease since few cases have been reported. It is expected that in future more patients will be recognised among children with unexplained hypoglycaemic episodes. The inheritance is autosomal recessive. In three families consanguinity has been

TABLE 10.4   Activity of fructose-1,6-diphosphatase (U/g tissue) in liver of controls, 2 patients with FDPase deficiency and their parents

	Gitzelmann et al.[54]	Saudubray et al.[41]
Controls	4.82, 4.98	4.4–5.8
Patient	0.0	0.0
Mother	0.80	2.6
Father	1.37	—

noted[37, 38, 40]. Of the 16 published children, 10 were female and 5 male; sex was not stated in one case[44].

The parents of patients with FDPase deficiency are healthy. Three parents had intermediate enzyme activity in liver[41, 54] (Table 10.4).

Intermediate enzyme activity has also been detected in leukocytes[42, 52]. In a recent report of Taunton et al.[55] a mother and her daughter with FDPase deficiency were described and dominant inheritance was suggested. Both had residual enzyme activity of about 30–40% of normal. This could well indicate either heterozygosity or the presence of a second enzyme variant.

SUMMARY AND COMMENTS

A synopsis of the three inborn errors of fructose metabolism is given in Table 10.5. Essential fructosuria has little clinical importance. Fructose, which is not utilized by liver, intestine and kidney in this disorder is cleared

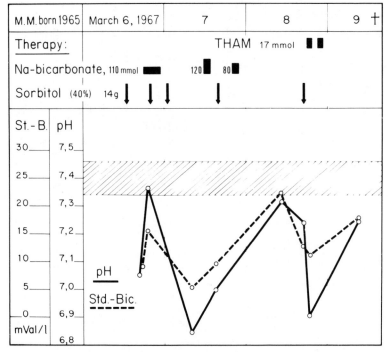

Figure 10.14 Final course of a 2-year-old girl with undiagnosed fructose-1,6-diphosphatase deficiency after repeated sorbitol infusions for cerebral oedema. Each time after sorbitol severe acidosis followed which was corrected by sodium-bicarbonate and Tris-buffer (Tham)[54]

TABLE 10.5 Synopsis of disorders of fructose metabolism

	Essential fructosuria (fructokinase-deficiency)	Hereditary fructose intolerance (fructaldolase-deficiency)	Fructose 1,6-diphosphatase deficiency
Incidence	~1 : 130 000	~1 : 20 000	
Inheritance	Autosomal recessive	Autosomal recessive	Autosomal recessive
Appearance of symptoms	After exposure (fructose, sucrose, sorbitol)	After exposure (Fructose etc.)	After prolonged fasting, especially in neonatal period and during infections, after exposure (fructose etc.)
Symptoms	None	Acute: vomiting, sweating, tremor, coma, convulsions. Chronic: failure to thrive, vomiting, hepatomegaly, jaundice, ascites, oedema, hypoglycaemic convulsions, aversion against sweets	Hyperventilation, apathy, unconsciousness, convulsions, hepatomegaly, hypotonia
Laboratory findings	Fructosaemia, -uria	Fructosaemia, -uria, hypoglycaemia, hypophosphataemia, liver dysfunction, tubular syndrome	Hypoglycaemia, lactic acidosis, ketone bodies, hyperalaninuria
Diagnosis	Fructose in blood or urine after exposure	Fructose-tolerance test (0.2–0.3 g/kg i.v.), enzyme activity in liver or intestine	Prolonged fasting, loading tests (fructose, glycerol), enzyme activity in liver (intestine)
Treatment	None	Fructose free diet	Fructose restricted diet
Course without treatment	Harmless	Episodic, possibly fatal	Episodic, possibly fatal
with treatment		Benign	Benign

by renal excretion as well as by metabolism in muscle and adipose tissue.

In contrast, patients with a defect of fructaldolase B or fructose-1,6-diphosphatase are intolerant of exogenous fructose, sucrose or sorbitol. The adverse reaction seems stronger in patients with HFI. By vomiting, patients protect themselves from further intake of fructose and, later in life, they develop an aversion against sweetened food. Fasting or infections do not evoke acute symptoms in children with HFI. On the other hand, in FDPase deficiency fasting and infections trigger acute episodes characterised by lactic acidosis (hyperventilation) and hypoglycaemia.

For paediatricians it is important to know that many milk formulae for infant nutrition contain fructose and sucrose which are harmful to patients with the two disorders. Most endangered are newborns and young infants. Some glucose substitutes such as fructose, sucrose or sorbitol, used either for parenteral nutrition or for treatment of cerebral oedema, cause great danger to patients with HFI or FDPase deficiency (Figure 10.14).

Reports of children and adults with known or unknown defects in fructose metabolism who died following fructose or sorbitol infusions are steadily appearing[23, 56, 57]. The pathophysiologic mechanism underlying the metabolic changes after fructose ingestion in these patients will be discussed in Chapter 11.

References

1. Bode, J. Ch., Ismail, T., Bode, Ch., Dürr, H. K. and Maroske D. (1978). Zur Frage der Verwendung von Glucose oder Fruktose für die parenterale Ernährung. *Schweiz. Med. Wochenschr.*, **108,** 816
2. Froesch, E. R. (1978). Parenterale Ernährung: Glucose oder Glucoseersatzstoffe? *Schweiz. Med. Wochenschr.*, **108,** 813
3. Nikkilä, E. A. and Juttunen, J. K. (eds.). (1972). Clinical and metabolic aspects of fructose. *Acta Med. Scand.*, 542 (Suppl.)
4. Zöllner, N. and Heuckenkamp, P. U. (eds.). (1975). Zucker und Zuckeraustauschstoffe. *Nutr. Metab.*, 18 (Suppl. 1)
5. Hue, L. (1974). The metabolism and toxic effects of fructose. In H. L. Sipple and K. W. McNutt (eds.). *Sugars in Nutrition*, pp. 357–371. (New York: Academic Press)
6. Ritzel, G. and Brubacher, G. (eds.). (1976). Monosaccharides and polyalcohols in nutrition, therapy and dietetics. *Int. J. Vitam. Nutr. Res.*, (Suppl. 15)
7. Woods, H. F. (1972). Hepatic accumulation of metabolites after fructose loading. *Acta Med. Scand.*, (Suppl. 542), 87
8. Odièvre, M., Poirier, C., Levillain, P., Modigliani, E. and Strauch, G. (1970). Etude des réponses glucosémiques, lactacidémiques et insulinémiques après administration intraveineuse rapide de doses variables de fructose chez l'enfant normal. *Arch. Fr. Pédiatr.*, **27,** 1057

9. Froesch, E. R. (1978). Essential fructosuria and hereditary fructose intolerance. In J. B. Stanbury, J. B. Wyngaarden and D. S. Fredrickson (eds.). *The Metabolic Basis of Inherited Disease*, pp. 121–136. (New York: McGraw-Hill)

10. Schapira, F., Schapira, G. and Dreyfuss, J. C. (1961–1962). La lésion enzymatique de la fructosurie bénigne. *Enzym. Biol. Clin.*, **1**, 170

11. Steinmann, B., Baerlocher, K. and Gitzelmann, R. (1975). Hereditäre Störungen des Fruktosestoffwechsels. Belastungsproben mit Fruktose, Sorbitol und Dihydroxyaceton. *J. Nutr. Metab.*, **18**, 115

12. Cook, G. C. (1971). Absorption and metabolism of D-fructose in man. *Am. J. Clin. Nutr.*, **24**, 1302

13. Zöllner, N., Neuckenkamp, P. U. and Nechwatal, W. (1968). Ueber die Verwertung und renale Ausscheidung von Fructose während ihrer langdauernden intravenösen Zufuhr. *Klin. Wochenschr.*, **46**, 1300

14. Froesch, E. R. (1972). Fructose metabolism in adipose tissue. *Acta Med. Scand.*, **542**, 37

15. Wick, A. N. and Drury, D. R. (1951). Action of insulin on the permeability of cells to sorbitol. *Am. J. Physiol.*, **166**, 421

16. Marble, A. (1947). Diagnosis of less common glycosurias including pentosuria and fructosuria. *Med. Clin. N. Am.*, **31**, 313

17. Sachs, B., Sternfeld, L. and Kraus, G. (1942). Essential fructosuria: Its pathophysiology. *Am. J. Dis. Child.*, **63**, 252

18. Leonidas, J. C. (1965). Essential fructosuria. *NY State J. Med.*, **65**, 2257

19. Chambers, R. A. and Pratt, R. T. (1956). Idiosyncrasy to fructose. *Lancet*, **2**, 340

20. Froesch, E. R., Prader, A., Labhart, A., Stuber, H. W. and Wolf, H. P. (1957). Die hereditäre Fructoseintoleranz, eine bisher nicht bekannte kongenitale Stoffwechselstörung. *Schweiz. Med. Wochenschr.*, **87**, 1168

21. Hers, H. G. and Joassin, G. (1961). Anomalie de l'aldolase hépatique dans l'intolérance au fructose. *Enzymol. Biol. Clin.*, **1**, 4

22. Kranhold, J. F., Loh, D. and Morris, R. C. Jr. (1969). Renal fructose metabolizing enzymes: significance in hereditary fructose intolerance. *Science*, **165**, 402

23. Baerlocher, K., Gitzelmann, R., Steinmann, B. and Gitzelmann-Cumarasamy, N. (1979). Hereditary fructose intolerance in early childhood: a major diagnostic challenge. Survey of 20 symptomatic cases. *Helv. Paediatr. Acta*, **33**, 465

24. Gitzelmann, R. (1974). Enzymes of fructose and galactose metabolism. In H. C. Curtius and H. Roth (eds.). *Clinical Biochemistry, Principals and Methods*. pp. 1236–1240. (Berlin: De Gruyter)

25. Odièvre, M. (1976). L'avenir des enfants atteints d'intolérance héréditaire au fructose. *Rev. Pédiatrie*, **12**, 449

26. Gitzelmann, R. and Baerlocher, K. (1973). Vorteile und Nachteile der Fructose in der Nahrung. *Pädiat. Fortbildiung Praxis*, **37**, 40

27. Perheentupa, J., Raivio, K. O. and Nikkilä, E. A. (1972). Hereditary fructose intolerance. *Acta Med. Scand.*, **542**, 65

28. Odièvre, M., Gentil, C., Gautier, M. and Alagille, D. (1978). Hereditary fructose intolerance in childhood. Diagnosis, management and course in 55 patients. *Am. J. Dis. Child.*, **132**, 605

29. De Barsy, Th., Froesch E. R. and Schaub, J. (Personal communication)
30. Wolf, H., Zschokke, F., Wedemeyer, R. and Hübner H. (1959). Angeborene
     hereditäre Fruktoseintoleranz. *Klin. Wochenschr.*, **37**, 693
31. Köhlin, P. and Mehlin, K. (1968). Hereditary fructose intolerance in four
     Swedish families. *Acta Paediatr. Scand.*, **57**, 24
32. Kurz, R., Hächl, G., Hohenwallner, W. and Berger, H. (1971). Hereditäre
     Fruktoseintoleranz mit vermutlich dominantem Erbgang. *Acta Kinder-
     heilkind*, **183**, 233
33. Raivio, K., Perheentupa, J. and Nikkilä, E. A. (1967). Aldolase activities in
     the liver in parents of patients with hereditary fructose intolerance. *Clin.
     Chim. Acta*, **17**, 275
34. Beyreiss, K., Willgerodt, H. and Theile, H. (1968). Untersuchungen bei
     heterozygoten Merkmalsträgern für Fruktoseintoleranz. *Klin. Wochenschr.*,
     9, 465
35. Pagliara, A. S., Karl, I. E., Hammond, M. and Dipnis, D. M. (1973).
     Hypoglycaemia in infancy and childhood, Parts I and II. *J. Pediatr.*, **82**, 365
     and 558
36. Baker, L. and Winegrad, A. I. (1970). Fasting hypoglycaemia and metabolic
     acidosis associated with deficiency of hepatic fructose-1,6-diphosphatase ac-
     tivity. *Lancet*, **2**, 13
37. Hülsmann, W. C. and Fernandes, J. (1971). A child with lactacidemia and
     fructose-diphosphatase deficiency in the liver. *Pediatr. Res.*, **5**, 633
38. Baerlocher, K., Gitzelmann, R., Nüssli, R. and Dumermuth, G. (1971). Infan-
     tile lactic acidosis due to hereditary fructose-1,6-diphosphatase deficiency.
     Helv. Paediatr. Acta, **26**, 489
39. Pagliara, A. S., Karl, I. E., Keating, J. P., Brown, B. J. and Kipnis, D. M.
     (1972). Hepatic fructose-1,6-diphosphatase deficiency. A cause of lactic
     acidosis and hypoglycaemia in infancy. *J. Clin. Invest.*, **51**, 2115
40. Greene, H. L., Stifel, F. B. and Herman, R. H. (1972). 'Ketotic
     hypoglycaemia' due to hepatic fructose-1,6-diphosphatase deficiency. Treat-
     ment with folic acid. *Am. J. Dis. Child.*, **124**, 415
41. Saudubray, J. M., Dreyfus, J. C., Cepanec, C., Le Lo'ch, H., Trung, P. H. and
     Mozziconacci, P. (1973). Acidose lactique, hypoglycémie et hépatomégalie
     par déficit héréditaire en fructose-1,6-diphosphatase hépatique. *Arch. Fr.
     Pédiatr.*, **30**, 609
42. Melançon, S. B., Khachardurian, A. K., Nadler, H. L. and Brown, B. I.
     (1973). Metabolic and biochemical studies in fructose-1,6-diphosphatase
     deficiency. *J. Pediatr.*, **82**, 650
43. De Rosas, R. J., Wapnir, R. A., Lifshitz, F., Silverberg, M. and Olson, M.
     (1974). Folic acid enhanced gluconeogenesis in glycerol induced
     hypoglycemia and fructose-1,6-diphosphatase deficiency. Presented at the
     56th Annual Meeting of the Endocrine Society, Atlanta.
44. Eagle, R. B., Macnab, A. J., Ryman, B. E. and Strang, L. B. (1974). Liver
     biopsy data on a child with fructose-1,6-diphosphatase deficiency that closely
     resembled many aspects of glucose-6-phosphatase deficiency (Von Gierke's
     type I glycogen-storage disease). *Biochem. Soc. Trans.*, **2**, 1118
45. Odièvre, M., Brivet, M., Moatti, N., Dreyfus, J. C., Beaufils, F., Lejeune, C.
     and Feffer, J. (1975). Déficit en fructose-1,6-diphosphatase chez deux soeurs.
     Arch. Fr. Pédiatr., **32**, 113

46. Retbi, J. M., Gabilan, J. C. and Marsac, J. (1975). Acidose lactique et hypoglycémie à début neonatal par déficit congénital en fructose-1,6-diphosphatase hépatique. *Arch. Fr. Pédiatr.*, **32**, 367

47. Corbeel, L., Eggermont, E., Eeckels, R., Jaeken, J., Casteels, M., Van Daele, H., Devlierger and Delmotte, B. (1976). Recurrent attacks of ketotic acidosis associated with fructose-1,6-diphosphatase deficiency. *Acta Paediatr. Belg.*, **29**, 29

48. Hopwood, N. J., Holzman, I. and Drash, A. L. (1977). Fructose-1,6-diphosphatase deficiency. *Am. J. Dis. Child.*, **131**, 418

49. Hug, H. and de Barsy, Th. (1978). (Personal communication)

50. Bakker, H. D., De Bree, P. K., Ketting, D., van Sprang, F. J. and Wadman, S. K. (1974). Fructose-1,6-diphosphatase deficiency: another enzyme defect which can present itself with the clinical features of 'Tyrosinosis'. *Clin. Chim. Acta*, **55**, 41

51. Steinmann, B. and Gitzelmann, R. (1976). Fruktose und Sorbitol in Infusionsflüssigkeiten sind nicht immer harmlos. In G. Ritzel and G. Brubacher (eds.). Monosaccharides and Polyalcohols in Nutrition, Therapy and Dietetics. *Int. J. Vitam. Nutr. Res.*, (Suppl. 15), 289

52. Schrijvers, J. and Hommes, F. A. (1975). Activity of fructose-1,6-diphosphatase in human leucocytes. *N. Engl. J. Med.*, **292**, 1298

53. Cahill, J. and Kirtley, M. E. (1975). FDPase activity in human leucocytes. *N. Engl. J. Med.*, **292**, 212

54. Gitzelmann, R., Baerlocher, K. and Prader, A. (1973). Hereditäre Störungen im Fruktose- und Galactose-Stoffwechsel. *Monatsschr. Kinderheilkind.*, **121**, 174

55. Taunton, O. D., Greene, H. L., Stifel, F. B., Hofeldt, F. D., Lufkin, E. G., Hagler, L., Herman, Y. and Herman, R. H. (1978). Fructose-1,6-diphosphatase deficiency, hypoglycemia, and response to folate therapy in a mother and her daughter. *Biochem. Med.*, **19**, 260

56. Schulte, M.-J. and Lenz, W. (1977). Fatal sorbitol infusion in patient with fructose-sorbitol intolerance. *Lancet*, **2**, 188

57. Hackl, J. M., Balogh, D., Kunz, F., Dworzak, E., Puschendorf, B., Decristoforo, A. and Maier, F. (1978). Postoperative Fruktoseinfusion bei wahrscheinlich hereditärer Fruktoseintoleranz. *Wien. Klin. Wochenschr.*, **90**, 237

11

Pathogenic mechanisms of disorders in fructose metabolism

H. F. Woods

Fructose is a normal constituent of the Western diet occurring in some fruits and vegetables and in honey. It is also a component of the disaccharide sucrose which is used extensively in the manufacture of confectionery. The usual daily intake has been estimated to be 50–100 grams. Three main types of metabolic defect involving fructose have been described in man:

> essential fructosuria (EF)
> hereditary fructose intolerance (HFI)
> fructose-1,6-diphosphatase deficiency (FDD)

All three are due to either a total or partial lack of an enzyme involved in the metabolic pathway of fructose utilization together with secondary enzyme blocks in HFI and FDD.

This paper will consider the mechanisms of the metabolic derangements in HFI.

FRUCTOSE METABOLISM

Fructose is absorbed from the gut lumen via a specific carrier transport mechanism and, once in portal blood, it is delivered to the liver which is the main site of fructose metabolism[1]. Other tissues have the capacity to metabolise fructose; these include the small intestine[2] and the kidney[3] but their capacity is small.

The first step in fructose metabolism is phosphorylation to fructose-1-phosphate. This reaction is catalysed by the enzyme ketohexokinase[4].

$$\text{Fructose} + \text{ATP} \quad \overset{ketohexokinase}{\rightleftharpoons} \quad \text{Fructose-1-phosphate} + \text{ADP} \qquad (1)$$

In mammalian liver this enzyme has a relatively high maximal rate and a low K_m (Table 11.1). Thus the phosphorylation of fructose is a rapid process.

TABLE 11.1   The properties of enzymes of fructose metabolism in rat liver

Enzyme	Maximal rate (μmol/min per g tissue at 25 °C at pH 7.4–7.5)	K_m (mmol/l)
Ketohexokinase	3.12^5	$0.2–0.4^8$
	$3.14 \pm 0.81(7)^6$	0.44
	$2.20 \pm 0.39(8)^7$	$<0.5^{10}$
Ketose 1-phosphate aldolase	$3.40 \pm 0.36(3)^6$	$0.35 \pm 0.18(8)^6$
	$1.63 \pm 0.11(5)^7$	

Results refer to normal well-fed rats but the strains and diets used were not identical. The results are expressed as Means or Mean $\pm$ S.D. The superscript numbers refer to the original references.

The phosphorylating molecule is adenosine triphosphate (ATP)[9] and the K_m for ATP in the reaction is also probably low because fructose-1-phosphate is formed rapidly in rat liver under anaerobic conditions when the ATP content of the tissue has fallen to 0.54 mM[11]. The further metabolism of fructose-1-phosphate is via the aldolase reaction to form dihydroxyacetone phosphate and D-glyceraldehyde[12].

$$\text{Fuctose-1-phosphate} \quad \overset{aldolase}{\rightleftharpoons} \quad \begin{array}{l} \text{Dihydroxyacetone phosphate} + \\ \text{D-glyceraldehyde} \end{array} \qquad (2)$$

Aldolase also has the property of splitting fructose-1,6-diphosphate into the triose phosphates, dihydroxyacetone phosphate and D-glyceraldehyde 3-phosphate. This latter reaction is reversible, the two triose phosphates also reacting to give fructose-1,6-diphosphate. Aldolase occurs in three forms which can be characterized by their relative capacities to cleave fructose-1, 6-diphosphate and fructose-1-phosphate (the activity ratio). Table 11.2 lists

TABLE 11.2 Tissue aldolase types

Type	Tissue in which the type is preponderant	Activity ratio (FDP cleared/F1P cleared)
A	Muscle	50
B	Liver	1
C	Brain	5–10

the aldolase isoenzymes together with their activity ratios and their site of occurrence.

Much discussion has concerned the metabolic pathways followed by triose D-glyceraldehyde. Three possible pathways exist:

(1) Phosphorylation to D-glyceraldehyde 3-phosphate by the enzyme triokinase. ATP provides the phosphate group in this reaction.
(2) Oxidation to glycerate by aldehyde dehydrogenase and subsequent metabolism via glycerate kinase to 2-phosphoglycerate.
(3) Reduction of D-glyceraldehyde to form glycerol via alcohol dehydrogenase followed by phosphorylation to glycerol 3-phosphate which can then be oxidised to give dihydroxyacetone phosphate.

The conversion of D-glyceraldehyde to glycerol can also take place via a reaction catalyzed by aldose reductase. All these possible reaction pathways are shown in Figure 11.1.

The first of these pathways is the main reaction route for D-glyceraldehyde. Sillero et al.[13] pointed out that the triokinase reaction is favoured because of the low K_m for D-glyceraldehyde (0.01 mM). They concluded that some 90% of the D-glyceraldehyde formed from fructose in the liver is metabolised in this way. In addition the activity of triokinase is high in mammalian liver[7]. Later work by Hue and Hers[14] using doubly labelled radioactive D-fructose confirmed the phosphorylation of D-glyceraldehyde in this way. The overall reaction for the initial stages of fructose utilization is therefore:

$$\text{Fructose} + 2\text{ATP} \underset{\text{triokinase}}{\rightleftharpoons} \text{D-glyceraldehyde 3-phosphate} +$$
$$\text{Dihydroxyacetone phosphate} + 2\text{ADP}$$

The triose phosphates can either be metabolised via the glycolytic sequence of reactions or to glucose. In man about 20% of the splanchnic fructose uptake can be accounted for as lactate production[15].

During metabolism of fructose by normal mammalian liver, fructose-1-phosphate accumulates[7, 16, 17]. The mechanisms involved in this accumulation will be discussed below.

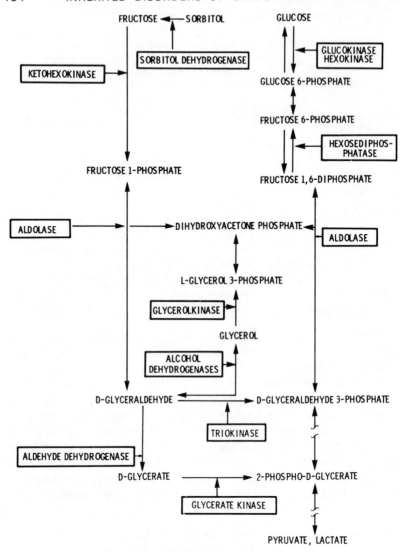

Figure 11.1   Fructose metabolism

In adipose tissue and muscle, which have a low ketohexokinase activity, fructose can be metabolised to fructose-6-phosphate by hexokinase[18]. In liver, hexokinase activity is low[7] and it has a K_m of 2.4–6.7 mM for fructose which is much higher than that of ketohexokinase[5, 8]. In addition, the formation of fructose-6-phosphate via the hexokinase reaction is slow in the presence of glucose[19].

METABOLIC AND STRUCTURAL CONSEQUENCES OF HFI

The subject of inherited defects of fructose metabolism is discussed elsewhere in this volume by Baerlocher (Chapter 10). It is necessary to consider briefly some of the signs and symptoms of the disorder as a preliminary to discussion of the pathogenic mechanisms involved.

The symptoms and signs of HFI can be divided into those which occur shortly after ingestion of D-fructose and those which are a result of long term ingestion of D-fructose usually starting during weaning. The effects can be divided into four main groups:

(1) Fructose accumulation with hypophosphataemia
(2) Hypoglycaemia
(3) Renal damage
(4) Liver damage leading to cirrhosis.

Thus the two organs most involved are those in which there is a considerable capacity to metabolise D-fructose via the ketohexokinase pathway; the liver and kidney.

The primary enzyme defect in HFI is a markedly lowered fructose-1-phosphate aldolase activity in liver as low as 5% of normal. The enzyme has the substrate specificities more typical of the type A and C (muscle and brain) enzyme. The defect also occurs in the small gut and the renal cortex[20, 21]. The aldolase activity towards fructose-1,6-diphosphate is high enough to maintain blood glucose concentrations during starvation.

When fructose is ingested by the patient with HFI, fructose-1-phosphate will accumulate in liver, kidney and small intestine because the tissue ketohexokinase activity is maintained; these organs suffer the main adverse effects of fructose in HFI. It has therefore been postulated that fructose-1-phosphate is the toxic metabolite in HFI. However fructose-1-phosphate accumulates in these organs in normal mammals who do not have the enzyme defect of HFI. Perheentupa et al.[22] first suggested that the metabolic consequences of fructose ingestion in HFI can be looked upon as marked exaggerations of metabolic events which occur in normal individuals.

The toxicity of fructose has been discussed by several authors[23, 24] and any mechanisms proposed must be capable of explaining the hypoglycaemia which is due to a decreased capacity of the liver to release glucose from glycogen rather than a defect in gluconeogenesis or an increase in insulin release. In additon the other biochemical abnormalities must be accounted for (see the review by Van den Berghe[25]).

THE ACCUMULATION OF FRUCTOSE-1-PHOSPHATE

If the postulate of Perheentupa et al.[22] is correct the mechanisms leading to fructose-1-phosphate accumulation are central to an understanding of the abnormalities in HFI. The accumulation has been known for some time but until 1970 the reasons for it were unclear. It could not be explained on the basis of the relative activities of ketohexokinase and fructose-1-phosphate aldolase in the normal liver which are comparable when assayed under physiological conditions (see Table 11.1). Experiments using the isolated perfused liver have partially elucidated the mechanisms. The accumulation of fructose-1-phosphate in liver occurs at the same time as a depletion of hepatic ATP and inorganic phosphate (P_i)[6, 17, 26], and the two processes are interconnected. The ATP and P_i depletion lead to an increased rate of adenine nucleotide degradation because the enzymes which mainly control the breakdown of adenine nucleotides, namely 5'-nucleotidase and adenosine deaminase are inhibited by ATP and P_i respectively. The products of AMP breakdown namely IMP and uric acid (allantoin in the rat) accumulate[6, 26]. The initial ATP depletion was explainable on the basis of the demand for ATP as the phosphate donor in the ketohexokinase reaction

Woods et al.[6] suggested that fructose-1-phosphate accumulates because IMP is a potent inhibitor of fructose-1-phosphate aldolase at concentrations which occur in liver after fructose loading. This explanation has not been universally acceptable; for example, Van den Berghe[25] has criticised it because IMP accumulation is itself dependent on ATP depletion which in part depends on fructose-1-phosphate accumulation because the lowered P_i concentration is caused by the sequestration of P_i in the phosphate group of fructose-1-phosphate.

Van den Berghe[25] suggested that the triokinase reaction may be the rate limiting step in fructose metabolism and the accumulation of fructose-1-phosphate is a result of the equilibrium position of the aldolase reaction. Some support for this latter postulate comes from the observation that the mass action ratio for the aldolase reaction calculated from the concentrations of the metabolites in liver is very close to the apparent equilibrium constant for the reaction $(2.8 \times 10^{-6} \text{ mol/l})$[27]. This observation also holds true for anaerobic liver after D-fructose loading[11], when the mass action ratio is also close to that quoted above.

Adenine nucleotide depletion after fructose loading is not a phenomenon unique to that substrate. It occurs after loading with both glycerol[28, 29] and xylitol[30] (Table 11.3). These substrates also cause a lowering of the hepatic P_i concentration and a large accumulation of a phosphorylated intermediate (a-glycerophosphate in both cases).

The relative importance of demand for ATP as a phosphate donor and consumption of ATP via the degradation pathways can be assessed[30] by calculating the rate of extra ATP consumption during the metabolism of the various substrates. Data for fructose, glycerol, xylitol and dihydroxyacetone are included in Table 11.4. All of these substrates are rapidly metabolised in liver via pathways which include an early phosphorylation step requiring ATP. The rates of additional ATP consumption are all of the same order of magnitude and there is no simple correlation between the extra ATP consumption and the depletion of adenine nucleotides. Fructose, glycerol and xylitol cause adenine nucleotide loss while dihydroxyacetone does not.

When the rate of additional ATP consumption is compared with the turnover rate of ATP in the liver, lack of correlation is to be expected. The turnover rate is 15 μmol/min per gram of wet liver which is more than five times the additional rate of ATP consumption. The results indicate a correlation between the accumulation of phosphorylated intermediates in liver and accompanying depletion of P_i on the one hand with the loss of adenine nucleotides on the other.

The fall in the P_i content must be taken as the main factor responsible for the adenine nucleotide depletion because dihydroxyacetone loading, which does not cause the accumulation of phosphorylated intermediates or P_i depletion, does not result in adenine nucleotide depletion although the additional ATP consumption is comparable with those seen after loading with substrates which do cause adenine nucleotide depletion (see Tables 11.3 and 11.4). Thus the de-inhibition of ATP-degrading enzymes resulting from the fall in the concentrations of ATP and P_i must be taken as a major cause of the adenine nucleotide depletion. Further support for this conclusion comes from experiments where a perfusion medium with a low phosphate concentration was used. When glycerol is the substrate, the use of a low phosphate medium results in a greater loss of adenine nucleotides than that found during perfusion with a standard medium[29]. It is not possible to prevent the depletion by using a medium containing a high phosphate concentration (10 mM)[11].

The objections to the interrelated mechanisms of ATP depletion and fructose-1-phosphate accumulation formulated by Van den Berghe[25] may be valid so far as the initiation of the ATP depletion process is concerned.

TABLE 11.3   Hepatic metabolite contents after substrate loading

Substrate	Metabolite content (μmol/g wet wt)						
	ATP	ADP	AMP	Total adenine nucleotides	P_i	F1P	αGP
Nil	2.22	0.78	0.26	3.27	4.25	0.23	0.13
Fructose	0.51	0.66	0.20	1.37	1.67	8.72	1.06
Glycerol	1.62	0.71	0.24	2.56	2.13	—	4.77
Xylitol	1.48	0.66	0.21	2.35	2.34	—	3.59
Dihydroxyacetone	2.05	0.70	0.26	3.01	3.78	—	0.44

The contents of metabolites have been determined in freeze-clamped tissue after 10 min perfusion with a medium containing an initial substrate concentration of 10 mmol/l. The animals were in the fed state and the figures are mean values for 2–4 observations.

TABLE 11.4 Hepatic ATP consumption after substrate loading

Substrate	Additional ATP consumption (μmol/min per gram wet liver)	
	Fed animal	48 h starved animal
Fructose	1.66	2.03
Glycerol	2.36	1.24
Xylitol	2.08	1.68
Dihydroxyacetone	3.04	2.77

The rates of additional ATP consumption in the perfused rat liver are given; they all refer to experiments in which the initial substrate concentration was 10 mmol/l. Adapted from Woods and Krebs[30]

SECONDARY METABOLIC EFFECTS OF FRUCTOSE-1-PHOSPHATE ACCUMULATION

The accumulation of fructose-1-phosphate has several secondary effects as it inhibits a number of metabolic steps. These are listed below (see also Perheentupa et al.[22]):

(a) An inhibition of ketohexokinase
(b) An inhibition of glycogen breakdown
(c) An inhibition of fructose-1-,6-diphosphate synthesis via the aldolase reaction
(d) Inhibition of the conversion of fructose-6-phosphate to glucose-6-phosphate via phosphohexose isomerase.

BIOCHEMICAL MECHANISMS IN HFI

From the previous sections it is clear that many of the acute effects of fructose loading in HFI result from exaggeration of the events following fructose loading in a normal individual. An intact adenine nucleotide system is a key factor in the maintenance of cell function and it is likely that some of the abnormalities are a consequence of the loss of adenine nucleotides. Energy requiring processes may be adversely affected by fructose infusion and the concomitant fall in hepatic ATP content. There is some experimental evidence to support this conclusion.

Protein synthesis, RNA synthesis and triglyceride synthesis are all inhibited in rat liver during fructose loading (Table 11.5) and ultrastructural studies have demonstrated intracellular oedema[31] together with disaggregation of liver polysomes[32]. These changes have also been described in normal

TABLE 11.5   Inhibition of synthetic processes following fructose loading

Metabolic process	Experimental system	Reference
(1) Protein synthesis	U-[14]C Leucine incorporation into rat liver protein	Mäenpää et al.[26]
(2) Triglyceride synthesis	Triglyceride synthesis from oleate in the isolated perfused rat liver	Walton et al.[37]
(3) RNA synthesis	Incorporation of 6-^{14}C-orotic acid into regenerating rat liver	Bode et al.[33]

human liver after fructose loading[33]. Tubular function in the kidney is also impaired under these conditions[34].

The hypoglycaemic response to fructose in HFI probably results from an inhibition of glycogenolysis because the interaction of phosphorylase *a* with its substrates glycogen and P_i is blocked (see review by Van der Berghe[25]). This block may result from a combination of ATP depletion and the inhibition of activation of α-phosphorylase by fructose-1-phosphate[35].

A parallel for the acute disturbances in liver function caused by fructose in HFI may be provided by the observations of Schumer[36] who infused large quantities of xylitol in normal subjects (4.8 g/h per kg). This caused abdominal pain, nausea, vomiting and a rise in the serum concentrations of uric acid, bilirubin, glutamate-oxaloacetate aminotransferase and alkaline phosphatase. These effects may have been connected with the hepatic ATP depletion caused by xylitol loading (see above and Table 11.3).

FINAL CONCLUSIONS

Fructose loading in normal man causes widespread metabolic changes in those tissues which metabolise fructose via the ketohexokinase reaction. It may be that the metabolic effects of fructose administration in patients with HFI are an exaggeration of those effects.

References

1. Mendeloff, A. I. and Weichselbaum, T. E. (1953). Role of the human liver in the assimilation of intravenously administered fructose. *Metabolism*, **2**, 450
2. Deuel, H. S. (1936). The intermediary metabolism of fructose and galactose. *Physiol. Rev.*, **16**, 173
3. Raivio, K. O., Kekomaki, M. P. and Mäenpää, P. H. (1969). Depletion of liver adenine nucleotides induced by D-fructose. Dose dependence and specificity of the fructose effect. *Biochem. Pharmacol.*, **18**, 2615
4. Leuthardt, F. and Testa, E. (1951). Die phosphorylierung der fructose in der leber. *Helv. Chim. Acta*, **34**, 931
5. Adelman, R. C., Ballard, F. J. and Weinhouse, S. (1967). Purification and properties of rat liver fructokinase. *J. Biol. Chem.*, **242**, 3360
6. Woods, H. F., Eggleston, L. V. and Krebs, H. A. (1970). The cause of hepatic accumulation of fructose-1-phosphate on fructose loading. *Biochem. J.*, **119**, 501
7. Heinz, F., Lamprecht, W. and Kirsch, J. (1968). Enzymes of fructose metabolism in human liver. *J. Clin. Invest.*, **47**, 1826
8. Parks, R. E., Ben-Gershom, E. and Lardy, H. A. (1957). Liver fructokinase. *J. Biol. Chem.*, **227**, 231
9. Hers, H. G. (1952). La fructokinase de foie. *Biochem. Biophys. Acta*, **8**, 416

10. Hers, H. G. (1952). Role du magnésium et du potassium dans la réaction fructokinasique. *Biochim. Biophys. Acta*, **8**, 424

11. Woods, H. F. (1972). Hepatic accumulation of metabolites after fructose loading. *Acta. Med. Scand.*, **542**, 87

12. Leuthardt, F., Testa, E. and Wolf, H. P. (1953). Der enzymatische Abban des fructose-1-phosphate in der leber. *Helv. Chim. Acta*, **36**, 227

13. Sillero, M. A. G., Sillero, A. and Sols, A. (1969). Enzymes involved in fructose metabolism in liver and the glyceraldehyde metabolic crossroads. *Eur. J. Biochem.*, **10**, 345

14. Hue, L. and Hers, H. G. (1972). The conversion of |4-³H| fructose and of |4-³H| glucose to liver glycogen in the mouse. An investigation of the glyceraldehyde crossroads. *Eur. J. Biochem.*, **29**, 268

15. Bergström, J., Fürst, P., Gallyas, F., Hultman, E., SonNilsson, L. H., Roch-Norlund, A. E. and Vinnas, E. (1972). Aspects of fructose metabolism in normal man. *Acta Med. Scand.*, **542**, 57

16. Kjerulf-Jensen, K. (1942). The phosphate esters formed in the liver tissue of rats and rabbits during assimilation of hexoses and glycerol. *Acta Physiol. Scand.*, **4**, 249

17. Burch, H. B., Max, P., Chyu, K. and Lowry, O. H. (1969). Metabolic intermediates in liver of rats given large amounts of fructose or dihydroxyacetone. *Biochem. Biophys. Res. Commun.*, **34**, 619

18. Hers, H. G. (1955). The conversion of fructose-1-C¹⁴ and sorbitol-1-C¹⁴ to liver and muscle glycogen in the rat. *J. Biol. Chem.*, **214**, 373

19. Sols, A. and Crane, R. K. (1954). Substrate specificity of brain hexokinase. *J. Biol. Chem.*, **210**, 581

20. Nissel, J. and Linden, L. (1968). Fructose-1-phosphate aldolase and fructose-1,6-diphosphate aldolase activity in the mucosa of the intestine in hereditary fructose intolerance. *Scand. J. Gastroenterol.*, **3**, 80

21. Kranold, J. F., Loh, D. and Morris, R. C. Jr. (1969). Renal fructose-metabolizing enzymes: significance in hereditary fructose intolerance. *Science*, **165**, 402

22. Perheentupa, J., Raivio, K. O. and Nikkilä, E. A. (1972). Hereditary fructose intolerance. *Acta Med. Scand.*, **542**, 65

23. Hers, H. G. (1970). Misuses for fructose. *Nature*, **227**, 421

24. Woods, H. F. and Alberti, K. G. M. M. (1972). Dangers of intravenous fructose. *Lancet*, **2**, 1354

25. Van den Berghe, G. (1975). Fructose metabolism. In F. A. Hommes and C. J. Van den Berghe (eds.). *Normal and Pathological Development of Energy Metabolism*, p. 211 (London: Academic Press)

26. Mäenpää, P. H., Raivio, K. O. and Kekomaki, M. P. (1968). Liver adenine nucleotides: fructose induced depletion and its effect on protein synthesis. *Science*, **161**, 1253

27. Lehninger, A. L., Sicé, J. and Jensen, E. V. (1955). Effect of substrate structure on the aldolase equilibrium. *Biochim. Biophys. Acta*, **17**, 285

28. Burch, H. B., Lowry, O. H., Meinhardt, L., Max, P. and Chyu, K. (1970). Effect of fructose, dihydroxyacetone, glycerol and glucose on metabolites and related compounds in liver and kidney. *J. Biol. Chem.*, **245**, 2092

29. Woods, H. F. and Krebs, H. A. (1973). The effect of glycerol and dihydroxyacetone on hepatic adenine nucleotides. *Biochem. J.*, **132**, 55

30. Woods, H. F. and Krebs, H. A. (1973). Xylitol metabolism in the isolated perfused rat liver. *Biochem. J.*, **134**, 437
31. Yu, D. T. and Phillips, M. J. (1971). Hepatic ultrastructural changes in acute fructose overload. *Ultrastructure Res.* **36**, 222
32. Mäenpää, P. H. (1972). Fructose induced alterations in liver polysome profiles and Mg^{2+} levels. *FEBS Lett.*, **24**, 37
33. Bode, J. Ch., Zelder, O., Rumpell, H. J. and Wittkamp, U. (1973). Depletion of liver adenosine phosphates and metabolic effects of intravenous infusion of fructose or sorbitol in man and in the rat. *Eur. J. Clin. Invest.*, **3**, 436
34. Morris, R. C. Jr., McSherry, E. and Sebastian, A. (1973). On the metabolic pathogenesis of the renal disorder of hereditary fructose intolerance (HFI). *J. Clin. Invest.*, **52**, 57
35. Van den Berghe, G. (1973). *Mémoires de l'Académie Royale de Médecine de Belgique*, **47**, 93
36. Schumer, W. (1971). Adverse effects of xylitol in parenteral alimentation. *Metabolism*, **20**, 345
37. Walton, I. G., Woods, H. F. and Hockaday, T. D. R. (1973). Inhibition by sucrose of triglyceride production by the perfused rat. *Proceedings of Spring Meeting of the Medical and Scientific Sections of the British Diabetic Association*

Discussion

DISCUSSION ON DISORDERS OF FRUCTOSE METABOLISM

HERS (Brussels): We have made calculations on the accumulation of fructose-1-phosphate which indicate that, although fructose-1-phosphate accumulates, the metabolites are in thermodynamic equilibrium with aldolase. One of the best ways to get a large increase in fructose-1-phosphate in the liver is to inject glyceraldehyde, which is converted to fructose-1-phosphate by aldolase. In our opinion fructose-1-phosphate accumulates because it is formed faster than it can be reutilised by the sum of its conversion to glucose and its conversion to lactate. In other words, what is limiting is the rate of glycolysis and of gluconeogenesis. Accumulation of fructose-1-phosphate then causes depletion of phosphate. I don't think aldolase is limiting at all.

WOODS (Sheffield): This is difficult because we have two diametrically opposed camps. Although we have used the arguments based on activity of aldolase versus the activity of fructokinase, it may be entirely wrong to transfer arguments based on kinetic properties measured under ideal conditions to what happens in the whole organ. Professor Hers, in his Milner Lecture (Chapter 1) pointed out that interpretation of metabolic disorders is very difficult because of the limits placed upon us by the particular system we use. I believe that the accumulation of breakdown products of adenine nucleotides may affect the subsequent metabolism of fructose-1-phosphate once it is formed; this is based on the inhibition of fructose-1-phosphate aldolase, which we have seen with inosine monophosphate (IMP) in particular. This occurs at concentrations of both fructose-1-phosphate as substrate and IMP as inhibitor found in our whole liver system. The basis of your argument is that the formation of IMP is dependent upon accelerated ATP breakdown. If I say that the acceleration of adenine nucleotide breakdown is consequent upon alterations in phosphate economy, secondary to fructose-1-phosphate accumulation, I am in a very nice Catch 22 circular chicken and egg argument. This is why I have said that I do not exclude the possibility that additional demand for ATP may well initiate the process of adenine nucleotide depletion.

I appreciate the argument about the influence of triokinase in diverting carbon in fructose-1-phosphate either up to glucose or down to lactate. I cannot answer you on that point because our interpretation of the kinetics of that particular part of fructose metabolism is very different from yours. In the final analysis it leaves us with you saying one thing and us saying another.

BLASS (White Plains): Since cyclic-AMP has manifold effects on the metabolism of proteins (including phosphorylation of ribosomal proteins), lipids, and carbohydrates, do you think that alterations in cyclic-AMP metabolism may play a role in the pernicious effects of fructose on the liver of patients with fructose intolerance?

WOODS: This question takes us into a discussion of the mechanism of the hypoglycaemia in hereditary fructose intolerance. There is some evidence that the AMP content of liver after stimulation by glucagon is lowered in the presence of fructose. I do not think that this necessarily gives the complete answer to the hypoglycaemia because we have shown that, even at a time when adenine nucleotide depletion is maximal, which is about 40 minutes in the perfused liver, the rate and quantity of $3',5'$-cyclic AMP efflux from that liver is the same in the presence or absence of fructose.

SECTION FIVE

Disorders of Pyruvate Metabolism

12

Pathways and regulation of pyruvate metabolism

R. M. Denton and A. P. Halestrap

Pyruvate occupies a central position in the metabolism of all animal cells, a fact easily confirmed by a cursory glance at a chart of metabolic pathways. Such is the obvious importance of pyruvate metabolism that it is surprising that so many inborn errors have been found in this area. Its metabolism has been studied extensively in recent years and a number of important advances made, especially in our understanding of its regulation.

The major pathways of pyruvate utilization are oxidation, lipogenesis and gluconeogenesis; tissue location is indicated in Table 12.1. Most of the enzymes of pyruvate metabolism are involved in more than one of the pathways (Figure 12.1); for this reason the properties of the individual enzymes will be considered first, followed by a discussion of some general aspects of the regulation of the pathways. Much of our research is concerned with the laboratory rat but we will try to indicate its implications for the study of inborn errors of metabolism in man. The role of pyruvate in the many aspects of amino acid metabolism is not fully covered.

COMPARTMENTATION OF PYRUVATE METABOLISM

Mitochondrial pyruvate transport

The mitochondrial inner membrane acts as a barrier to charged molecules unless some specific transport mechanism is available. Since pyruvate (pK_a

TABLE 12.1   Tissue location of the major metabolic pathways involving pyruvate

Tissue	Glucose→ pyruvate	Pyruvate → lactate	Pyruvate → CO_2	Pyruvate → glucose	Pyruvate → lipids
Heart and skeletal muscle	111	11	111	–	1
Brain and central nervous system	111	111	111	–	–
Red blood cells	111	111	–	–	–
Liver	1	1	11	111	11
Kidney	111	111	111	11	–
Adipose tissue	111	11	1	111	111

The activity of each pathway is expressed in relative terms: 1 (slow); 111 (fast). A dash means that the pathway is absent. Data is given only for the rat, but much the same pattern may be expected for the human with the exception that human adipose tissue converts glucose to lipids very much slower than the rat tissue. Rates shown under pyruvate to CO_2 represent the rates of complete oxidation of pyruvate via pyruvate dehydrogenase and the citrate cycle

2.49) exists almost totally as the negatively charged anion at physiological pH, it is not surprising to find a specific carrier to transport pyruvate into the mitochondria where it may act as a substrate for pyruvate dehydrogenase and pyruvate carboxylase. This transport mechanism has been investigated in some detail in recent years by several workers[1-8].

Inhibition Studies have been made easier by the discovery that α-cyanocinnamate and its derivatives are specific and potent inhibitors of mitochondrial pyruvate transport[9, 10]. These compounds act as analogues of pyruvate, binding to the active site where they form a reversible covalent bond with an essential thiol group and effectively trap the carrier molecule on the matrix side of the mitochondrial membrane[3]. Because the active site of the carrier is no longer exposed to externally added pyruvate, inhibition is effectively noncompetitive. However, some analogues of pyruvate, such as monochloroacetate, may enter the mitochondria independently of the carrier and displace the inhibitor from the inside of the membrane[3]. The K_i for α-cyanocinnamate inhibition depends on the energy state of the mitochondria and the pH gradient across the inner membrane. Inhibition is greatest in uncoupled mitochondria when the K_i for inhibition is less than 1 μmol/l[3] whilst in energized mitochondria inhibition increases as the pH gradient (alkaline inside) increases[11].

The potency and specificity of α-cyanocinnamate inhibition has allowed its extensive use in studying the metabolic implications of mitochondrial pyruvate transport. For example, it has been shown that the substrate bin-

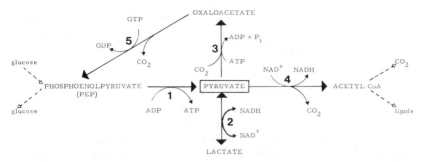

Figure 12.1 General outline of the major enzymes of pyruvate metabolism. Location of the enzymes within cells are as follows: (Cytoplasmic) 1 – Pyruvate kinase (PK); 2 – Lactate dehydrogenase (LDH): (Intramitochondrial) 3 – Pyruvate carboxylase (PC); 4 – Pyruvate dehydrogenase (PDH): (Cytoplasmic and intramitochondrial) 5 – Phosphoenolpyruvate carboxykinase (PEPCK). Pathways involved in amino acid metabolism are not shown

ding sites of both pyruvate dehydrogenase and pyruvate carboxylase as well as the regulatory site for pyruvate of pyruvate dehydrogenase kinase are all exposed to only intramitochondrial pyruvate[12]. This inhibitor is particularly useful in intact tissue preparations, where those metabolic processes involving mitochondrial pyruvate transport are inhibited. Lipogenesis from glucose and fructose, but not acetate, is inhibited in rat epididymal fat pads and gluconeogenesis from pyruvate and lactate, but not from glutamate, is inhibited in kidney cortex slices and isolated rat liver cells[12, 13]. For metabolic pathways whose exact details are not clear, α-cyanocinnamate has proved useful in establishing whether or not mitochondrial pyruvate transport is required. For example, during gluconeogenesis in the adult rat liver, alanine transamination to pyruvate may occur in the mitochondria rather than in the cytoplasm, whereas serine must be converted to pyruvate by serine dehydratase in the cytoplasm rather than by transamination to hydroxypyruvate in the mitochondria[13]. Unfortunately, α-cyanocinnamate derivatives possess little activity in the intact animal probably because they bind extremely tightly to albumin[12].

Pathological conditions exist in which the accumulation of naturally occurring inhibitors of pyruvate transport may cause severe disturbances of pyruvate metabolism. Two examples are phenylketonuria and maple syrup urine disease. In these diseases the build up in the bloodstream of phenylpyruvate and α-ketoisocaproate respectively causes derangement of carbohydrate and lipid metabolism and it has been suggested that mitochondrial pyruvate and ketone body transport are the major sites of action of these compounds[14–16]. Both of these metabolites are pyruvate analogues with a hydrophobic moiety attached and both are reversible inhibitors of pyruvate transport[2]. The effects of these compounds on isolated mitochondria suggest that during metabolism, inhibition is not easily reversed by addition of excess pyruvate[15, 17]. Like α-cyanocinnamate, these compounds may trap the pyruvate carrier on the inner surface of the mitochondrial membrane, preventing their easy displacement by externally added pyruvate. This theory awaits kinetic proof.

Kinetics   The kinetic properties of mitochondrial pyruvate transport have been studied in most detail in rat liver, although the presence of the carrier has been shown in all mitochondria studied[1]. Various experimental techniques have been used, notably the 'inhibitor stop' techniques[2, 7], rapid multiple layer centrifugation[4–6] and membrane filtration[7]. For a more detailed account of the results obtained and the discrepancies between various workers the reader is directed elsewhere[1]. Only those properties pertinent to the control of pyruvate metabolism are discussed below.

The K_m of the carrier for pyruvate is between 0.2 and 0.6 mmol/l, the exact value depending on the conditions used for the determination[1–7]. The carrier has a broad specificity for short chain carboxylates substituted in the 2 or 3 position with a keto group or halide[2–5]. Thus in the physiological situation the carrier may be important for the transport of ketone bodies as well as for pyruvate[3, 5, 6, 16, 18] and pharmacologically it is important for dichloroacetate entry into the mitochondria[2]. The V_{max} for transport is dependent on the conditions used for measuring pyruvate uptake. If net uptake is measured, transport of pyruvate occurs with a proton and the V_{max} depends on the pH gradient across the membrane, increasing as the matrix becomes more alkaline. There is an apparent pK for the uptake process of 8.3 which may be the pK of an essential histidine or lysine residue[3]. Under conditions similar to those to be expected physiologically, the V_{max} for transport at 37 °C is between 40 and 100 nmoles/min per mg mitochondrial protein[2, 3, 7]. This rate is slow compared with most other mitochondrial transport mechanisms and may be rate limiting under certain circumstances providing a potential site of control. Pyruvate may be transported very much faster by exchange with another carboxylate[3] and it has been suggested that during rapid gluconeogenesis pyruvate entry into the mitochondria may be stimulated by exchange with outgoing ketone bodies[3, 5].

Pyruvate transport across the plasma membrane

Pyruvate and lactate are known to enter and leave most cells without difficulty. The efflux of lactate is of obvious importance for those tissues with high rates of anaerobic glycolysis whilst its influx into liver cells for gluconeogenesis is also essential. Loss of pyruvate from cells is known to occur, although the physiological reason for this is unclear and it may be a secondary consequence of a carrier for the transport of lactate.

Data on the transport of pyruvate across the cell membrane (most notably of the red blood cell) has only recently become available[1, 9, 19-27]. In the red blood cell two carriers exist which are both inhibited by α-cyanocinnamate derivatives[9, 19, 26]. One carrier has been identified as the anion transporter of the red blood cell and is probably not of physiological importance since its K_m for both pyruvate and L-lactate is very high (> 100 mmol/l). The other carrier is powerfully inhibited by p-chloromercuribenzene sulphonate[22, 26] and has a K_m for pyruvate of about 2 mmol/l and for L-lactate of about 10 mmol/l[19, 26]. A similar carrier exists on the plasma membrane of Erhlich ascites cells[22] and intestinal epithelial cells[20, 21]. Experiments in this laboratory suggest that this carrier is physiologically important in both kidney cortex and diaphragm and there is circumstantial evidence for a similar carrier in heart and liver[19, 26]. Like the mitochondrial pyruvate carrier, the plasma membrane carrier catalyses both net transport of pyruvate or lactate with a proton and exchange of one carboxylate for another[19, 22, 23, 26]. The carrier has a broad specificity for short chain carboxylates[19, 22] and may also transport ketone bodies in the physiological situation[19, 28].

Phenomena related to the compartmentation of pyruvate metabolism

The existence of two compartments of pyruvate metabolism, the cytoplasmic and mitochondrial, demands not only transport of pyruvate across the mitochondrial membrane, but also movement of other substances. Most notably, there must be transport of reducing power between the two compartments, and in gluconeogenesis transport of four carbon intermediates from mitochondria to cytoplasm occurs. These two processes are intimately linked in the liver[29].

In the majority of tissues such as liver and heart the transfer of reducing power occurs by means of the aspartate malate shuttle depicted in Figure 12.2(I). This shuttle relies on the fact that oxaloacetate itself does not cross the inner mitochondrial membrane to any significant extent whereas both aspartate and malate do, aspartate by exchange with glutamate and malate by exchange for oxoglutarate[30]. The electrogenic nature of aspartate–glutamate exchange (aspartate is exchanged with glutamate + H+)

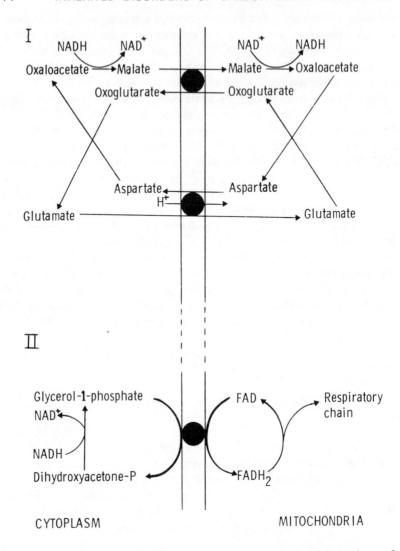

Figure 12.2 Transfer of reducing power across the mitochondrial membrane. I. The aspartate–malate shuttle occurs in many tissues and normally operates in heart, brain and other peripheral tissues in the direction shown. In liver and kidney the direction may be reversed so that reducing power is transferred from mitochondria to the cytoplasm for gluconeogenesis. II. The glycerol phosphate shuttle is important in skeletal muscle for the transfer of reducing power into mitochondria

causes aspartate to be actively driven out of the mitochondria with the consequence that the cytoplasm is oxidised relative to the mitochondria. This aids the oxidation of NADH produced by glycolysis and so tends to diminish lactate formation from pyruvate. In skeletal muscle an alternate redox shuttle involving α-glycerol phosphate may operate as shown in Figure 12.2(II). Any perturbation in these redox shuttles will be reflected in the output of lactate by the cell.

Gluconeogenesis   Gluconeogenesis involves, in the majority of animals including man, the mitochondrial formation of a four carbon unit which must cross the mitochondrial membrane before being converted to phosphoenolpyruvate by cytoplasmic phosphoenolpyruvate carboxykinase. Since the conversion of phosphoenolpyruvate to glucose requires NADH to reverse glyceraldehyde-3 phosphate dehydrogenase, the way oxaloacetate crosses the membrane will depend on the availability of cytoplasmic NADH. Where lactate is the gluconeogenic substrate, pyruvate production in the cytoplasm produces NADH which may be used for the reduction of 1,3-diphosphoglycerate. Under these conditions pyruvate crosses the mitochondrial membrane, is converted to oxaloacetate by pyruvate carboxylase and then leaves the mitochondria as aspartate after transamination with glutamate. In the cytoplasm the transamination is reversed to regenerate oxaloacetate; reducing power does not cross the mitochondrial membrane in this pathway. However, gluconeogenesis from other substrates does not generate cytoplasmic NADH directly and here oxaloacetate must cross the mitochondrial membrane as malate, which leads to the coincident transport of reducing power from the mitochondria to the cytoplasm. For a fuller treatment of these pathways and the effects of inhibitors on them, the reader is directed elsewhere[29, 30].

PRINCIPLE FEATURES OF THE KEY ENZYMES INVOLVED IN PYRUVATE METABOLISM

Pyruvate kinase (EC 2.7.1.40)

Pyruvate kinase catalyses the final step in the formation of pyruvate from glucose via the glycolytic pathway. The enzyme is exclusively cytoplasmic and is present in all cells. Thermodynamically the reaction it catalyses is extremely favourable. From a number of considerations including the measurement of the intracellular concentration of substrates and products, it is evident that the step is very far from equilibrium in cells. The reaction is thus a potential site of regulation and changes in pyruvate formation will be brought about either by alterations in the concentrations of the substrates phosphoenolpyruvate (PEP) and ADP or by changes in enzyme activity. Another consequence of the step being essentially irreversible in cells is that the synthesis of PEP from pyruvate in gluconeogenesis must occur by another pathway; this is the route involving pyruvate carboxylase and phosphoenolpyruvate carboxykinase.

At least three different isoenzymes of pyruvate kinase have been recognised in mammalian tissues. These are: the M_1 type, found in muscle and brain; the L type, found as the major isoenzyme in liver and as a minor one in kidney; and the M_2 type (also called the K type or A type) which is the major isoenzyme in kidney and probably in many other tissues including adipose tissue and lung. The isoenzymes can be differentiated by their kinetic and regulatory properties, antisera cross-reactivity, isoelectric point, and precipitation by ammonium sulphate and most definitively by clear differences in amino acid composition[31-34]. All isoenzymes occur predominantly as tetramers made up of subunits of molecular weight between 50 000 and 60 000. The pyruvate kinase in erythrocytes may represent a fourth isoenzyme (Type R)[31], but may be a proteolytically modified L type enzyme[35]. Deficiencies of erythrocyte pyruvate kinase are a well recognized cause of hereditary haemolytic anaemia. They comprise a heterogeneous group of disorders characterised by both quantitative and qualitative abnormalities in pyruvate kinase activity[36-38].

The M_1 type isoenzyme has the most straightforward kinetic properties. The enzyme shows essentially hyperbolic Michaelis-Menten kinetics with respect to both substrates with a low K_m of about 0.1 mmol/l for pyruvate. Its activity is largely unaffected by fructose-1,6-diphosphate, alanine and ATP which have marked effects on the activity of the M_2 and L type isoenzymes. In the absence of these compounds, the M_2 and L isoenzymes show sigmoid kinetics with respect to PEP with a K_m of up to 1.0 mmol/l. After exposure to fructose-1,6-diphosphate the V_{max} of these isoenzymes is not altered but the K_m is very markedly decreased to about 0.1 mmol/l; thus at the low concentrations of PEP found in cells, fructose-1,6-diphosphate is a potent activator. Fructose-1,6-diphosphate binds extremely tightly to the liver isoenzyme and is bound to freshly extracted preparations unless precautions are taken to remove it. Full activation of the liver enzyme is observed with concentrations of about 1.0 μmol/l fructose-1,6-diphosphate. Alanine and ATP inhibit activity by increasing the K_m for PEP of the liver enzyme. Recently it has been demonstrated that the activity of the L type isoenzyme is markedly altered by phosphorylation catalysed by cyclic adenosine monophosphate (cAMP) dependent protein kinase[39,40]. Phosphorylation has also been shown to occur in liver cells in which the cAMP levels have been increased by glucagon[41]. Phosphorylation converts the enzyme into a less active form with a markedly higher K_m for PEP, an enhanced sensitivity to alanine and ATP but a decreased sensitivity to fructose-1,6-diphosphate. Dephosphorylation and reversal of these changes has been demonstrated in the presence of a protein phosphatase extracted from liver.

The M_2 or K isoenzyme is not a substrate for cAMP dependent protein kinase[42] but the M_2 isoenzyme from chicken liver may also be converted to a less active form by phosphorylation which is catalysed by a cAMP independent protein kinase[43]. Two interconvertible forms of the adipose tissue enzyme have been described[44] but it is not clear whether these represent forms with and without bound fructose-1,6-diphosphate or whether a phosphorylation–dephosphorylation cycle is involved.

Lactate dehydrogenase (EC 1.1.1.27)

This cytoplasmic enzyme is present in most mammalian tissues at high activity. The reaction is almost certainly close to equilibrium in cells and thus will readily interconvert lactate and pyruvate. It seems unlikely that changes in the activity of lactate dehydrogenase are important in the regulation of pyruvate metabolism. Instead, the cytoplasmic concentration ratio of lactate/pyruvate is largely determined by the cytoplasmic $NADH/NAD^+$ ratio. When the cytoplasmic redox state increases (as for example in anoxia), the cytoplasmic lactate/pyruvate ratio increases and *vice versa*. Such changes are often reflected in the ratio of lactate to pyruvate released by tissues.

Lactate dehydrogenase in mammalian tissues is a tetramer of four subunits of molecular weight 35 000. In most tissues, the subunits are of two types (M and H) in varying proportions[45]. Heart and kidney contain predominantly H type while skeletal muscle and liver contain the M type. The two types of subunits form hybrid tetramers i.e. H_4, H_3M, M_2H_2, M_3H and M_4. The physiological importance or rationale of the separate isoenzymes remains a mystery. The H_4 form is inhibited by high concentrations of pyruvate and this may be important in retaining high cell concentrations of pyruvate for oxidation[45]. However, the level of pyruvate required is well above that reached in cells and such inhibition would have effect only if the step was not in equilibrium. As emphasised above, there is no evidence for this in cells.

The structure and enzymology of lactate dehydrogenase has recently been extensively reviewed elsewhere[46].

Pyruvate dehydrogenase (EC 1.2.4.1.)

This exclusively intramitochondrial enzyme complex catalyses the oxidative decarboxylation of pyruvate to give acetyl CoA. As with pyruvate kinase the overall reaction catalysed by pyruvate dehydrogenase is effectively irreversible in animal cells, but unlike the pyruvate kinase reaction there is no energetically feasible by-pass which would allow acetyl CoA to be reconverted to pyruvate and thence to glucose. Since the activity of pyruvate dehydrogenase regulates the point of no return in the utilization of carbohydrate, its control is of crucial importance in animal cells. Flux through pyruvate dehydrogenase must be diminished to near zero during starvation to ensure that the meagre carbohydrate reserves in animals are preserved, whereas following feeding on a carbohydrate rich diet the activity of pyruvate dehydrogenase must be stimulated so that acetyl CoA can again be formed from pyruvate. In many tissues, including muscle and brain, acetyl CoA so formed is nearly all oxidised via the citrate cycle; but in other tissues, such as adipose tissue, liver and mammary gland, a substantial proportion of the acetyl CoA is utilized in the synthesis of fatty acids and steroids. Pyruvate dehydrogenase thus serves both bioenergetic and biosynthetic roles. As the enzyme complexes isolated from all mammalian tissues have very similar if not identical properties, it is perhaps not surprising that a range of different regulatory mechanisms are involved in ensuring appropriate modulation of activity under a wide variety of circumstances.

The pyruvate dehydrogenase complex is made up of three enzymes which catalyse the series of reactions shown in Figure 12.3. The total number of separate polypeptide chains is close to 150 and the overall molecular weight in the range 7–10 million. The core of the complex is composed of acetyl

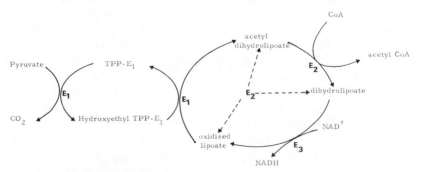

Figure 12.3 Sequence of reactions catalysed by the pyruvate dehydrogenase complex: E_1 – pyruvate decarboxylase; E_2 – dihydrolipoate acetyl transferase; E_3 – dihydrolipoate dehydrogenase

transferase (enz$_2$) units to which are bound the other enzymes, pyruvate decarboxylase (enz$_1$) which appears to be a tetramer of subunit composition $\alpha_2\beta_2$ and dihydrolipoyl dehydrogenase (enz$_3$). Interaction of the three enzymes is brought about by the lipoyl groups which move to the active sites on the three enzymes sequentially. Many questions about the molecular architecture and enzymology remain to be answered[47-49].

Regulation of activity of the enzyme complex   Regulation of the activity of the whole complex is almost certainly brought about through alterations in the activity of pyruvate decarboxylase (enz$_1$) since the first step is by far the most thermodynamically favourable and the only partial reaction which cannot be reversed[48]. Two mechanisms of regulation have been recognised. Firstly, the activity of the enzyme complex becomes progressively diminished as the ratios of acetyl CoA/CoA and NADH/NAD$^+$ are increased[50, 51]. This can be considered as an example of end product inhibition in which the end products acetyl CoA and NADH are competitive inhibitors with respect to CoA and NAD$^+$ respectively.

The second type of regulation is by phosphorylation-dephosphorylation and was first reported by Linn *et al.*[52, 53]. Pyruvate dehydrogenase exists in an inactive phosphorylated form and an active non-phosphorylated form. Interconversion between the two forms is catalysed by an ATP requiring kinase and a phosphatase. The kinase is tightly bound to the complex and catalyses the transfer of the terminal phosphate from ATP to serine groups in the α-subunits of pyruvate decarboxylase (enz$_1$)[54]. Studies on the effects of phosphorylation on the partial reactions catalysed by pyruvate dehydrogenase have shown that all reactions involving the enzyme bound intermediate 2-α-hydroxyethyl TPP are inhibited whereas reactions in which this intermediate is not involved are unaffected[48]. The properties of the kinase and phosphatase have been extensively studied[47, 55-57], and those of potential physiological significance are summarised in Figure 12.4. It should be noted that there are no known effects of cyclic AMP or cyclic AMP dependent protein kinase on the pyruvate dehydrogenase system.

Pyruvate dehydrogenase phosphatase from a number of sources requires both Mg^{2+} and Ca^{2+} for full activity[56]. In the presence of saturating Mg^{2+} (the K_a for Mg^{2+} is about 1 mmol/l) the further addition of Ca^{2+} causes up to a fivefold increase in activity (the K_a for Ca^{2+} is about 1 μmol/l).

In general the kinase appears to be inhibited by the substrates of pyruvate dehydrogenase (pyruvate, NAD$^+$, CoA, TPP) and activated by its products (NADH, acetyl CoA). Physiologically the most important type of regulation of the kinase may be through changes in the NADH/NAD$^+$ and acetyl CoA/CoA ratios[57]. By this means phosphorylation and thus inactivation of

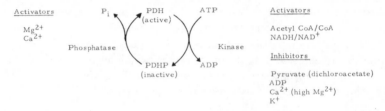

Figure 12.4 Summary of the properties of pyruvate dehydrogenase phosphate (PDHP) phosphatase and pyruvate dehydrogenase (PDH) kinase

the complex may be promoted under conditions when end product inhibition occurs.

Dichloroacetate is a potent inhibitor of the kinase[58] probably because it is an analogue of pyruvate. Exposure of tissues to dichloroacetate *in vivo* and *in vitro* leads to dephosphorylation of pyruvate dehydrogenase and increased pyruvate oxidation[59]. Dichloroacetate and its analogues have recently attracted much attention as possible therapeutic agents in the treatment of diabetes and lactic acidosis. It has to be emphasised that dichloroacetate also inhibits gluconeogenesis and lipogenesis by mechanisms which are not understood except that they are independent of pyruvate dehydrogenase activity[59, 60].

Studies using purified pyruvate decarboxylase preparations have indicated that three different serine residues of the α-chain can be phosphorylated sequentially by pyruvate dehydrogenase kinase[54]. Phosphorylation of only one site correlates with inactivation. The physiological role of phosphorylation at the other sites remains to be established. There is evidence that all three sites are phosphorylated in the intact complex[49, 54] both within mitochondria[61] and in whole cells[61]. It is possible that phosphorylation of the second pair of sites inhibits the dephosphorylation of the site linked to enzyme activity[62].

Pyruvate carboxylase (EC 6.4.1.1.)

Pyruvate carboxylase catalyses the ATP dependent carboxylation of pyruvate to oxaloacetate and is now accepted as an exclusively mitochondrial enzyme[63, 64]. The enzyme is important for the production of oxaloacetate in gluconeogenesis and lipogenesis and as part of a mechanism for topping up the citric acid cycle intermediates. The reaction occurs in two steps, the first being the carboxylation of biotin attached to an ϵ-amino group of a lysine on the enzyme and the second being the transfer of this activated CO_2 group on to pyruvate:

(i) Enzyme–Biotin + ATP + HCO_3^- $\xrightleftharpoons{Mg^{2+}}$

$\qquad\qquad\qquad\qquad\qquad$ Enzyme–Biotin–CO_2 + ADP + P

(ii) Enzyme–Biotin –CO_2 + Pyruvate $\xrightleftharpoons{Mn^{2+}}$

$\qquad\qquad\qquad\qquad\qquad$ Enzyme–Biotin + Oxaloacetate

The detailed structural, kinetic and regulatory properties of pyruvate carboxylase are reviewed in detail elsewhere[65–69].

Mammalian and avian liver pyruvate carboxylase is active only when present as a tetramer of identical monomers (Mol. Wt. 130 000–150 000)[70–72]. The monomers may be split under more extreme conditions to give smaller peptides which may show partial enzyme activities of biotin carboxylation, biotin binding and transcarboxylation[71, 73]. The activity of the enzyme at low pyruvate concentrations (< 0.5 mmol/l) is almost totally dependent on the presence of acetyl CoA whose activation shows a sigmoidal concentration dependence; at higher (unphysiological) pyruvate concentrations some acetyl CoA independent activity is obtained[71, 74, 75]. The K_a for acetyl CoA activation is highly dependent on the conditions of the assay[67, 76–78] but under physiological conditions the apparent K_a value would appear to be 200–340 μmol/l, a value well within the physiological range[67, 78–80].

Under conditions of rapid fatty acid oxidation the mitochondrial acetyl CoA concentration is raised and this may be important for the activation of pyruvate carboxylase and thus gluconeogenesis. Similarly activation of pyruvate dehydrogenase in adipose tissue by insulin may lead to an increase in mitochondrial acetyl CoA, thus stimulating the production by pyruvate carboxylase of oxaloacetate for citrate formation (see below). Various acyl CoA molecules act as competitive inhibitors with respect to acetyl CoA[65], but it is unlikely that many of these have a physiological regulatory function. Methylmalonyl CoA may be an exception for in ruminants propionate is a major source of glucose and the presence of propionate inhibits gluconeogenesis from lactate[81]. This is thought to be due to a build up in methylmalonyl CoA which is an intermediate in the metabolism of propionate. Any inborn error associated with methylmalonyl CoA mutase may show an inhibition of gluconeogenesis from lactate and a consequent increase in blood lactate levels.

Other kinetic parameters[65–71, 78] for pyruvate carboxylase are of less interest. The K_m for pyruvate in the presence of acetyl CoA is about 0.1 mmol/l which is near the expected physiological concentration of pyruvate[82]. It is possible that pyruvate carboxylase activity is limited by the supply of pyruvate so that pyruvate transport may limit the rate of gluconeogenesis[11, 12]. The K_m for HCO_3^- is 2–3 mmol/l, thus the enzyme is fully active with respect to this substrate under physiological conditions.

The enzyme exhibits a K_m for ATPMg of 0.1 mmol/l or less but ADP acts as a competitive inhibitor. Thus the enzyme could be regulated by the ATP/ADP ratio within the mitochondria. *In vitro* experiments with isolated rat liver mitochondria have demonstrated this possibility[83, 84], but *in vivo* evidence for significant changes in mitochondrial ATP/ADP ratios is lacking.

Pyruvate carboxylase shows relatively little change in concentration during starvation and refeeding and this may reflect the requirement for the enzyme in both lipogenic (fed) and gluconeogenic (starved) conditons[67].

Phosphoenolpyruvate carboxykinase (EC 4.1.1.32)

Phosphoenolpyruvate carboxykinase (PEPCK) is responsible for the production of phosphoenolpyruvate required for the reversal of glycolysis in gluconeogenesis and glyceroneogenesis. The enzyme catalyses the GTP dependent decarboxylation and phosphorylation of oxaloacetate to give phosphoenolpyruvate (Figure 12.1).

$$\text{Oxaloacetate} + \text{GTP} \underset{\text{or Fe}^{2+}}{\overset{\text{Mn}^{2+}}{\rightleftharpoons}} \text{Phosphoenolpyruvate} + \text{GDP} + CO_2$$

The subcellular distribution of the enzyme varies from species to species, being almost fully cytoplasmic in rat liver, almost fully mitochondrial in the pigeon and in both compartments in many other species such as the guinea pig and man[85]. The two forms of the enzyme are immunologically distinct[86] and where cytoplasmic and mitochondrial enzymes co-exist it is the cytoplasmic form of the enzyme which shows adaptive changes to diet[87, 88]. The compartmentation of the enzyme affects the path taken by gluconeogenesis since the mitochondrial enzyme produces intramitochondrial phosphoenolpyruvate which must leave the mitochondria on the carrier normally used to transport citrate[89, 90].

PEPCK is a monomeric enzyme (Mol. Wt. about 70 000) whose kinetic properties have been studied extensively[86, 91, 92]. Pertinent to this article are the K_m values for oxaloacetate and GTP and the metal ion requirements of the enzyme. The K_m for GTP is about 16 μmol/l; this is far less than intracellular GTP concentration in liver of about 100–600 μmol/l indicating that enzyme regulation through GTP concentrations is unlikely. The K_m value for oxaloacetate has been in dispute with values ranging from 4 mmol/l to 1.5 μmol/l, but the most recent data on the purified enzyme suggests a value of 9 μmol/l compared to physiological cytoplasmic concentrations of about 5 μmol/l [92]. Mitochondrial oxaloacetate concentrations are more than an order of magnitude lower than cytoplasmic concentrations because the highly reduced state of the mitochondria shifts the equilibrium of malate dehydrogenase towards malate. How the mitochondrial enzyme works at these low oxaloacetate concentrations is not fully understood. It appears probable that the major short term control of PEPCK may be through oxaloacetate supply, since the physiological oxaloacetate concentration is close to, or below, the K_m value, but an alternative mechanism has been proposed involving the divalent metal ion requirement.

In vitro assays of the purified enzyme require Mn^{2+} or a similar divalent cation for full activity[93], but in recent years Lardy and his colleagues have shown that in the cell activation is achieved not by Mn^{2+} but by Fe^{2+}, bound to a protein termed the ferroactivator protein[94-96]. This protein occurs in all gluconeogenic tissues and in some non-gluconeogenic tissues such as erythrocytes and brain. It is capable of totally activating phosphoenolpyruvate carboxykinase by transporting Fe^{2+} into the active site of the enzyme. The tryptophan metabolite quinolinate appears to inhibit gluconeogenesis by specifically chelating the Fe^{2+} bound to the enzyme. The presence of the ferroactivator protein has led to the suggestion that it may be important in short term regulation of the enzyme[96], but there is little evidence to support this theory at present.

The best established control mechanism for PEPCK activity is through changes in the enzyme concentration, brought about by alteration of the rate of enzyme synthesis. Induction and repression of the enzyme in liver is caused by long term dietary and hormonal changes such as occur in starvation and refeeding. Glucagon and the glucocorticoids stimulate enzyme production and insulin antagonises this[85]. In the kidney, enzyme synthesis is rapidly induced by acidosis[97, 98]. Induction effects appear to be caused by an increased production of mRNA[99], and in the case of glucagon action are related to a rise in cyclic AMP production[100]. This rise in cyclic AMP is thought to cause the catalytic subunit of protein kinase to dissociate from its regulator protein and to migrate into the nucleus where it phosphorylates histone proteins[101]. These appear to enhance the transcription of mRNA, but it has been suggested that there may be a further site of action of cAMP to stimulate protein synthesis at the translocational level, possibly by ribosomal protein phosphorylation[97].

REGULATION OF THE MAJOR PATHWAYS OF PYRUVATE UTILIZATION

Pyruvate utilization in muscle

Pyruvate derived from glucose or glycogen via glycolysis in muscle may be converted to lactate or alanine, or oxidised within the mitochondria to CO_2

via pyruvate dehydrogenase and the citrate cycle. The proportion of pyruvate lost from muscle cells as lactate is probably determined largely by the extent to which pyruvate and cytoplasm reducing equivalents formed by glycolysis, can be oxidised by the mitochondria. In anoxia, oxidation of both these end products is necessarily restricted and lactate is the major end product of glycolysis. Lactate is also the principle end product of the high rates of glycolysis associated with contraction of fast-acting or white muscle which contain relatively few mitochondria. Conversion of pyruvate to alanine is an important means whereby amino groups derived from the oxidation of certain amino acids (including valine, isoleucine and leucine) are transferred out of muscle[102, 103]. A substantial proportion of both lactate and alanine released from muscle may be converted to glucose in the liver completing the well known Cori and alanine cycles. Alanine is also converted to urea.

Oxidation of pyruvate in muscle depends on the activity of pyruvate dehydrogenase. When respiration is not limited by the availability of oxygen, the rate of pyruvate oxidation changes in parallel with alterations in ATP utilization associated with muscle contraction. However, the proportion of oxygen consumption accounted for by the oxidation of pyruvate is dependent on the availability of other fuels for respiration. Under conditions of lipid mobilization such as starvation and diabetes, fatty acids and ketone bodies are available and are oxidised in preference to pyruvate. The principal questions of regulation are: what are the mechanisms whereby the activity of pyruvate dehydrogenase is linked to changes in respiration on the one hand and to the availability of the preferred fat fuels on the other?

The first question has received surprisingly little attention. In heart and gastrocnemius muscle, changes in work load are associated with parallel changes in the proportion of pyruvate dehydrogenase in its active non-phosphorylated form[104, 105]. The mechanism has not been established but there are at least two possibilities. One is that changes in mitochondrial $NADH/NAD^+$ ratio are involved. Increase in respiration may well result in a decrease in this ratio and thus an increase in pyruvate dehydrogenase activity (see Figure 12.4). The other plausible mechanism is via regulation of pyruvate dehydrogenase phosphatase by changes in the mitochondrial concentration of Ca^{2+}. This mechanism requires that changes in mitochondrial concentrations of Ca^{2+} are parallel and secondary to changes in Ca^{2+} concentration in the cytoplasm.

The inhibition of pyruvate oxidation by fat fuels has been extensively studied[105-108]. It has become clear from studies in heart muscle that the activity of pyruvate dehydrogenase is decreased by a combination of phosphorylation and end-product inhibition. Since there is a very marked increase in the tissue acetylCoA/CoA ratio under these conditions, it seems likely that this forms the basis of both types of inhibition. Recent studies by Randle and colleagues[108] indicate that this is not the complete answer since they found that the kinase becomes insensitive to inhibition by pyruvate and the phosphorylated pyruvate dehydrogenase complex a poorer substrate for the phosphatase. A possible explanation of these observations is that there are changes in the relative degree of phosphorylation at the three different sites[108].

Pyruvate utilisation in lipogenesis

In animals, the major sites of fat synthesis are adipose tissue (both white and brown), liver and, when appropriate, mammary tissue. The synthesis of fatty acids involves two cytoplasmic enzymes, acetyl CoA carboxylase and fatty acid synthetase, and requires a supply of cytoplasmic acetyl units (as acetyl CoA) and reducing power (as NADPH). When fatty acids are synthesised from glucose, acetyl CoA is formed from pyruvate within mitochondria by pyruvate dehydrogenase; thus there must be a means of transferring acetyl units across the mitochondrial membrane as this membrane is impermeable to acetyl CoA itself. Much evidence indicates that the major pathway involves formation of citrate from acetyl CoA and oxaloacetate within mitochondria, transfer of citrate across the membrane and then cleavage of citrate to yield acetyl CoA and oxaloacetate in the cytoplasm by ATP-citrate lyase (Figure 12.5). Continuous transfer of acetyl units as citrate requires regeneration of mitochondrial oxaloacetate from that formed in the cytoplasm. This is probably accomplished, as least in rat adipose tissue, by the conversion of oxaloacetate to pyruvate via cytoplasmic NAD^+-dependent malate dehydrogenase and the $NADP^+$-linked malic enzyme,

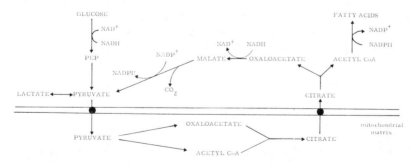

Figure 12.5 Pathways of pyruvate metabolism associated with lipogenesis in mammalian tissues

followed by the entry of pyruvate into the mitochondria and regeneration of oxaloacetate by pyruvate carboxylase. In one turn of the complete pyruvate–malate–citrate cycle one acetyl unit is transported out of the mitochondrial compartment and reducing power is transferred from one molecule of cytoplasmic NADH to NADP$^+$. This transfer accounts for most of the reducing power generated by glycolysis and produces sufficient NADPH to satisfy approximately half that required for fatty acid synthesis. The remainder is probably supplied by the pentose cycle.

Action of Insulin   Fatty acid synthesis in tissues is regulated in the long and short term largely by changes in the plasma concentration of a wide spectrum of hormones including insulin, catecholamines and glucocorticoids[109]. We will restrict discussion to the most studied example of hormonal regulation, namely the prompt and substantial increase in the conversion of glucose to fatty acids in adipose tissue in the presence of insulin. It is now evident that this increase is brought about by the stimulation of a series of key steps in the pathway. These include glucose transport and acetyl CoA carboxylase and in addition pyruvate kinase and pyruvate dehydrogenase (Figure 12.6).

Very recently it has been found that brief exposure of adipose tissue to insulin leads to a form of pyruvate kinase with a lower K_m for PEP[110] but little is understood of the mechanism involved. The effect persists in extracts containing EDTA and fluoride incubated at 0 °C or 30 °C for some hours and is thus likely to be due to some stable covalent modification. One possibility is

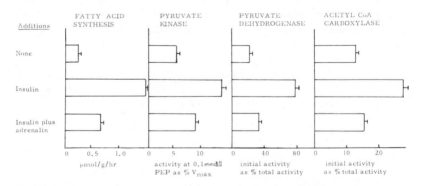

Figure 12.6   Effects of insulin and adrenalin on fatty acid synthesis in adipose tissue is brought about by parallel changes in the proportion of pyruvate kinase, pyruvate dehydrogenase and acetyl CoA carboxylase in their respective active forms[110, 111]

that the effects of insulin are brought about by dephosphorylation of the enzyme. So far, regulation of the pyruvate kinase isoenzyme present in adipose tissue (probably the so called M_2 or K type) by a phosphorylation–dephosphorylation mechanism has only been described for the isoenzyme from chicken liver[43].

The activation of pyruvate dehydrogenase by insulin was first demonstrated in the early 1970s[47]. Insulin causes the proportion of pyruvate dehydrogenase in its active dephosphorylated form to be greatly increased. The intriguing problem of how the interaction of insulin with receptors on the outside of the cell membrane can lead to acute changes in the phosphorylation of this wholly intramitochondrial enzyme has received much attention. As no really satisfactory explanation of the actions of insulin on a number of other intracellular processes such as glycogen synthesis, lipolysis and protein synthesis exists, it is hoped that an understanding of the mechanism of activation of pyruvate dehydrogenase may offer a clue to the mode of insulin action in general. Some progress towards this goal has been made.

The effect of insulin on pyruvate dehydrogenase is not secondary to the effects of insulin on glucose transport or triglyceride metabolism; its action persists during preparation of mitochondria from adipose tissue and is still evident after 10–20 min incubation of the mitochondria with respiratory substrates other than pyruvate[110]. Thus the factors which were responsible for the change in phosphorylation of pyruvate dehydrogenase in the intact tissue must remain in isolated mitochondria.

The rate of the kinase reaction can be measured in isolated mitochondria by observing the rate of incorporation of ^{32}P from inorganic phosphate into the α-subunits of pyruvate dehydrogenase[112]. It was found to be greater in mitochondria from insulin-treated tissue. Clearly the increase in the proportion of the complex in the active nonphosphorylated form was not brought about by an inhibition of the kinase. This suggests that insulin acts through an increase in phosphatase activity. The observed elevation in kinase activity is secondary to the increase in the concentration of its substrate, the nonphosphorylated form of pyruvate dehydrogenase[112].

Since no persistent changes in phosphatase activity have been detected in extracts of adipose tissue mitochondria[112], it seems reasonable to conclude that insulin acts through changes in the mitochondrial concentration of one or more effectors of the phosphatase, i.e. the bivalent metal ions Mg^{2+} and Ca^{2+}. The possibility that insulin alters the activity of the phosphatase through changes in the mitochondrial Ca^{2+} concentration remains the most plausible hypothesis.[113]

There are also long term effects of insulin on adipose tissue pyruvate dehydrogenase. The proportion in the active form is greatly diminished in adipose tissue from starved or diabetic rats. This diminution is not reversed by incubation with excess insulin *in vitro* and appears to be brought about by mechanisms similar to those involved in bringing about the decreased activities in muscle of such animals[113].

Pyruvate utilization in gluconeogenesis

In the liver, many metabolic pathways involve pyruvate but, in general, in the fed state pyruvate will tend to be directed towards fatty acid synthesis whilst in starvation; when blood glucagon levels are high for other reasons, pyruvate is converted largely into glucose and glycogen. An outline of the pathways of gluconeogenesis is shown in Figure 12.7. It has been established for some time that glucagon acting via cyclic AMP stimulates

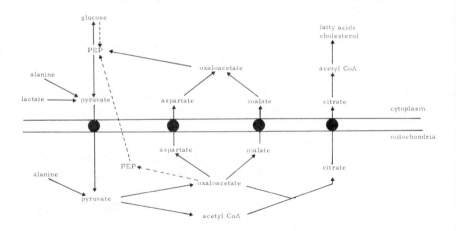

Figure 12.7 General outline of pyruvate metabolism in liver. (Note: The pathway taken from mitochondrial oxaloacetate to cytoplasmic phosphoenolpyruvate (PEP) in gluconeogenesis depends on the substrate and on the animal species concerned[29])

gluconeogenesis between pyruvate and phosphoenolpyruvate[114], but only recently have mechanisms been discovered to account for this effect.

In 1969 Adams and Haynes[115] suggested that liver mitochondria isolated from glucagon treated animals were able to metabolise pyruvate faster than mitochondria from untreated animals. Although they indicated that this might be due to an increased rate of pyruvate entry into mitochondria, this has only recently been confirmed[8, 11]. It appears that pyruvate transport into the mitochondria is stimulated after glucagon treatment by the production of a more alkaline mitochondrial matrix[11]. Pyruvate transport is highly pH dependent[3]. The rise in mitochondrial pH can be accounted for by the increased rate of respiratory chain activity found in glucagon treated mitochondria[11, 116, 117]. This increased respiratory chain activity is caused by an activation of electron flow in the cytochrome b region of the chain[117]; it has the secondary effect of increasing the supply of mitochondrial ATP for pyruvate carboxylase (Figure 12.8). This enzyme shows no direct hormonal activation and may be regulated by the supply of pyruvate from the

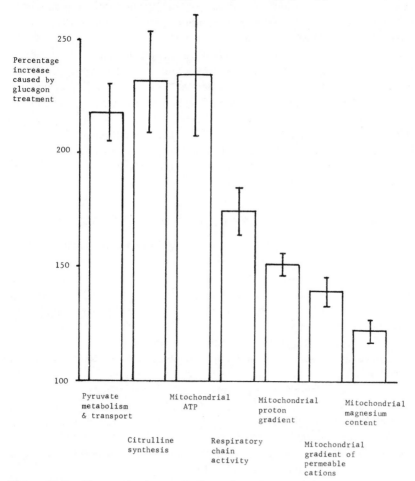

Figure 12.8 Changes in the metabolism of rat liver mitochondria induced by glucagon[11, 121]

pyruvate transporter and by high acetyl CoA levels found in some gluconeogenic conditions because of enhanced fatty acid oxidation[67, 80].

PEPCK is probably not regulated hormonally in the short term as discussed earlier, but it does appear to be of key importance in the medium and long term regulation of gluconeogenesis. It is probable that hormonally induced short term regulation of gluconeogenesis is most directly involved in lactate utilisation in the Cori cycle. For this process mitochondrial pyruvate transport may be the major regulatory step. In the longer term regulation of gluconeogenesis, amino acids such as glutamate and alanine are of greater importance as substrates and these do not require the mitochondrial pyruvate transporter[13]. Under these conditions induction of PEPCK would seem to be the site of regulation[85].

Many metabolic pathways which have the potential of 'futile' cycling show regulation of the metabolic flux in both directions. Thus in gluconeogenesis from pyruvate the potential 'futile' cycle of PEP being converted back into pyruvate is prevented by control of pyruvate kinase. It is found that glucagon treatment of liver cells enhances the phosphorylation of this enzyme and, as was discussed in the earlier section, this leads to an inhibition of its activity. Glucagon may thus stimulate pyruvate conversion to PEP both by a stimulation of pyruvate transport into the mitochondria and by an inhibition of pyruvate kinase.

INBORN ERRORS AND PYRUVATE METABOLISM

Perturbations of pyruvate metabolism in animals and man usually result in changes in circulating plasma levels of both lactate and pyruvate. Such changes are associated with many diseases including a number of inborn errors of metabolism. Unfortunately, identification of the underlying biochemical fault for observed changes in lactate and pyruvate is difficult. The complexity of pyruvate metabolism, which has become apparent from animal systems, means that a large number of possible reasons for alterations in blood lactate and pyruvate can be envisaged. The ethical restraints which necessarily apply to human investigations further magnifies the problem of distinguishing between the many possibilities.

When considering inborn errors of pyruvate metabolism, it is important to distinguish between those diseases where there is a primary change in an enzyme or transporter directly involved in pyruvate metabolism and those diseases where the changes in pyruvate metabolism are secondary to a metabolic disturbance in an associated pathway.

The first group of diseases would include the loss of activity of pyruvate carboxylase and pyruvate dehydrogenase discussed in Chapters 13 and 14.

The changes which have been observed in these enzymes so far are essentially in the V_{max} capacity. Inborn errors may also result in quite subtle but important changes in the kinetic constants for substrates and effectors. In the case of erythrocyte pyruvate kinase deficiencies, abnormalities of this type have been described[37, 38]. With pyruvate kinase and pyruvate dehydrogenase, the possibility also exists that errors may occur in the kinase and phosphatase enzymes involved in the interconversion of the phosphorylated and nonphosphorylated forms. Recently a fructose load test has been devised which may assist in discriminating between subjects with disorders of the catalytic components of the pyruvate dehydrogenase complex from those with defects in the regulatory mechanisms concerned with interconversion of the active and inactive forms of the complex[118]. Inborn errors resulting from direct changes in the activity of PEPCK and lactate dehydrogenase have not yet been found.

Since pyruvate metabolism is closely linked to cell reqirements, it follows that derangements which are associated with hereditary deficiencies of enzymes in other pathways often lead to secondary changes in lactate and pyruvate metabolism. Clearly any disruption of respiration, including hypoxia, will result in lactate acidosis. The oxidation of pyruvate in muscle, nerve and other tissues requires the parallel transfer of cytoplasmic reducing power into mitochondria; any defect in the processes involved in this transfer will cause an increased release of lactate from the tissues. Increases in blood lactate will also arise if liver metabolism is severely disturbed as for example in glycogen storage disease type 1 (glucose 6-phosphatase deficiency) and fructose 1-phosphate aldolase deficiency.

The accumulation of metabolic intermediates associated with certain inborn errors may have quite specific effects on pyruvate metabolism leading to hyperlactataemia. Thus in phenylketonuria and maple syrup urine disease (branched-chain α-keto acid dehydrogenase deficiency) the accumulation of keto acids (phenylpyruvate and α-ketoisocaproate respectively) appear to interfere with pyruvate utilisation, possibly at the level of pyruvate transport into mitochondria[14-16]. In methylmalonic acidaemia a deficiency of methylmalonyl CoA mutase leads to a build up of methylmalonyl CoA from odd chain fatty acids and those amino acids which are metabolised through propionyl CoA[119]. One result of this is an inhibition of pyruvate carboxylase[18, 120].

References

1. Halestrap, A. P. (1978). Pyruvate transport across mitochondrial and plasma membranes. In V. Esmann (ed.). *Regulatory Mechanisms of Car*

bohydrate Research, pp. 61–70. (Oxford: Pergamon Press)

2. Halestrap, A. P. (1975). The mitochondrial pyruvate carrier: kinetics and specificity for substrates and inhibitors. *Biochem. J.*, **148**, 85

3. Halestrap, A. P. (1978). Pyruvate and ketone body transport across the mitochondrial membrane. Exchange properties, pH dependence and mechanism of the carrier. *Biochem. J.*, **172**, 377

4. Papa, S. and Paradies, G. (1974). On the mechanism of translocation of pyruvate and other monocarboxylic acids in rat liver mitochondria. *Eur. J. Biochem.*, **49**, 265

5. Paradies, G. and Papa, S. (1975). The transport of mono carboxylic oxo acids in rat liver mitochondria. *FEBS Lett.*, **52**, 149

6. Paradies, G. and Papa, S. (1976). Substrate regulation of the pyruvate transporting system in rat liver mitochondria. *FEBS Lett.*, **62**, 318

7. Titheradge, M. A. and Coore, H. G. (1975). Initial rates of pyruvate transport in mitochondria determined by an inhibitor stop technique. *Biochem. J.*, **150**, 553

8. Titheradge, M. A. and Coore, H. G. (1976). The mitochondrial pyruvate carrier, its exchange properties and its regulation by glucagon. *FEBS Lett.*, **63**, 45

9. Halestrap, A. P. and Denton, R. M. (1974). Specific inhibition of pyruvate transport in rat liver mitochondria and human erythrocytes by α-cyano-4-hydroxycinnamate. *Biochem. J.*, **138**, 313

10. Halestrap, A. P. (1976). The mechanism of the inhibition of the mitochondrial pyruvate transporter by α-cyanocinnamate derivatives. *Biochem. J.*, **156**, 181

11. Halestrap, A. P. (1978). The stimulation of pyruvate transport in metabolizing mitochondria through changes in the transmembrane pH gradient induced by glucagon treatment of rats. *Biochem. J.*, **172**, 389

12. Halestrap, A. P. and Denton, R. M. (1975). The specificity and metabolic implications of the inhibition of pyruvate transport in isolated mitochondria and intact tissue preparations by α-cyano-4-hydroxycinnamate and related compounds. *Biochem. J.*, **148**, 97

13. Mendes-Mourão, J., Halestrap, A. P., Crisp, D. M. and Pogson, C. I. (1975). The involvement of mitochondrial pyruvate transport in the pathways of gluconeogenesis from serine and alanine in isolated rat and mouse liver cells. *FEBS Lett.*, **53**, 29

14. Halestrap, A. P., Brand, M. D. and Denton, R. M. (1974). Inhibition of mitochondrial pyruvate transport by phenylpyruvate and α-keto-isocaproate. *Biochim. Biophys. Acta*, **367**, 102

15. Clark, J. B. and Land, J. M. (1974). Differential effects of 2-oxo-acids on pyruvate utilization and fatty acid synthesis in rat brain. *Biochem. J.*, **140**, 25

16. Land, J. M., Mowbray, J. and Clark, J. B. (1976). Control of pyruvate and β-hydroxybutyrate utilization in rat brain mitochondria and its relationship to phenylketonuria and maple syrup urine disease. *J. Neurochem.*, **26**, 823

17. Patel, M. S. (1972). The effect of phenylpyruvate on pyruvate metabolism in rat brain. *Biochem. J.*, **128**, 677

18. Patel, T. B., Booth, R. F. G. and Clark, J. B. (1977). Inhibition of acetoacetate oxidation by brain mitochondria from the suckling rat by phenylpyruvate and α-keto-isocaproate. *J. Neurochem.*, **29**, 1151

19. Halestrap, A. P. (1976). Transport of pyruvate and lactate into human

erythrocytes: evidence for the involvement of the chloride carrier and a chloride-independent carrier. *Biochem. J.*, **156**, 193

20. Lamers, J. M. J. and Hulsman, W. C. (1975). Inhibition of pyruvate transport by fatty acids in isolated cells from rat small intestine. *Biochim. Biophys. Acta*, **394**, 31

21. Lamers, J. M. J. (1975). Some characteristics of monocarboxylic acid transfer across the cell membrane of epithelial cells from rat small intestine. *Biochim. Biophys. Acta*, **413**, 265

22. Spencer, T. L. and Lehninger, A. L. (1976). L-Lactate transport in Ehrlich ascites tumour cells. *Biochem. J.*, **154**, 405

23. Deuticke, B., Rickert, I. and Beyer, E. (1978). Stereoselective SH dependent transfer of lactate in mammalian erythrocytes. *Biochim. Biophys. Acta*, **507**, 137

24. Rice, W. and Steck, T. L. (1976). Pyruvate flux into resealed ghosts from human erythrocytes. *Biochim. Biophys. Acta*, **433**, 39

25. Rice, W. and Steck, T. L. (1977). Pyruvate transport into inside-out vesicles isolated from human erythrocyte membranes. *Biochim. Biophys. Acta*, **468**, 305

26. Leeks, D. L. and Halestrap, A. P. (1979). Chloride-independent transport of pyruvate and lactate across the red blood cell membrane. *Biochem. Soc. Trans.* (In press)

27. Sies, H., Noack, G. and Halder, K-H. (1973). Carbon dioxide concentration and the distribution of monocarboxylate and H^+ ions between intracellular and extracellular spaces of haemoglobin-free perfused rat liver. *Eur. J. Biochem.*, **38**, 247

28. Andersen, B. L., Tarpley, H. L. and Regan, D. M. (1978). Characterization of β-hydroxybutyrate transport in rat erythrocytes and thymocytes. *Biochim. Biophys. Acta*, **508**, 525

29. Denton, R. M. and Pogson, C. I. (1976). *Metabolic Regulation*. (London: Chapman and Hall)

30. Williamson, J. R. (1976). Role of anion transport in the regulation of metabolism. In R. W. Hanson and M. A. Mehlman (eds.). *Gluconeogenesis: Its Regulation in Mammalian Species*, pp. 165–220 (New York: Wiley Interscience)

31. Imamura, K. and Tanaka, T. (1972). Multimolecular forms of pyruvate kinase from rat and other mammalian tissues. *J. Biochem.*, **71**, 1043

32. Eigenbrodt, E. and Schoner, W. (1977). Purification and properties of the pyruvate kinase isoenzymes type L and M_1 from chicken liver. *Hoppe-Seyler's Z. Physiol. Chem.*, **358**, 1033

33. Harada, K., Saheki, S., Wada, K. and Tanaka, T. (1978). Purification of four pyruvate kinase isoenzymes of rats by affinity elution chromatography. *Biochim. Biophys. Acta*, **524**, 327

34. Seubert, W. and Schoner, W. (1971). The regulation of pyruvate kinase. *Curr. Top. Cell. Regul.*, **3**, 237

35. Dahlquist-Edberg, U. (1978). Lack of phosphorylatable site and some kinetic properties of erythrocyte pyruvate kinase from the rat. *FEBS Lett.*, **88**, 139

36. Rose, I. A. and Warms, J. V. B. (1966). Control of glycolysis in the human red blood cell. *J. Biol. Chem.*, **241**, 4848

37. Munro, G. F. and Miller, D. R. (1970). Mechanism of fructose diphosphate

activation of a mutant pyruvate kinase from human red cells. *Biochim. Biophys. Acta*, **206**, 89

38. Adachi, K., Ghory, P., Asakura, T. and Schwartz, E. (1977). A monomeric form of pyruvate kinase in human pyruvate kinase deficiency. *Proc. Natl. Acad. Sci. USA*, **74**, 501

39. Ljungström, O., Hjelmquist, G. and Engström, L. (1974). Phosphorylation of purified liver pyruvate kinase by cyclic AMP stimulated protein kinase. *Biochim. Biophys. Acta*, **358**, 289

40. Engström, L. (1978). The regulation of liver pyruvate kinase by phosphorylation-dephosphorylation. *Curr. Top. Cell. Regul.*, **13**, 29

41. Feliu, J. E., Hue, L. and Hers, H-G. (1976). Hormonal control of pyruvate kinase activity and of gluconeogenesis in isolated hepatocytes. *Proc. Natl. Acad. Sci. USA*, **73**, 2762

42. Berglund, L., Ljungström, O. and Engström, L. (1977). Purification and characterization of pig kidney pyruvate kinase (Type A). *J. Biol. Chem.*, **252**, 6108

43. Eigenbrodt, E., Abdel-Fattah Mostafa, M. and Schoner, W. (1977). Inactivation of a pyruvate kinase type M_2 from chickem liver by phosphorylation catalyzed by a cAMP-independent protein kinase. *Hoppe-Seyler's Z. Physiol. Chem.*, **358**, 1047

44. Pogson, C. I. (1968). Adipose tissue pyruvate kinase. Properties and interconversion of two active forms. *Biochem. J.*, **110**, 67

45. Fine, I. H., Kaplan, N. O. and Kuftinec, D. (1963). Developmental changes of mammalian lactic dehydrogenases. *Biochemistry*, **2**, 116

46. Holbrook, J. J., Liljas, A., Steindel, S. J. and Rossman, M. G. (1975). Lactate dehydrogenase. In P. D. Boyer (ed.). *The Enzymes, vol. XI*, pp. 191–292. (New York: Academic Press)

47. Denton, R. M., Randle, P. J., Bridges, B. J., Cooper, R. H., Kerbey, A. L., Pask, H. T., Severson, D. L., Stansbie, D. and Whitehouse, S. (1975). Regulation of mammalian pyruvate dehydrogenase. *Mol. Cell. Biochem.*, **9**, 27

48. Walsh, D. A., Cooper, R. H., Denton, R. M., Bridges, B. J. and Randle, P. J. (1976). The elementary reactions of the pig heart pyruvate dehydrogenase complex. A study of the inhibition by phosphorylation. *Biochem. J.*, **157**, 41

49. Sugden, P. H. and Randle, P. J. (1978). Regulation of pig heart pyruvate dehydrogenase by phosphorylation. Studies on the subunit and phosphorylation stoichiometries. *Biochem. J.*, **173**, 659

50. Garland, P. B. and Randle, P. J. (1964). Control of pyruvate dehydrogenase in perfused heart by the intracellular concentration of acetyl CoA. *Biochem. J.*, **91**, 6

51. Tsai, C. S., Burgett, M. W. and Reed, L. J. (1973). α-keto acid dehydrogenase complexes. XX. A kinetic study of the pyruvate dehydrogenase complex from bovine kidney. *J. Biol. Chem.*, **248**, 8348

52. Linn, T. C., Pettit, F. H. and Reed, L. J. (1969). α-keto acid dehydrogenase complexes. X. Regulation of the activity of the pyruvate dehydrogenase complex from beef kidney mitochondria by phosphorylation and dephosphorylation. *Proc. Natl. Acad. Sci. USA*, **62**, 234

53. Linn, T. C., Pettit, F. H., Hucho, F. and Reed, L. J. (1969). α-keto acid dehydrogenase complexes. XI. Comparative studies of regulatory properties of the pyruvate dehydrogenase complexes from kidney, heart and liver

mitochondria. *Proc. Natl. Acad, Sci. USA*, **64**, 227

54. Yeaman, S. J., Hutcheson, E. T., Roche, T. E., Pettit, F. H., Brown, J. R., Reed, L. J., Watson, D. C. and Dixon, G. H. (1978). Sites of phosphorylation on pyruvate dehydrogenase from bovine kidney and heart. *Biochemistry*, **17**, 2364

55. Reed, L. J. (1974). Multienzyme complexes. *Accts. Chem. Res.*, **7**, 40

56. Denton, R. M., Randle, P. J. and Martin, B. R. (1972). Stimulation by calcium ions of pyruvate dehydrogenase phosphate phosphatase. *Biochem. J.*, **128**, 161

57. Cooper, R. H., Randle, P. J. and Denton, R. M. (1975). Stimulation of phosphorylation and inactivation of pyruvate dehydrogenase by physiological inhibitors of the pyruvate dehydrogenase reaction, *Nature*, **257**, 808

58. Whitehouse, S. and Randle, P. J. (1973). Activation of pyruvate dehydrogenase in perfused rat heart by dichloroacetate. *Biochem. J.*, **134**, 651

59. Whitehouse, S., Cooper, R. H. and Randle, P. J. (1974). Mechanism of activation of pyruvate dehydrogenase by dichloroacetate and other halogenated carboxylic acids. *Biochem. J.*, **141**, 761

60. Lacey, J. H. and Randle, P. J. (1978). Inhibition of lactate gluconeogenesis in rat kidney by dichloroacetate. *Biochem. J.*, **170**, 551

61. Hughes, W. A. and Denton, R. M. (1979). Evidence for multi-site phosphorylation of pyruvate dehydrogenase within intact mitochondria. *Biochem. Soc. Trans.* (In press)

62. Sugden, P. H., Hutson, N. J., Kerbey, A. L. and Randle, P. J. (1978). Phosphorylation of additional sites on pyruvate dehydrogenase inhibits its reactivation by pyruvate dehydrogenase phosphatase. *Biochem. J.*, **169**, 433

63. Ballard, F. J., Hanson, R. W. and Reshef, L. (1970). Immunochemical studies with soluble and mitochondrial pyruvate carboxylase activities from rat tissues. *Biochem. J.*, **119**, 735

64. Walter, P. and Anabitarte, M. (1973). The use of glutamate dehydrogenase as a mitochondrial marker for the determination of intracellular pyruvate carboxylase distribution in rat liver. *FEBS Lett.*, **37**, 170

65. Utter, M. F. and Scrutton, M. C. (1969). Pyruvate carboxylase. *Curr. Top. Cell. Regul.*, **1**, 253

66. Utter, M. F., Barden, R. E. and Taylor, B. L. (1975). Pyruvate carboxylase: an evaluation of the relationships between structure and mechanisms and between structure and catalytic activity. *Adv. Enzymol.*, **42**, 1

67. Barrit, G. J., Zander, G. L. and Utter, M. F. (1976). The regulation of pyruvate carboxylase activity in gluconeogenic tissues. In R. W. Hanson and M. A. Mehlman (eds.). *Gluconeogenesis: Its Regulation in Mammalian Species*, pp. 3–46. (New York: Wiley)

68. McClure, W. R., Lardy, H. A., Wagner, M. and Cleland, W. W. (1971). Rat liver pyruvate carboxylase. II. Kinetic studies of the forward reaction. *J. Biol. Chem.*, **246**, 3579

69. Warren, G. B. and Tipton, K. F. (1974). Pig liver pyruvate carboxylase. The reaction pathway for the carboxylation of pyruvate. *Biochem. J.*, **139**, 311

70. Scrutton, M. C. and Utter, M. F. (1965). Pyruvate carboxylase: some physical and chemical properties of the highly purified enzyme. *J. Biol. Chem.*, **240**, 1

71. McClure, W. R., Lardy, H. A. and Kneifel, H. P. (1971). Rat liver pyruvate

carboxylase. Preparation, properties and cation specificity. *J. Biol. Chem.*, **246,** 3569

72. Barden, R. E., Taylor, B. L., Isohashi, F., Frey, W. H., Zander, G., Lee, J. C. and Utter, M. F. (1975). Structural properties of pyruvate carboxylases from chicken liver and other sources. *Proc. Natl. Acad. Sci. USA*, **72,** 4308

73. Warren, G. B. and Tipton, K. F. (1974). Pig liver pyruvate carboxylase. Purification, properties and cation specificity. *Bicchem. J.*, **139,** 297

74. Ashman, L. K., Keech, D. B., Wallace, J. C. and Nielsen, J. (1972). Sheep kidney pyruvate carboxylase. Studies on its activation by acetyl coenzyme A and characteristics of its acetyl coenzyme A independent reaction. *J. Biol. Chem.*, **247,** 5818

75. Scrutton, M. C. and White, M. D. (1972). Pyruvate carboxylase from rat liver. Properties in the absence and at four concentrations of acetyl CoA. *Biochem. Biophys. Res. Comm.*, **48,** 85

76. Scrutton, M. C. (1974). Pyruvate carboxylase studies of the activator-independent catalysis and of the specificity of activation by acyl derivatives of coenzyme A for the enzyme from rat liver. *J. Biol. Chem.,* **249,** 7057

77. Seufert, D., Herlemann, E. M., Albrecht, E. and Seubert, W. (1971). Purification and properties of pyruvate carboxylase from rat liver. *Hoppe-Seyler's Z. Physiol. Chem.*, **352,** 459

78. Halestrap, A. P. (1974). *Ph.D. Thesis*, University of Bristol

79. McClure, W. R. and Lardy, H. A. (1971). Rat liver pyruvate carboxylase. IV. Factors effecting the regulation *in vivo. J. Biol Chem.*, **246,** 3591

80. Von Glutz, G. and Walter, P. (1976). Regulation of pyruvate carboxylation by acetyl CoA in rat liver mitochondria. *FEBS Lett.*, **72,** 299

81. Chan, T. M. and Freedland, R. A. (1972). The effect of propionate on the metabolism of pyruvate and lactate in the perfused rat liver. *Biochem. J.*, **127,** 539

82. Greenbaum, A. L., Gumaa, K. A. and McLean, P. (1971). The distribution of hepatic metabolites and the control of the pathways of carbohydrate metabolism in animals of different dietary and hormonal status. *Arch. Biochem. Biophys.*, **143,** 617

83. Walter, P. and Stucki, J. W. (1970). Regulation of pyruvate carboxylase in rat liver mitochondria by adenine nucleotides and short chain fatty acids. *Eur. J. Biochem.*, **12,** 508

84. Stucki, J. W., Braurand, F. and Walter, P. (1972). Regulation of pyruvate metabolism in rat liver mitochondria by adenine nucleotides and fatty acids. *Eur. J. Biochem.*, **27,** 181

85. Tilgham, S. M., Hanson, R. W. and Ballard, F. J. (1976). Hormonal regulation of phosphoenolpyruvate carboxykinase (GTP) in mammalian tissues. In R. W. Hanson and M. A. Mehlman (eds.). *Gluconeogenesis: Its Regulation in Mammalian Species*, pp. 47–91. (New York: Wiley)

86. Ballard, F. J. and Hanson, R. W. (1969). Purification of phosphoenolpyruvate carboxykinase from the cytosol fraction of rat liver and the immunochemical demonstration of differences between this enzyme and the mitochondrial phosphoenolpyruvate carboxykinase. *J. Biol. Chem.*, **244,** 5625

87. Nordlie, R. C. and Lardy, H. A. (1963). Mammalian liver phosphoenolpyruvate carboxykinase activities. *J. Biol. Chem.*, **238,** 2259

88. Hanson, R. W. and Garber, A. J. (1972). Phosphoenolpyruvate car-

boxykinase. I. Its role in gluconeogenesis. *Am. J. Clin. Nutr.*, **25**, 1010

89. Robinson, B. (1971). Transport of phosphoenolpyruvate by the tricarboxylate transporting system in mammalian mitochondria. *FEBS Lett.*, **14**, 309

90. Robinson, B. (1971). The role of the tricarboxylate transporting system in the production of phosphoenolpyruvate by ox liver mitochondria. *FEBS Lett.*, **16**, 267

91. Utter, M. F. and Kolenbrander, H. M. (1972). Formation of oxaloacetate by CO_2 fixation on phosphoenolpyruvate. In P. D. Boyer (ed.). *The Enzymes*, Vol. 6, pp. 117–168. (London: Academic Press)

92. Jomain-Baum, M., Schramm, V. L. and Hanson, R. W. (1976). Mechanism of 3-mercaptopicolinic acid inhibition of hepatic phosphoenolpyruvate carboxykinase (GTP). *J. Biol. Chem.*, **251**, 37

93. Snoke, R. E., Johnston, J. B. and Lardy, H. A. (1971). Response of phosphopyruvate carboxylase to tryptophan metabolites and ions. *Eur. J. Biochem.*, **24**, 342

94. Bentle, L. A., Snoke, R. E. and Lardy, H. A. (1976). A protein factor required for activation of phosphoenolpyruvate carboxykinase by ferrous ions. *J. Biol. Chem.*, **251**, 2922

95. Bentle, L. and Lardy, H. A. (1977). Phenolpyruvate carboxykinase ferroactivator. Purification and some properties. *J. Biol. Chem.*, **252**, 1431

96. MacDonald, M. J., Bentle, L. A. and Lardy, H. A. (1978). Phosphoenolpyruvate carboxykinase ferroactivator. Distribution and the influence of diabetes and starvation. *J. Biol. Chem.*, **253**, 116

97. Alleyne, G. A. O. and Scullard, G. H. (1969). Renal metabolic response to acid base changes. I. Enzymatic control of ammoniagenesis in the rat. *J. Clin. Invest.*, **48**, 364

98. Iynedjian, P. B., Ballard, F. J. and Hanson, R. W. (1975). The regulation of phosphoenolpyruvate carboxykinase (GTP) synthesis in rat kidney cortex. The role of acid base balance and glucocorticoids. *J. Biol. Chem.*, **250**, 5596

99. Iynedjian, P. B. and Hanson, R. W. (1977). Increase in level of functional messenger RNA coding for phosphoenolpyruvate carboxykinase (GTP) during induction by cyclic adenosine 3'5'-monophosphate. *J. Biol., Chem.*, **252**, 655

100. Wicks, W. D. (1969). Induction of hepatic enzymes by adenosine 3'5'-monophosphate in organ culture. *J. Biol. Chem.*, **244**, 3941

101. Castagna, M., Palmer, W. K. and Walsh, D. A. (1975). Nuclear protein kinase activity in perfused rat liver stimulated with dibutyryl-adenosine cyclic 3'5'-monophosphate. *Eur. J. Biochem.*, **55**, 193

102. Felig, P. (1975). Amino acid metabolism in man. *Ann. Rev. Biochem.*, **44**, 933

103. Chang, T. W. and Goldberg, A. L. (1978). The origin of alanine produced in skeletal muscle. *J. Biol. Chem.*, **253**, 3677

104. Illingworth, J. A. and Mullings, R. (1976). Pyruvate dehydrogenase activation after an increase in cardiac output. *Biochem. Soc. Trans.*, **4**, 291

105. Henning, G., Löffler, G. and Wieland, O. H. (1975). Active and inactive forms of pyruvate dehydrogenase in skeletal muscle as related to the metabolic and functional state of the muscle cell. *FEBS Lett.*, **59**, 142

106. Wieland, O., Siess, E., Schulze-Wethmar, F. H., von Funcke, H. G. and Winton, B. (1971). Active and inactive forms of pyruvate dehydrogenase in rat heart and kidney: effect of diabetes, fasting and refeeding on pyruvate dehydrogenase interconversion. *Arch. Biochem. Biophys.*, **143**, 593

107. Kerbey, A. L., Randle, P. J., Cooper, R. H., Whitehouse, S., Pask, H. T. and Denton, R. M. (1976). Regulation of pyruvate dehydrogenase in rat heart. *Biochem. J.*, **154**, 327

108. Hutson, N. J., Kerbey, A. L., Randle, P. J. and Sugden, P. H. (1978). Conversion of inactive (phosphorylated) pyruvate dehydrogenase complex into active complex by the phosphate reaction in heart mitochondria is inhibited by alloxan-diabetes or starvation in the rat. *Biochem. J.*, **173**, 669

109. Jeanrenaud, B. and Hepp, D. (eds.). (1970). *Adipose tissue: Regulation and Metabolic Functions*. (New York: Academic Press)

110. Denton, R. M., Edgell, N., Bridges, B. J. and Poole, G. (1979). Regulation of pyruvate kinase activity in rat epididymal adipose tissue by insulin and adrenalin. (Submitted for publication)

111. Denton, R. M., Bridges, B. J., Brownsey, R. W., Evans, G. L., Hughes, W. A. and McCormack, J. (1978). Acute hormonal regulation of fatty acid synthesis in mammalian tissues. In R. Dils and J. Knudsen (eds.). *Regulation of Fatty Acid and Glycerolipid Metabolism*, pp. 21–30. (Oxford: Pergamon Press)

112. Hughes, W. A. and Denton, R. M. (1976). Incorporation of $^{32}P_i$ into pyruvate dehydrogenase phosphate in mitochondria from control and insulin-treated adipose tissue. *Nature*, **264**, 471

113. Denton, R. M., Hughes, W. A., Bridges, B. J., Brownsey, R. W., McCormack, J. G. and Stansbie, D. (1978). Regulation of mammalian pyruvate dehydrogenase by hormones. *Horm. Cell Regul.*, **2**, 191

114. Exton, J. H. and Park, C. R. (1969). Effects of L-lactate, pyruvate, fructose, glucagon, epinephrine and adenosine 3′5′-monophosphate on gluconeogenic intermediates in the perfused rat liver. *J. Biol. Chem.*, **244**, 1424

115. Adams, P. A. J. and Haynes, R. C. (1969). Control of hepatic mitochondrial CO_2 fixation by glucagon, epinephrine and cortisol. *J. Biol. Chem.*, **244**, 6444

116. Yamazaki, R. K. (1975). Glucagon stimulation of mitochondrial respiration. *J. Biol. Chem.*, **250**, 7924

117. Halestrap, A. P. (1978). Stimulation of the respiratory chain of rat liver mitochondria between cytochrome c_1 and cytochrome c by glucagon treatment of rats. *Biochem. J.*, **172**, 399

118. Stansbie, D., Sherriff, R. J. and Denton, R. M. (1979). Fructose load test – an *in vivo* screening test designed to assess pyruvate dehydrogenase activity and interconversion. (In press)

119. Williams, D. L., Spray, G. H. and Williamson, B. H. (1971). Metabolic effects of propionate administration to normal and vitamin B_{12} deficient rats. *Biochem. J.*, **121**, 16

120. Lindblad, G., Lindblad, B. S., Olin, P., Svanberg, G. and Zetterström, R. (1968). Methylmalonic acidaemia – a disorder associated with acidosis, hyperglycinaemia and hyperlactataemia. *Acta Paediatr. Scand.*, **57**, 417

121. Yamazaki, R. K. and Graetz, G. S. (1977). Glucagon stimulation of citrulline formation in isolated hepatic mitochondria. *Arch. Biochem. Biophys.*, **178**, 19

13

Pyruvate dehydrogenase deficiencies

J. P. Blass

INTRODUCTION

The extraordinary complexity of the pyruvate dehydrogenase complex (PDHC) is clearly documented in Chapter 12. PDHC contains three catalytic and two regulatory enzymes. It is subject to an intricate array of controls, including phosphorylation and dephosphorylation of the α-subunit of its thiamin-dependent component, end-product inhibition by NADH and acetyl-coenzyme A, and the action of a number of effectors. Furthermore, there is relatively little excess of this enzyme compared to the normal flux of its substrate, both in brain[1] and in other tissues[2]. The control of PDHC in health and disease is a subject of intense research in a number of laboratories at the present time, particularly in relation to diabetes and the mechanism of action of insulin. Even subtle changes in the structure of one of the proteins in PDHC could lead to metabolically significant impairment of its activity. Conversely, one can conceive of a wide variety of metabolic alterations which could lead to secondary impairment of the activity of PDHC and present clinically as deficiencies of PDHC. In view of this complexity, it is not surprising that the deficiencies of PDHC which have been described have not yet been fully characterized in biochemical detail.

Several points about PDHC deficiencies can be well documented and are the subject of this article. First, the existence of such deficiencies is in accord with a large body of work on hereditary diseases of the nervous system. Second, there is overwhelming evidence that genetically determined deficiencies in the activity of PDHC exist and are associated with disease in humans. Thirdly, there is substantial evidence that a significant proportion of patients with hereditary spinocerebellar ataxias have hereditary deficiencies of pyruvate oxidation, although whether these oxidative abnormalities are primary or secondary to other abnormalities of metabolism is controversial. Fourth, there is increasing evidence that rational biochemical approaches to ameliorating the biochemical and even clinical consequences of PDHC deficiencies are possible. Finally, there are a number of pressing technical problems, relating particularly to the diagnosis of these disorders.

HISTORICAL BACKGROUND

In the 1920s, 1930s, and 1940s there was great interest in the possibility that constitutional abnormalities in carbohydrate metabolism might underlie the development of a number of neurological or psychiatric disorders in which there was a hereditary component[3]. One reason for this interest was that the pathways of carbohydrate metabolism were then on the frontier of research, and it was natural to question whether those recent discoveries were relevant to brain disease. A second and more important reason was the recognition that even very mild impairment of cerebral carbohydrate oxidation leads to profound impairment of brain function, particularly of higher mental function[4]. Much research in this area was supported by the military in many countries, since it was realized that the performance of military aircraft in the Second World War was likely to be limited less by the hardware than by the supply of oxygen and blood sugar to the brains of the pilots and crew. The classical studies of Sir Rudolph Peters[5] demonstrating a biochemical lesion in carbohydrate oxidation in the brains of thiamine deficient pigeons were another stimulus to research in this area. The reasoning leading to studies of carbohydrate metabolism in patients with neurological or psychiatric disease has been elegantly summarized by Quastel[6].

A massive amount of work on carbohydrate metabolism in patients with neuropsychiatric disorders was done between 1930 and 1954[7]. Unfortunately, the techniques available were limited and nonspecific, often being limited to glucose tolerance tests. The diagnoses were also nonspecific, and subsequent studies have shown that the concordance in clinical diagnosis between different observers examining these patients at that time was only slightly better than random[8]. Consequently it is not surprising that the abnormalities which were detected were also nonspecific. Sourkes[3] has summarized the results of these studies, stressing their lack of reproducibility and specificity, and the need to develop more discriminating techniques to study the problem. With the elucidation of other pathways of metabolism and discrete inborn errors, interest in hereditary abnormalities of carbohydrate oxidation diminished sharply. However, the earlier results were never disproven, and the existence of abnormalities of glucose utilization in a large proportion of patients with a variety of hereditary disorders of the nervous system is one of the best documented observations in clinical neurochemistry[3].

In the middle 1960s, several patients were described who presented with profound and generalized disease of the nervous system, elevated levels of lactate and pyruvate in the blood and often other physiological fluids, and usually with metabolic acidosis. On the basis of clinical and chemical studies, it was suggested that these patients had inborn deficiencies in the oxidation of glucose to CO_2 and H_2O, and specifically in the oxidation of pyruvate (derived from glucose by glycolysis) to CO_2 and acetylcoenzyme-A by PDHC[9-16]. Direct confirmation of this possibility by direct assay for PDHC was, however lacking.

In 1970, a patient was reported with intermittent ataxia and mild acidosis and persistent hyperpyruvicaemia, in whose tissues a deficiency of PDHC activity was demonstrated by direct enzyme assay[17]. Subsequently more than fifty patients have been described in whom there is substantial evidence for a genetically determined deficiency of the activity of PDHC.

DOCUMENTATION OF PDHC DEFICIENCIES

Demonstration of PDHC deficiencies rests on four lines of evidence. The most important is direct demonstration of PDHC deficiencies in biopsied or cultured tissues from suspected cases, using assays designed to measure the activity of PDHC or of one of its components in disrupted cells. Demonstration of defective oxidation of pyruvate but not of other substrates by intact cells provides strong confirmatory evidence. Accumulation of excessive amount of pyruvate and of related metabolites in blood, urine or CSF is in accord with PDHC deficiency, although it is of course not a specific finding. Finally, the beneficial effects of a diet enriched in fat and low in carbohydrate, compared to the marked deterioration on a high carbohydrate diet, strongly suggests a block in the oxidation of carbohydrate to acetylcoenzyme-A.

All of the four types of evidence have not been accumulated for all of more than fifty patients with PDHC deficiency studied so far[16-41]. However, at least eight patients have been described in each of whom detailed studies demonstrated deficient PDHC activity, deficient pyruvate oxidation by intact cells, and accumulation of pyruvate and related metabolites in physiological fluids[16-22].

Deficient PDHC activity

Demonstration of deficient PDHC activity requires a reliable assay for the complex, and if possible of its components, which can be applied to the small amounts of human tissues available from biopsies or from cell cultures. This is not a trivial problem and has not been completely solved. Most studies have depended on radiochemical modifications of standard enzyme assays, following the conversion of [1-^{14}C]pyruvate to $^{14}CO_2$ by disrupted tissues in the presence of the appropriate cofactors[16-41]. Deficiency of the lipoamide dehydrogenase component (EC 1.2.4.1) of PDHC has been demonstrated by direct spectrophotometric assay[27, 30]. In unpublished studies, Stansbie and Denton[42] used a coupled enzyme assay which follows the pyruvate-dependent formation of acetylcoenzyme-A to demonstrate low PDHC activity in cultured fibroblasts from a boy with hyperlactataemia. Thus PDHC deficiency has been documented in human patients by three independent assay techniques.

Deficiency of PDHC has been demonstrated in a number of tissues. Most studies have used cultured skin fibroblasts, platelets or leukocytes from peripheral blood, because of the availability of these tissues. PDHC deficiency has also been demonstrated in biopsied muscle[17, 27] and liver[36], and in autopsied brain, liver, kidney, and muscle[25-27, 34]. In general when a deficiency has been demonstrable in one tissue it has been demonstrable in all[17, 25-27]. One exception is the patient studied by Willems et al.[36], in whom there was low activity of PDHC in biopsied liver but not in cultured fibroblasts. In this patient there was a possible defect in the activation of PDHC by PDHC-phosphatase.

The severity of the deficiencies in PDHC activity has varied, and there has been a rough correlation between the severity of the clinical disorder and the degree of metabolic deficiency[40, 41]. The most severely affected patients were a Dutch child studied by Hommes[43] and an American child studied by Farrell and coworkers[25, 26], both of whom presented in the first few days of life with profound lactic acidosis and severe, generalized neurological disease; in both of them activity of PDHC was virtually undetectable. The most mildly affected patients developed signs and symptoms of hereditary spinocerebellar degeneration in their late teens. The activity of PDHC in their tissues was about 40–50% of normal, as measured under conventional conditions of assay[37, 39]. Patients with disease of intermediate severity and age of onset have been found to have an intermediate level of

PDHC activity (Figure 13.1). While this rough correlation between the extent of the biochemical and clinical abnormalities is gratifying, its importance can be very easily overestimated. All assays of PDHC are carried out under specified and nonphysiological conditions. It is unsafe to assume that the extent to which a mutation expresses itself under artificial conditions necessarily reflects the affects of the mutation under physiological conditions. This point has been clearly demonstrated by Yoshida for mutations of glucose-6-phosphate dehydrogenases[44]. It is even more likely to be true for PDHC, which is a complicated system acting within the inner mitochondrial space.

It should be emphasized that the large majority of hereditary abnormalities of PDHC reduce but do not abolish its activity. By analogy with mutations in bacteria, they are 'leaky' mutations. PDHC has a critical role in the central pathway of carbohydrate catabolism, and it seems unlikely that mutations which completely abolish the activity of this critical enzyme would be compatible with extrauterine life, at least for very long.

Inheritance   Available data are in general consistent with PDHC deficiency being inherited as an autosomal recessive. Detailed family studies were done in the first five patients in whom the enzyme defect was demonstrated. In each instance, PDHC activity in the parents was intermediate between those of the patients and the control mean, i.e. at or below the lower end of the range for controls[17-21]. These observations strongly suggest that these patients inherit one abnormal gene from each of their parents. In agreement with this conclusion, there appears to be an approximately equal incidence in males and females. Parents have relatively subtle or no clinical abnormalities, compared to their affected offspring. In one family the parents of a patient with PDHC deficiency were known to be consanguineous[19]. Preliminary kinetic studies in the first patient in whom PDHC deficiency was demonstrated are consistent with that patient inheriting a different abnormal gene from each of his parents, i.e. being an affected 'double heterozygote'[17]. This observation has not been pursued as yet in greater detail.

Family studies have indicated a close link between the biochemical and clinical abnormality. In the three families with more than one affected sibling studied by the authors, a close link was shown; all affected siblings had the enzyme defect and no unaffected sibling had the deficiency[40,41]. A number of other families have been identified in whom some of the affected siblings had died before the clinical assays for PDHC were introduced. In these families, all affected siblings had the clinical chemical abnormalities of hyperlactataemia and hyperpyruvicaemia, and none of the unaffected siblings had excessive levels of pyruvate or lactate in their blood. However, Filla et al.[45] have mentioned the existence of families in which they were able to demonstrate low activities of PDHC in platelets from some members with clinical spinocerebellar disorders but not other clinically affected siblings. The assays are difficult and it is always possible that discrepancies are due to technical factors. Also, in some patients deficiency of PDHC may be a primary genetic abnormality and demonstrable while in others it is secondary to some other aberration and not invariably demonstrable, by current techniques.

Vitamin dependency   The reactions catalyzed by PDHC involve five cofactors derived from vitamins, so that vitamin dependent forms of PDHC deficiency are in principle possible. Wick et al.[23] in Basle have studied a 20 month old boy who responded clinically and biochemically to treatment with 1.8 g of oral thiamine daily. His hypotonia improved dramatically and his developmental quotient (DQ) increased from 64 to 90. When thiamine was discontinued, ataxia developed promptly, which regressed when thiamine was reinstituted. Simultaneously with the clinical improvement, blood lactate and pyruvate levels, which had been elevated, returned to normal. Addition of a large excess of thiamine to fibroblasts cultured *in vitro* also ameliorated the deficiency in PDHC.

Another child, described by Clayton et al.[11] before the introduction of clinical assays for PDHC activity, improved both clinically and biochemically when treated with lipoate, although the underlying disease progressed and the child died. Definitive demonstration of a lipoate dependent form of PDHC deficiency would be of great interest. Lipoate is covalently bound to the transacetylase component of PDHC. It is not immediately obvious how increased concentrations of this compound would increase PDHC activity; one possibility is that of protecting the enzyme from degradation.

In ten other patients, addition of large excesses of cofactor did not ameliorate the deficiency *in vitro*. No other patients with PDHC deficiency have been shown to be clinically vitamin dependent.

Complex activation   Since PDHC is inactivated by phosphorylation and reactivated by dephosphorylation, it is entirely possible that apparent deficiencies of PDHC are due to deficiencies in the reactivation of the complex, but data on this point is limited. Incubation of disrupted fibroblasts or platelets with 10 mmol/l Mg^{2+} and 0.5 mmol/l Ca^{2+}, with or without added beef heart PDHC phosphatase (i.e. under conditions which are normally used to reactivate the phosphorylated PDHC) did not increase PDHC activity in preparations from controls or from either of the two patients in whom this aspect has been studied[20, 46].

Robinson and Sherwood[34] described a male infant with lactic acidosis in whose liver PDHC activity did not increase as rapidly as in control liver, under conditions of incubation which normally activate (dephosphorylate) PDHC, and they proposed that their patient has a deficiency of the reactivating phosphatase. The patient described by Willems et al.[36] might also have had a deficiency in the activity of PDHC phosphatase, since PDHC activity was normal in fibroblasts, in which it is normally fully activated, but not in liver, in which it is normally largely inactivated and must be reactivated by dephosphorylation. As emphasized by Denton in the preceding contribution (Chapter 12), the control of the inactivation and reactivation of PDHC is very complex. The relationship between deficiencies of PDHC activity in humans and possible alterations in the inactivation–reactivation system for this complex needs more intensive study by better methods than have been applied up to now.

Secondary deficiencies   There is no evidence at all that any cases of hereditary PDHC deficiency are due to the accumulation of an inhibitor of the enzyme. The conventional biochemical mixing experiments have been done with cells from at least ten patients[17–21]. This is not to say that secondary deficiencies of PDHC do not occur. Among classical examples of metabolic disorders which cause secondary deficiency of PDHC are thiamine deficiency and heavy metal toxicity[47, 48]. Robinson et al.[48] reported PDHC activity less than 12% of normal in autopsy liver from six patients with Reye's syndrome, presumably secondary to mitochondrial damage and a general decrease of mitochondrial enzyme activity in this disorder.

Powerful evidence that deficiencies of PDHC are genetically determined is their persistence in cultured skin fibroblasts through serial passages. After n passages in culture, the material in the original biopsy has been diluted by a factor of at least 2^n–3^n. After 20 passages in culture, the dilution is so large that only the genetic material of the cells and their genetic properties have been conserved.

Summary   Summarizing the results of enzyme assays, deficient activity of PDHC has been demonstrated by direct enzyme assays in tissues of over fifty patients, studied by ten groups of workers from three continents, using three different enzyme assays, in a variety of tissues, notably cultured skin fibroblasts. Typically, deficiencies are partial (i.e. leaky) rather than total loss of activity. Family studies indicate that the patients usually inherit an abnormal gene for PDHC from each of their parents, and in general there is a close link between occurrence of the biochemical and of the clinical abnormality. Although one patient with a thiamine dependent form of PDHC deficiency has been described, in most patients there is no evidence for vitamin dependency. Available results suggest that deficiencies of PDHC may sometimes be secondary to deficiencies in reactivation of PDHC, but more often are not; data on this point is inadequate. The persistence of PDHC deficiency in cultured skin fibroblasts provides strong evidence that it is genetically determined.

Deficient pyruvate oxidation

Demonstration of deficient oxidation of pyruvate by intact cells from these patients is important even though it is less specific than demonstration of deficient PDHC activity. Since the control of PDHC activity is complex, one cannot assume that a partial deficiency of PDHC activity, demonstrated with cell extracts under specific artifical conditions, is significant under more physiological conditions in intact cells with intact mitochondria.

Impaired oxidation of pyruvate has been demonstrated in intact cell preparations from at least ten patients in whom PDHC deficiency has been demonstrated by enzyme assay[17-21, 23, 24, 37, 40, 41, 49]. The basic technique is to incubate intact cultured skin fibroblasts, intact white blood cells, or intact slices of biopsied muscle with [1-^{14}C] pyruvate or with [2-^{14}C] pyruvate and to measure the $^{14}CO_2$ evolved. Defective conversion of radioactive pyruvate to CO_2 may reflect defective PDHC activity but it can result from a defect in the further oxidation of acetylcoenzyme-A in the Krebs tricarboxylic acid cycle, a defect in the transport of pyruvate into mitochondria by the monocarboxylate acid carrier, or even just an increase in the size of the intracellular pyruvate pool. The possibility of defects in the oxidation of acetylcoenzyme-A has been largely ruled out, not only by the demonstration of a deficiency of PDHC itself, but also because oxidation of substrate other than pyruvate was normal. These other substrates included the fatty acid palmitate and the ketone body β-hydroxybutyrate, which are converted to acetylcoenzyme-A before their conversion to CO_2. Normal oxidation of palmitate and β-hydroxybutyrate provides strong evidence against a deficiency in the oxidation of acetylcoenzyme-A.

In one unusual patient[19], disrupted cells were shown to be deficient in PDHC activity but intact cells were deficient in the oxidation not only of pyruvate but also of palmitate and citrate, although not of isocitrate or glutamate. The cause of these surprising and anomalous findings has not been clarified.

It should be emphasized that deficient oxidation of [1-^{14}C] pyruvate by intact cells does not necessarily reflect deficient activity of PDHC, while deficient oxidation of [2-^{14}C] pyruvate or of [3-^{14}C] pyruvate can reflect a defect in PDHC, or in the Krebs tricarboxylic acid cycle, or in electron transport. Any metabolic abnormality which increases the intracellular pools of pyruvate and/or impairs the net transport of pyruvate into the mitochondrion can impair the production of $^{14}CO_2$ from [1-^{14}C] pyruvate, [2-^{14}C] pyruvate, or [3-^{14}C] pyruvate. For instance, a-cyano-4-hydroxycinnamic acid and other experimental inhibitors of the monocarboxylate carrier clearly reduce the oxidation of [1-^{14}C] pyruvate in animal tissues[50, 51]. Specification of enzymatic abnormalities clearly requires direct study of the enzymes. However, the demonstration of low oxidation of pyruvate by intact cells from patients with PDHC deficiency provides valuable support for the physiological significance of the abnormalities in PDHC activity demonstrated in disrupted cells.

Accumulation of metabolites *in vivo*

Further evidence for the physiological significance of the observed abnormalities in PDHC activity *in vitro* is provided by the accumulation of pyruvate and related metabolites in physiological fluids of PDHC deficient patients. The existence of hereditary PDHC deficiencies was first suspected because of the accumulation of pyruvate, of lactate (the product of reduction of pyruvate), and of alanine (the product of transamination of pyruvate). Although the finding of elevated levels of these compounds is not specific for PDHC deficiency, it is often the clue that leads to more intensive investigation of patients.

The levels of pyruvate which accumulate in the blood of patients are usually only moderately elevated to 0.15–0.3 mmol/l compared to a normal upper limit of 0.1 mmol/l (approximately 10 mg/dl). The level of pyruvate can be normal intermittently, depending in part on diet[21, 23]. The finding of a single normal blood pyruvate in a patient does not rule out the possibility of PDHC deficiency[20]. Measurement of pyruvate in urine is less reliable, not only because of the existence of a renal threshold for pyruvate but also because this compound is not very stable in urine. Like other 2-keto acids, it undergoes aldol condensation and other complex reactions at the neutral or slightly alkaline pH often found in urine samples, particularly by the time they have reached the analytical laboratory. Levels of pyruvate were higher in CSF than in blood in one patient with PDHC deficiency in whom they were measured simultaneously[17, 52], but studies of CSF pyruvate in these patients have been limited.

Lactate levels in blood generally rise in parallel with pyruvate in patients with PDHC deficiency, although the rise in lactate may be less marked[17, 52]. Since the lactate–pyruvate equilibrium appears to be normally maintained in the absence of changes in the NADH/NAD ratio, and since there is no evidence that these patients have an abnormality in the oxidation of NADH, this observation is not surprising. Urinary lactate levels may be more reliable than urinary pyruvate, and have been suggested to be a good screening test for disorders of carbohydrate catabolism[29]. When these patients deteriorate, urinary lactate levels may rise very high indeed[20].

The elevation of blood or urine alanine in PDHC deficient patients is often modest, but can be important because of the widespread use of amino acid analyses to detect inborn errors of metabolism. Abnormal elevation of L-alanine on a urinary chromatogram led Derek Lonsdale et al. to discover the syndrome of intermittent ataxia with hyperpyruvicaemia[16]. Transamination of pyruvate to alanine converts an acidic compound to a zwitterion, and alanine is an important means of transporting 3-carbon fragments to the liver, in gluconeogenesis.

Elevation of pyruvate and related metabolites in physiological fluids is not a specific finding for PDHC deficiency. Such elevations also occur in other disorders of pyruvate metabolism (such as pyruvate carboxylase deficiency, discussed by Hommes, Schrijver and Dias in the next chapter) and in any disorder in which there is a primary or secondary metabolic abnormality which leads the rate of pyruvate and lactate production to exceed the rate of pyruvate utilization. Raised levels of blood lactate characteristically occur in one of the glycogen storage diseases, glucose-6-phosphatase deficiency. The finding of excess lactate or pyruvate in body fluids is analogous not to the finding of an excess of a specific amino acid, but rather to an elevation of α-amino nitrogen. It indicates that an abnormality exists somewhere in a large area of metabolism and is not specific, even for a particular pathway.

Dietary studies

The effects of high fat and high carbohydrate diets provide strong support for the significance of the abnormalities in PDHC observed in vitro. It has become clear within the last ten years that the brain can utilize the ketone bodies acetoacetate and β-hydroxybutyrate effectively when their concentration in the blood rises to 1–2 mmol/l[53]. The oxidation of ketone bodies provides an alternate source of acetylcoenzyme-A to the otherwise obligatory oxidation of pyruvate by the brain. By replacing pyruvate in part with another substrate, the residual PDHC activity may more nearly suffice for the metabolic needs of the tissue. These considerations suggest that a diet enriched in fat and reduced in carbohydrates, to a degree which makes the patients ketonaemic but not hypoglycaemic or acidotic, might ameliorate both the metabolic and even the clinical abnormalities. Conversely, a diet enriched in carbohydrates and low in fat might increase metabolic demands on the defective pathway and lead to clinical deterioration. Both these predictions have been borne out in a number of these patients.

The first published studies of the effects of a ketogenic diet in PDHC deficiency concerned two brothers with PDHC deficiency documented in both fibroblasts and platelets[21]. When they were switched from a standard diet containing 40% of the energy as carbohydrate, 40% as fat, and 20% as protein, to a diet containing 50% of the energy as fat, 30% as carbohydrate, and 20% as protein, the levels of pyruvate in their blood fell and they seemed stronger and better coordinated (Table 13.1). When a diet containing 60% of the energy as carbohydrate, 20% as fat, and 20% as protein was tried, the patients promptly deteriorated. Levels of pyruvate and lactate in their blood rose and they became so weak that the study was terminated. The boys were maintained on the high fat diet over the next three months and showed marked improvement. One of them who had not been able to take more than a few steps was able to walk more than 15 metres. However, after surgery to lengthen a heel cord, this patient began to deteriorate and eventually died. It was not clear whether the unpalatable ketogenic diet was beneficial during this deterioration. His brother is reported to continue to do reasonably well although there have been no marked improvements since the spurt in weight during the first three months on the ketogenic diet.

A number of other patients have been studied, who showed both clinical and biochemical amelioration on a ketonaemic diet. The general picture which appears to be emerging is that the institution of a ketonaemic diet slows but does not stop the progression of the disease in children with PDHC deficiency.

These patients can be exquisitely sensitive to a dietary carbohydrate load. Before this sensitivity was recognized, a child with minimal and intermittent hyperlactataemia was put on a 60% carbohydrate diet preparatory to a glucose tolerance test[20]. One day later he developed profound lactate acidosis, dropping his blood pH to 7.14, pouring 30 g of lactate into his urine (Table 13.2), and requiring the replacement of twice his calculated total body HCO_3^-, with his serum Na^+ eventually rising above 180 mmol/l. These studies have not been repeated in other patients, now that the danger of a high carbohydrate diet is appreciated. Even a relatively slight and gradual increase in dietary carbohydrate has led to clear, although mild and transient, deterioration in other PDHC deficient patients, as noted in the brothers described above[21].

TABLE 13.1   Effects of a ketonaemic diet

	Blood pyruvate (mg/100 ml and μmol/l in brackets)		
	Normal diet	*High fat diet*	*High carbohydrate diet*
Patient No. 1			
Fasting	1.0, 1.5 (114, 170)	1.2, 0.9 (136, 102)	1.5 (170)
Post-prandial	1.8, 2.2 (204, 250)	1.2, 1.1 (136, 125)	4.5, 6.5 (511, 738)
Patient No. 2			
Fasting	1.4 (159)	1.3 (148)	—
Post-prandial	1.9 (216)	1.1 (125)	3.7 (420)
Controls			
Fasting	0.3–1.0 (34–114)	—	—
Post-prandial	0.5–1.2 (57–136)	—	—

	Blood lactate (mg/100 ml and μmol/l in brackets)		
Patient No. 1			
Fasting	7.5, 16.2 (833, 1800)	9.2, 16.0 (1022, 1778)	15.6 (1733)
Post-prandial	28.2, 16.0 (3133, 1778)	7.7, 19.1 (855, 2122)	33.5, 64.5 (3722, 7166)
Patient No. 2			
Fasting	14.8 (1644)	10.0 (1111)	—
Post-prandial	29.4 (3266)	10.3 (1144)	16.8 (1866)
Controls			
Fasting	5.0–12.0 (556–1333)	—	—
Post-prandial	5.0–15.0 (556–1667)	—	—

Two brothers with PDHC deficiency were fed either a normal diet (20% protein, 40% carbohydrate, 40% fat, as calories), and a high fat diet (20% protein, 15% carbohydrate, 65% fat), or a high carbohydrate diet (20% protein, 65% carbohydrate, 15% fat). The normal and high fat diets were given for 7 days, while the high carbohydrate diet was given for only 30 h, because the patients deteriorated clinically on that diet. Values for patient No. 1 are for 2 trials, 5 months apart; values for patient No. 2 are for only 1 trial.

For details, including measurements of other metabolites, see Falk *et al.*[21]

Three patients have been reported who did not respond to the ketonaemic diet. One was the patient reported by Robinson and Sherwood[34] to have a deficiency of PDHC phosphatase. The other was a patient with deficiency of a component common to both the PDHC and the ketoglutarate dehydrogenase complexes, so that they were deficient not only in the oxidation of pyruvate to acetylcoenzyme-A but also in the further oxidation of acetylcoenzyme-A itself[22, 27].

The effects of ketonaemic and high carbohydrate diets in patients with PDHC deficiencies are important both theoretically and clinically. Theoretically, the development of lactic acidosis on a carbohydrate load and

TABLE 13.2 Urinary lactate on a high carbohydrate diet

	Urinary lactate	
	(g/g creatinine)	(mmol/g creatinine)
Day 1	9.6	107
Day 2	15.5	172
Day 3	130.8	1453
Day 4	6.7	74
Control	0.1–0.7	1–8

Urinary lactate was determined after institution of a diet containing 60% of energy as carbohydrate in a boy with mild, intermittent elevations of blood lactate[20], due to PDHC deficiency. On a diet containing 50% of energy as fat, urinary lactate has been normal

its amelioration when fat is provided as an alternate substrate argues for a deficiency in the oxidation of carbohydrate to acetylcoenzyme-A, i.e. in the reaction catalyzed by PDHC, but not in the oxidation of acetylcoenzyme-A. It provides strong evidence for the existence of deficiencies of PDHC activity *in vivo* and therefore for the significance of the deficiencies of PDHC which have been demonstrated in these patients' tissues *in vitro*. Clinically, it provides a relatively easily available procedure to test for PDHC deficiency. If a patient appears better on a high fat than on a normal or a high carbohydrate diet, it is clearly in order to prescribe a high fat diet, whatever the detailed enzymatic deficiency may turn out to be.

PDHC DEFICIENCY AND SPINOCEREBELLAR DISORDERS

In considering the role of abnormalities of PDHC in spinocerebellar degeneration, there is both a clinical and a biochemical problem. The hereditary spinocerebellar disorders have been defined originally on clinical and then on pathological grounds. In investigating these conditions by biochemical means, it is important to group the patients into biologically meaningful categories and to specify the criteria for these categories.

Clinical classification of spinocerebellar degenerations

In his original article on Friedreich's ataxia, it was pointed out that there exists a group of patients with ataxia and long tract signs with a hereditary basis, distinct from patients with syphilis of the central nervous system or with multiple sclerosis[54, 55].

Subsequently, extensive studies were carried out in an attempt to further classify and characterize patients with hereditary ataxias[56-59]. The literature in the area is large, and over forty types of hereditary ataxia have been reported, some occurring in only one family[58, 59]. Systems of classification are not only complex but inconsistent: for instance, the classifications used in the new American textbook by Adams and Victor[58] and in the new British textbook by Brain and Walton[59] differ strikingly. Furthermore, although the clinical pattern in any single family often breeds true, it certainly does not always appear to do so. There are well documented instances where one sibling has one of the commonly accepted syndromes, while a second sibling, with presumably the same genetic abnormality, has another of the 'classic' spinocerebellar degenerations.

In the face of this complexity, we have assumed that if current clinical techniques allow the elucidation of biologically distinct forms of spinocerebellar degenerations, we do not know what they are. We assume that the situation is analogous to that in the early days of the lipidoses, and that combined clinical and laboratory studies will eventually clarify the biology of these disorders. In the absence of clear biological differences, we classify these disorders into the single category of 'spinocerebellar disorder'. Our operational definition of a hereditary spinocerebellar disorder is the disorder in a patient referred with that diagnosis by a physician competent in neurology.

Biochemical studies of spinocerebellar degenerations

The general topic of biochemical abnormalities in spinocerebellar disorders has been the subject of a recent symposium[60] and is beyond the scope of this article. It is worth noting that many inborn errors have been reported to present as spinocerebellar disease, at least in rare cases (Table 13.3). These are clearly a heterogeneous group of disorders.

Pyruvate metabolism in spinocerebellar disorders

Several considerations led to a systematic study of pyruvate oxidation in patients with spinocerebellar disorders. First of all, the first patient in whom PDHC deficiency was demonstrated had cerebellar ataxia as his most prominent clinical abnormality[17]. He has subsequently developed frank optic atrophy and probably reduced vibratory sense in his ankles and mild pes cavus, and must be classified as having a spinocerebellar degeneration[52]. Secondly, it was recognized that disorders in which there is a secondary deficiency of PDHC activity, notably thiamine deficiency[46] and mercurial poisoning[60], can typically present with ataxia and neuropathy as cardinal

TABLE 13.3 Inborn errors which have presented as spinocerebellar disorders[60, 101]

I. *Oxidative disorders*
  A. Pyruvate dehydrogenase complex
  1. Pyruvate dehydrogenase (EC 1.2.4.1)
  2. Lipoate acetyltransferase (EC 2.3.1.12)
  3. Lipoamide dehydrogenase (EC 1.6.4.3)
  B. Cytochrome-b

II. *Lipid disorders*
  A. Phytanic acid hydroxylase – 'Refsum's disease'
  B. ApoLPser – 'Bassen–Kornzweig syndrome'
  C. Arylsulphatase-A (EC 3.1.6.1) – 'Juvenile metachromatic leukodystrophy'
  D. β-galactosidase (EC 3.2.1.23) – 'Juvenile GM_1 gangliosidosis'
  E. Hexosaminidase-A – 'Sandhoff Variant'

III. *Disorders of nitrogenous compounds*
  A. γ-Glutamyl-cysteine synthetase (EC 6.3.2.2)
  B. Hypoxanthine-guanine phosphoribosyl transferase (EC 2.4.2.8) – 'Variant form of Lesch–Nyhan syndrome'
  C. Branched-chain α-keto acid decarboxylases – 'Intermittent maple syrup urine disease'
  D. Neutral amino acid transporter – 'Hartnup disease'

---

clinical findings. Finally, the high frequency of diabetes in patients with spinocerebellar disorders suggests that they might have some primary abnormality of carbohydrate metabolism[58, 59].

To test the hypothesis that abnormalities of pyruvate metabolism occur in a significant proportion of patients with hereditary spinocerebellar degenerations, the ability of small slices of biopsied muscle from a series of such patients to oxidize pyruvate and several other substrates was compared to that from controls[49]. Muscle from patients with hereditary spinocerebellar degenerations oxidized pyruvate to CO_2 more slowly than did muscle from normal controls, or from controls with various myopathies. Low oxidation of pyruvate was also found in muscle from patients with neuropathies of unknown aetiology, but this has not yet been pursued further. Low oxidation of pyruvate was confirmed in intact cultured skin fibroblasts from patients with spinocerebellar degeneration, indicating that the abnormalities were genetically determined rather than secondary to the disease.

Studies with intact fibroblasts required two years to demonstrate the deficiency in cells from three patients. Up to sixteen replicate cultures were studied from each patient and control subject, since high variance otherwise obscured the relatively small differences between patients und controls. Deficiencies of PDHC were demonstrated in disrupted fibroblasts from four patients in the original series[49] and in one other[37]. Activities were about 40–50% of the control mean, just below those in 'asymptomatic' parents of patients with lactate acidosis and PDHC deficiency (Figure 13.1). PDHC activity has also been measured in platelets from fourteen unselected patients who presented to the ataxia clinic at UCLA, and found to be low in six cases[39], in agreement with earlier evidence indicating the existence of abnormalities in pyruvate oxidation in 25–50% of patients with spino-cerebellar degenerations (Figure 13.2). Kark and Rodriguez-Budelli[30] have reported low activities of the lipoamide dehydrogenase (LAD) component of

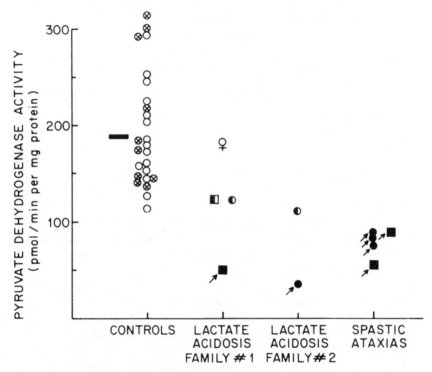

Figure 13.1 PDHC activity in fibroblasts from patients with lactic acidosis and spastic ataxias was measured in disrupted cultured skin fibroblasts by a published radiochemical procedure[93]. Each symbol represents the mean values for up to 14 replicate cultures for a single individual, patient or control: ▬ – mean value for all controls; ○ – clinically normal controls; ⊗ – disease controls; ■ – male patients; – female patients; ▯ – fathers of patients; ◐ – mothers of patients; ♀ – asymptomatic sister of a patient. Family No. 1[20]; family No. 2[19]; spastic ataxias[37]

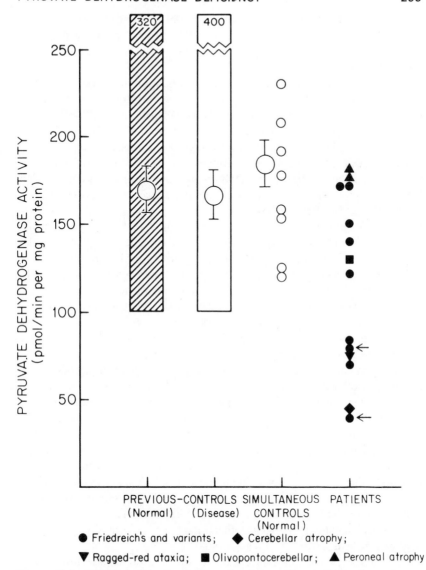

Figure 13.2 PDHC activity in platelets of patients with spastic ataxias and controls was measured radiochemically in platelet-enriched preparations, exactly as described elsewhere[93]. Controls included individuals of both sexes, varying in age from 4 to over 70 years, and included clinically normal individuals as well as individuals with psychiatric and neurological disorders other than hereditary ataxias. The 'previous controls' are those described previously[93]. For more detailed descriptions of the patients and 'simultaneous controls,' see Blass *et al.*[93]

the PDHC and ketoglutarate complexes in about a third of an unselected series of patients with spinocerebellar degenerations and have presented kinetic evidence consistent with a structural mutation of LAD in two of these patients[35].

The existence of deficiencies of pyruvate oxidation in a large proportion of patients with hereditary spinocerebellar degenerations has been confirmed, but whether these reflect hereditary deficiencies of PDHC is controversial[60]. Scott, Farrell and colleagues[61] in Seattle have found low activities of PDHC in 2 of 6 patients with hereditary spinocerebellar degeneration, in agreement with the results discussed above. Stumpf and Parks[62] in Denver have found activity of PDHC within the normal range in platelets from seven patients with 'Friedreich's ataxia'. However, the lowest of their 'controls' was a patient with a 'different form' of spinocerebellar degeneration, namely olivopontocerebellar atrophy (OPCA). If this patient with OPCA is considered a patient with a PDHC deficient spinocerebellar degeneration, then they found low PDHC activity in 3 of 8 patients with hereditary spinocerebellar degenerations, in good agreement with the results reported above. This difference in interpretation is obviously not trivial.

Barbeau and coworkers[63] have studied pyruvate metabolism in a large series of patients with spinocerebellar degenerations. They found reduced clearance of pyruvate in about half of their patients. The clinically normal parents also cleared pyruvate abnormally, at rates midway between the patients and the controls. These studies provide very strong evidence that deficiencies of pyruvate utilization occur in a large proportion of patients with hereditary spinocerebellar degenerations, and that these deficiencies are determined genetically. These investigators also found low activities of PDHC in platelets from 5 of 11 ataxics and low activity of the lipoamide dehydrogenase component of PDHC in the serum of their patients[45]. However, they did not confirm the decrease in PDHC activity and in lipoamide dehydrogenase in cultured fibroblasts. Also, they did not find platelet PDHC deficiency consistently in all affected siblings within the families. They have put forward the view that the deficiency in pyruvate oxidation is secondary to some other metabolic abnormality, perhaps in lipid metabolism, at least in their patients[64].

Several groups have described patients with the clinical syndrome of an unusual spinocerebellar disorder, pathological findings suggestive of both 'Freidreich's ataxia' and 'Leigh's subacute necrotizing encephalo-myelopathy', and elevated levels of pyruvate and related metabolites in blood[65-67].

The consensus at the present time would probably include three statements. First, the spinocerebellar syndromes can be associated with a number of inborn metabolic abnormalities, but deficiencies of pyruvate oxidation are particularly common, occurring in a quarter to a half of these patients. Second, there are at least rare patients in whom these disorders are due to primary genetic abnormalities of PDHC. Third, there is intense controversy over how large a proportion of the 'pyruvate abnormal' patients with hereditary ataxias have primary abnormalities of PDHC.

APPROACHES TO THERAPY

At least nine approaches to the therapy of patients with PDHC deficiency have been suggested[11, 16, 17, 20, 21, 23, 25–27, 32, 34, 52, 68–79], primarily in individual case reports. None has been subjected to the type of double-blind crossover trial in a relatively large series of patients which would be necessary to allow definitive statements about their efficacy and side effects.

Ketonaemic diets

Ketonaemic diets are discussed above, including the rationale and results of initial trial. There are both published and unpublished reports of patients in whom they had a definite if limited effect[21, 25, 26] and of patients in whom they were useless or even deleterious[27, 34, 68]. It is crucial that the diet be adjusted to the particular patient. There should be a high enough proportion of fat and a low enough proportion of carbohydrate in the diet to make the patient ketonaemic, with blood ketones of 1.5–2.0 but not acidotic or hypoglycaemic. In our experience, this is a diet with about 50% of the energy provided by fat, 30% by carbohydrate, and 20% by protein. Any patient in whom there is substantial evidence for a primary deficiency of pyruvate utilization deserves a trial of a high fat diet; this should be done in hospital with careful monitoring of the patient's clinical condition and of blood glucose, pH, and ketones, and the trial should be stopped if the patient deteriorates.

Thiamine

Large doses of thiamine have often been tried in patients with PDHC deficiency, with very variable results. Oral doses of as much as 1–2 g/day have been used[16, 23, 52]. Two rationales have been used to justify this approach.

First, PDHC requires thiamine pyrophosphate as a cofactor, and it is possible that there are patients with low PDHC activity secondary to inadequate binding of the cofactor. Wick and coworkers[23] studied a toddler, who showed a dramatic clinical and biochemical response to oral thiamine (600 mg, 3 i.d.). This patient may have a mutation in PDHC which leads to inadequate binding of thiamine pyrophosphate at normal concentrations of thiamine in tissue, but which becomes normal when tissue levels of thiamine are increased by feeding pharmacological doses. In other words, this patient may have a true 'thiamine-dependent' form of PDHC deficiency. It is problematical whether or not other patients have been identified in whom feeding large doses of thiamine significantly increased saturation of PDHC with thiamine pyrophosphate with resultant increases in PDHC activity[16, 17]. Experimental studies of PDHC from both animals and humans indicate that the enzyme is normally saturated with thiamine pyrophosphate which remains bound to the enzyme very tightly at physiological pH[80].

The second rationale for treatment with pharmacological doses of thiamine is that thiamine pyrophosphate inhibits the regulatory kinase which inactivates PDHC; thus high doses of thiamine might be expected to increase the general level of activity of the complex[23, 81]. This reasoning requires the assumption, as yet untested, that hereditary deficiency of PDHC does not of itself lead to an increase in the proportion of PDHC in the active form. The general efficacy of large doses of thiamine in patients with PDHC deficiency remains unproven, but any patient with PDHC deficiency deserves a trial of high dose thiamine, since the patients of Wick et al.[23] are probably not unique. It should be remembered that the older literature contains reports of significant toxicity associated with the use of large doses of thiamine, including cardiac abnormalities and such neurological signs as convulsions, tremors, and profound weakness[78].

The possible value of thiamine, or thiamine derivatives such as thiamine tetrafurfuryl disulphide, in patients with the clinical diagnosis of 'Leigh's subacute necrotizing encephalomyelopathy' is an extremely complicated issue[82, 83], which is distinct from the possible utility of thiamine and derivatives in patients with the biochemical diagnosis of PDHC deficiency; this topic is outside the scope of this article.

Other treatments

Citrate, in a dose of 500 mg/day orally, was given by Oka et al.[32] to a 5 year old boy with a $2\frac{1}{2}$ year history of episodic vomiting, stupor, and ataxia, and low pyruvate oxidation demonstrated in intact WBC. Treatment with citrate was reported to nearly abolish the incidence of attacks, which recurred immediately citrate was withdrawn. Pyruvate levels remained elevated during treatment with citrate. The quantity of citrate given was very small compared to the normal daily metabolic flux through pyruvate, and no reports replicating this observation have appeared. If this low oral dose of a normal metabolite does prove useful in PDHC deficiency, it provides a very attractive approach to therapy, whatever the mechanism[84].

Steroids were found to reduce the length and severity of attacks of ataxia in the first patient in whom PDHC deficiency was subsequently demonstrated[52]. In this patient, only short courses of steroids were used (3.2 mg of decadron/day for 3 days). Others have confirmed the efficacy of steroids in at least some of their patients[85] and also in patients with other abnormalities of oxidative metabolism[86]. The mechanism of action of steroids in these disorders is unknown. The profound side effects of steroids, particularly in children, makes their use undesirable but they are worth a trial in any patient with PDHC deficiency who appears to be undergoing life threatening deterioration.

Cholinergic agonists were introduced into the care of patients with spinocerebellar degenerations and PDHC deficiency because of studies of pathophysiology, which indicated that cholinergic systems were exquisitely sensitive to conditions which impair pyruvate oxidation[87, 88]. Double-blind crossover studies by Kark and colleagues[69, 70] indicated that there was a small but distinct improvement in coordination in patients treated with the cholinesterase inhibitor physostigmine[69]. This occurred in all patients with hereditary ataxia and PDHC deficiency, but also in some of the ataxic patients with no demonstrated abnormalities of pyruvate metabolism. Barbeau[71, 72] found that treatment with choline or lecithin, which appear to be cholinergic agonists by virtue of their potential role as precusors of acetylcholine[89], was of benefit. These studies are in an early stage, which, it is hoped, is analogous to the earliest use of L-Dopa in Parkinsonism[72]. Neither the optimal drug nor the optimal dosage have been determined nor have truly objective criteria been used for measuring changes in the coordination of the patients. Nevertheless, the possibility of another avenue of treatment in this group of diseases deserves exploration.

The compound dichloroacetate was found in experimental studies to inhibit the kinase which inactivates PDHC[73] and in clinical studies to lower lactate and pyruvate levels in patients with diabetes[74]. Anecdotally, it has been reported to stabilize patients with PDHC deficiency[75, 76]. However, it has been reported to have significant neurotoxicity[90] and its ultimate clinical utility remains questionable.

Evans et al.[77] recently reported beneficial results of treatment with acetozolamide in two boys with attacks of periodic weakness and elevated levels of lactate after a glucose load. Concomitant with treatment with acetozolamide, the frequency of attacks decreased and glucose/lactate tests became normal. Acetozolamide was originally used to treat these patients because they were diagnosed as having periodic paralysis. Its apparent efficacy in these children, both clinically and metabolically, is interesting and indicates that further study of this drug in these disorders is warranted.

The alkalinizing agent THAM, tris(tris(hydroxy)aminomethane), has been used both experimentally and clinically to treat conditions in which carbohydrate oxidation is impaired[79, 91]. Recent experimental studies indicate that pretreatment with THAM can delay the onset of seizures and partially reverse the changes in acetylcholine and cyclic GMP in the brains of animals with anaemic anoxia induced with $NaNO_2$[92]. Clinically, THAM has been extensively studied and reported to mitigate the effects of pulmonary insufficiency, perhaps in part by its effects on removal of CO_2[79, 91]. Infusion of THAM has been tried in one child with PDHC deficiency in terminal coma, but the results were unimpressive[90]. THAM does appear to be relatively safe clinically, and its use in patients with PDHC deficiency, and in particular those with concomitant lactate acidosis, seems worth further investigation.

The use of lipoate in a patient who may have had PDHC deficiency has been discussed above[11]. All of these approaches to the therapy of PDHC deficiency are supported primarily by anecdotal evidence; for all of them, further studies are needed. PDHC deficiency typically represents a partial lesion in a highly regulated and relatively well understood pathway; this disorder therefore represents an opportunity to try to develop rational and effective dietary or medicinal therapy.

DIAGNOSTIC AND OTHER PROBLEMS

There are a number of pressing problems in the study of PDHC deficiencies, particularly in relation to making the diagnosis and specifically in relation to the assay of PDHC activity in small samples of human tissue. As noted above, diagnosis may be suspected on the basis of the response to a carbohydrate load and specifically to a high fat, low carbohydrate diet compared to a high carbohydrate diet. However, definite diagnosis requires demonstration of low PDHC activity in some tissue. Discrepancies have been found in the results of these assays, even among groups studying the same patients. These have led to re-examination of the assays used with a view to identifying potential problems.

One potential difficulty is the marked instability of the [1-^{14}C] pyruvate used as substrate[93, 94]. Silverstein and Boyer[94] demonstrated this instability dramatically. They repurified a sample of [1-^{14}C] pyruvic acid and stored it at $-15\,°C$ in solution for 6 days, thawing it once during that time; at the end of this period less than 2% of the original radioactivity was still associated with pyruvic acid (Table 13.4).

In the author's experience[93], the only way to keep [1-^{14}C] pyruvate reasonably stable is as the bone dry (sodium) salt, stored in a vacuum desiccator over P_2O_5 and KOH (to trap any $^{14}CO_2$ produced by deterioration of the [1-^{14}C] pyruvate). We tested the effects of leaving [1-^{14}C] pyruvate overnight either in solution (frozen at $-20\,°C$) or in the refrigerator at $4\,°C$ as the putatively 'dry' powder in the screw-cap vial provided by the manufacturer. Both of these common ways of storing the pyruvate led to a marked decrease in the apparent activity (Table 13.5). In our experience failure to demonstrate radioactive impurities in [1-^{14}C]

TABLE 13.4   Instability of pyruvic acid

	Radioactivity in pyruvate	
Prior to freezing	54 000 cpm	(100%)
Sample frozen 6 days without thawing	10 335 cpm	(19%)
Sample thawed on days 5 and 6	720 cpm	(1.3%)

Silverstein and Boyer[94] repurified a sample of [1-^{14}C] pyruvate by silicic acid chromatography and stored it in solution at $-15\,°C$ for up to 6 days. They thawed and refroze one portion at 5 days, and then thawed and studied that aliquot and a portion which had been kept frozen for 6 days

pyruvate by thin layer or paper chromatography is not an adequate criterion of purity for these radiochemical assays. Failure to take adequate precautions to maintain the purity of the substrate is, in our experience, the most common cause of difficulties with these assays.

A second potential difficulty is contamination of cultured fibroblasts with mycoplasma (PPLO). These micro-organisms typically have higher specific activity of PDHC than the mammalian cells in the culture[93, 95]. Thus relatively mild contamination with PPLO can obscure PDHC deficiency in a culture. In our experience, contamination of human fibroblast lines is extremely common and is often unrecognized. A large proportion of the cell lines sent to us for study prove to have PPLO, usually unrecognized by the investigator who sent the cells. We now routinely screen cultures for PPLO by fluorescent stains[96] and by the uridine/uracil incorporated method[97]. Testing the cells is tedious but necessary to obtain reliable results. Contaminated lines are discarded or, if no other sample from the patient is available, treated to kill the PPLO[98], passed through at least three passages

TABLE 13.5   Effect of conditions of storage of [1-¹⁴C] pyruvate substrate on apparent PDHC activity

	Apparent PDHC activity	
	(pmol/min per mg protein)	(per cent)
1.		
Standardized substrate	200	100
Refrigerated substrate	89	45
2.		
Standardized substrate	120	100
Aqueous substrate	46	38

The apparent activity of PDHC was measured radiochemically in platelet-enriched preparation from two clinically normal controls[93] using three different types of substrate.
Standardized substrate was stored in a vacuum desiccator at 4 °C over P_2O_5 and KOH, as the bone-dry powder. *Refrigerated substrate* was stored overnight in the refrigerator in the vial supplied by the manufacturer. *Aqueous substrate* was stored overnight at 4 °C in solution at pH 4.0. For details, see Blass *et al.*[93]. Note that with inadequately stored pyruvate, the apparent activity in these normal controls fell into the range for patients with spinocerebellar disease (Figure 13.2)

in culture to reduce the effects of treatment, and then studied if they prove free of PPLO on repeated testing. In our experience, it is not safe to assume that a line is free of PPLO contamination unless it is tested.

A third and very disturbing difficulty is suggested by recent experiments by Gibson and coworkers[92, 99]. They found that relatively mild alterations in growth conditions could increase the ability of the intact cells to oxidize [1-¹⁴C] pyruvate almost three fold. PDHC activity itself was not measured in the experiments. However, these experiments raise the disturbing possibility that even in control cells, we have been measuring only 35% of maximal PDHC activity. If so, then PDHC deficiencies have been identified by comparing 5–15% of maximal normal activity in the patients to 35% of maximal normal activity in the controls. If this is true, it is easy to understand that discrepancies have arisen. The possible permutations of growth conditions for cultured cells are vast, and determining the optimal conditions for maximal expression of PDHC activity in cultured human fibroblasts is a challenging problem.

Finally, study of the protein structure of PDHC will provide the ultimate evidence of inherited defects in the enzyme complex. Thus, purification and study of human PDHC is a challenging problem, but again one which needs to be attacked directly[100].

CONCLUSIONS

It is apparent that studies of inborn errors of carbohydrate catabolism in general and of PDHC deficiency in particular are at an early stage, i.e. about the stage that the study of lipidoses was a quarter century ago. The brain is uniquely dependent on carbohydrate catabolism. Once again, it now appears possible that an assumption held widely 30 years ago is correct, and that constitutional abnormalities in carbohydrate catabolism are not rare in patients with neuropsychiatric disorders with major genetic components. Tools to examine this possibility have been developed by those studying inborn errors. Furthermore, studies of inborn aberrations of carbohydrate catabolism may relate to common forms of diabetes, in which there appear to be abnormalities of the regulation of PDHC and a strong genetic component. There is the exciting prospect that major discoveries in this area may be made in the years ahead.

Acknowledgements

This work was supported by grants from the NIH (HD 06576), the Dystonia Medical Research Foundation, and the Winifred Masterson Burke Relief Foundation.

References

1. Reynolds, S. F. and Blass, J. P. (1976). A possible mechanism for selective cerebellar damage in partial PDH deficiency. *Neurology*, **26**, 625
2. Wieland, O. H., Siess, E. A., Weiss, L., Löffler, G., Patzelt, C., Portenhauser, R., Hartmann, U. and Shirmann, A. (1973). Regulation of the mammalian pyruvate dehydrogenase complex by covalent modification. *Symp. Soc. Exp. Biol.*, **27**, 371
3. Sourkes, T. L. (1962). *Biochemistry of Mental Disease*, pp. 151–155. (New York: Hober-Harper)
4. Siesjö, B. K., Johannnsson, H., Ljunggren, B. and Norberg, K. (1974). Brain dysfunction in cerebral hypoxia and ischemia. In F. Plum (ed.). *Brain Dysfunction in Metabolic Disorders*, pp. 75–112. (New York: Raven Press)
5. Peters, R. A. (1969). Biochemical lesion and its historical development. *Br. Med. Bull.*, **25**, 223
6. Quastel, J. H. (1974). Fifty years of biochemistry. A personal account. *Can. J. Biochem.*, **52**, 71
7. Henneman, D. H., Altschule, M. D. and Goncz, R. M. (1954). Carbohydrate metabolism in brain disease. II. Glucose metabolism in schizophrenic manic depressive and involutional psychoses. *Arch. Intern. Med.*, **54**, 402
8. Kendell, R. E. (1975). *The Role of Diagnosis in Psychiatry*, p. 176. (London: Blackwell Scientific Publications)

9. Erickson, R. J. (1965). Familial infantile lactic acidosis. *J. Pediatr.*, **66,** 1005
10. Israels, S., Haworth, J. C., Courley, B. and Ford, J. D. (1964). Chronic acidosis due to an error in lactate and pyruvate metabolism. *Pediatrics*, **34,** 346
11. Clayton, B. E., Dobbs, R. H. and Patrick, A. D. (1967). Leigh's subacute necrotizing encephalopathy: clinical and biochemical study; therapy with lipoate. *Arch. Dis. Child.*, **42,** 467
12. Hartman, A. F., Wohltmann, H. J., Puckerson, M. C. and Wesley, M. E. (1962). Lactate metabolism-studies of a child with a serious congenital deviation. *J. Pediatr.*, **61,** 165
13. Haworth, J. C., Ford, J. D. and Younoszai, M. K. (1967). Familial chronic acidosis due to an error in lactate and pyruvate metabolism. *Can. Med. Assoc. J.*, **97,** 773
14. Greene, H. L., Schubert, W. K. and Hug, G. (1970). Chronic lactic acidosis of infancy. *J. Pediatr.*, **76,** 853
15. Eastham, R. D. and Jancar, J. (1968). *Clinical Pathology in Mental Retardation*, pp. 159–161. (Bristol: John Wright & Sons)
16. Lonsdale, D., Faulkner, W. R., Price, J. W. and Smeby, R. R. (1969). Intermittent cerebellar ataxia associated with hyperpyruvic acidemia and hyperalaninuria. *Pediatrics*, **43,** 1025
17. Blass, J. P., Avigan, J. and Uhlendorf, B. W. (1970). A defect in pyruvate decarboxylase in a child with an intermittent movement disorder. *J. Clin. Invest.*, **49,** 423
18. Blass, J. P., Lonsdale, D., Uhlendorf, B. W. and Hom, E. (1971). Intermittent ataxia with pyruvate decarboxylase deficiency. *Lancet*, **1,** 1302
19. Blass, J. P., Schulman, J. D., Young, D. S. and Hom, E. (1972). An inherited defect affecting the tricarboxylic acid cycle in a patient with congenital lactic acidosis. *J. Clin. Invest.*, **51,** 1845
20. Cederbaum, S. D., Blass, J. P. and Minkoff, N. *et al.* (1976). Sensitivity to carbohydrate in a patient with familial intermittent lactic acidosis and pyruvate dehydrogenase deficiency. *Pediat. Res.*, **10,** 713
21. Falk, R. E., Cederbaum, S. D., Blass, J. P., Pruss, R. J. and Carrell, R. E. (1976). Ketonic diet in the management of pyruvate dehydrogenase deficiency. *Pediatrics*, **58,** 713
22. Haworth, J. C., Perry, T. L., Blass, J. P., Hansen, S. and Urquhart, N. (1976). Lactic acidosis in three sibs due to defects in both pyruvate dehydrogenase and α-ketoglutarate dehydrogenase complexes. *Pediatrics*, **58,** 564
23. Wick, H., Schweizer, K. and Baumgartner, R. (1977). Thiamine dependency in a patient with congenital lacticacidemia due to pyruvate dehydrogenase deficiency. *Agents Actions*, **7,** 405
24. Strömme, J. H., Borud, O. and Moe, P. J. (1976). Fatal lactic acidosis in a newborn attributable to a congenital defect of pyruvate dehydrogenase. *Pediatr. Res.*, **10,** 60
25. Farrell, D. F., Clark, A. F., Scott, C. R. and Wennberg, R. P. (1975). Absence of pyruvate decarboxylase activity in man: a cause of congenital lactic acidosis. *Science*, **187,** 1082
26. Farrell, D. F. (1977). Pyruvate dehydrogenase (E$_1$) deficiency associated with congenital lactic acidosis. In P. Mittler (ed.). *Research to Practice in Mental Retardation: Biomedical Aspects*, Vol. 3, pp. 147–155. (New York: IASSMD)

27. Robinson, B. H., Taylor, J. and Sherwood, W. G. (1977). Deficiency of dihydrolipoyl dehydrogenase (a component of the pyruvate and α-ketoglutarate dehydrogenase complexes): a cause of congenital chronic lactic acidosis in infancy. *Pediatr. Res.*, **11**, 1198

28. Farmer, T. W., Veath, L., Miller, A. L., O'Brien, J. S. and Rosenberg, R. M. (1973). Pyruvate decarboxylase deficiency in a patient with subacute necrotizing encephalomyelopathy. *Neurology*, **23**, 429

29. Fernandes, J. and Blom, W. (1976). Urinary lactate excretion in normal children and in children with enzyme defects of carbohydrate metabolism. *Clin. Chim. Acta.*, **66**, 345

30. Kark, R. A. P. and Rodriguez-Budelli, M. (1977). The spectrum of ataxia syndromes due to lipoamide dehydrogenase deficiency. *Neurology*, **27**, 359

31. Kuroda, Y., Sweetman, L., Nyhan, W. L., Kling, J. J. and Groshong, T. D. (1978). Abnormal pyruvate and α-ketoglutarate dehydrogenases in a patient with lactic acidemia. *Clin. Res.*, **26**, 176

32. Oka, Y., Matsuda, I., Arashima, S., Anakura, M., Mitsuyama, T. and Nagamatsu, I. (1976). Citrate treatment in a patient with pyruvate decarboxylase deficiency. *Tohoku J. Exp. Med.*, **118**, 131

33. Oka, Y., Matsuda, I., Arashima, S., Anakura, M., Mitsuyama, T. and Nambu, H. (1975). Transient hyperalaninuria and hyperpyruvic acidemia. *Neuropaediatrie*, **6**, 202

34. Robinson, B. H. and Sherwood, W. G. (1975). Pyruvate dehydrogenase phosphatase deficiency. Cause of congenital chronic lactic acidosis in infancy. *Pediatr. Res.*, **9**, 935

35. Rodriguez-Budelli, M. and Kark, R. A. P. (1977). Analysis of a defect in lipoamide dehydrogenase in Friedreich's Ataxia. *Trans. Am. Soc. Neurochem.*, **8**, 116

36. Willems, J. L., Monnens, L. A. H., Trijbels, J. M. F., Sengers, R. A. C. and Veerkamp, J. H. (1974). Pyruvate decarboxylase deficiency in liver. *N. Engl. J. Med.*, **290**, 406

37. Blass, J. P., Kark, R. A. P., Menon, N. and Harris, S. H. (1976). Decreased activities of the pyruvate and ketoglutarate dehydrogenase complexes in fibroblasts from five patients with Friedreich's ataxia. *N. Engl. J. Med.*, **295**, 62

38. Blass, J. P., Cederbaum, S. D. and Dunn, H. G. (1976). Biochemical defect in Leigh's disease. *Lancet*, **1**, 1237

39. Kark, R. A. P. and Rodriguez-Budelli, M. (1979). Pyruvate dehydrogenase deficiencies in six of fourteen unselected patients with spinocerebellar degenerations. *Neurology*, **29**, 126

40. Blass, J. P., Cederbaum, S. D. and Kark, R. A. P. (1976). Pyruvate dehydrogenase deficiency: summary of results with 25 patients. *Trans. Am. Soc. Neurochem.*, **7**, 167

41. Blass, J. P., Cederbaum, S. D. and Kark, R. A. P. (1978). Pyruvate dehydrogenase deficiency. In Sperling, O., deVries, A. (eds.) *Monographs in Human Genetics*. Vol. 9, 12–15. (Basel: S. Karger)

42. Stansbie, D. and Denton, R. M. (Personal communication)

43. Hommes, F. A. (Personal communication)

44. Yoshida, A. (1973). Hemolytic anemia and G6PD deficiency. *Science*, **179**, 532

45. Filla, A., Butterworth, R. F., Geoffrey, G., Lemieux, B. and Barbeau, A. (1978). Serum and platelet lipoamide dehydrogenase in Friedreich's ataxia. *Can. J. Neurol. Sci.*, **5,** 111

46. Blass, J. P., Cederbaum, S. D. and Gibson, G. E. (1976). Clinical and metabolic abnormalities accompanying deficient oxidation of pyruvate. In F. A. Hommes and C. J. Van Den Berg (eds.). *Normal and Pathological Development of Energy Metabolism*, p. 193. (New York: Academic Press)

47. Moncrieff, A. A., Koumides, O. P., Clayton, B. E., Patrick, A. D., Renwick, A. G. G. and Roberts, G. E. (1964). Lead poisoning in children. *Arch. Dis. Child.*, **39,** 1

48. Robinson, B. H., Gall, D. G. and Cutz, E. (1977). Deficient activity of hepatic pyruvate dehydrogenase and pyruvate carboxylase in Reye's syndrome. *Pediatr. Res.*, **11,** 279

49. Kark, R. A. P., Blass, J. P. and Engel, W. K. (1974). Pyruvate oxidation in neuromuscular disease: evidence of a genetic defect in two families with the clinical syndrome of Friedreich's ataxia. *Neurology,* **24,** 964

50. Halestrap, A. P. (1975). Mitochondrial pyruvate carrier. Kinetics and specificity for substrates and inhibitors. *Biochem. J.*, **148,** 85

51. Land, J. M., Mowbray, J. and Clark, J. B. (1976). Control of pyruvate and β-hydroxybutyrate utilisation in rat brain mitochondria and its relevance to phenylketonuria and maple-syrup-urine disease. *J. Neurochem.*, **26,** 823

52. Blass, J. P., Kark, R. A. P. and Engel, W. K. (1971). Clinical studies of a patient with pyruvate-decarboxylase deficiency. *Arch. Neurol.*, **25,** 449

53. Sokoloff, L. (1973). Metabolism of ketone bodies by the brain. *Annu. Rev. Med.*, **24,** 271

54. Friedreich, N. (1863). Ueber degenerative atrophie der spinalen hinterstränge. *Virchows Arch. (Pathol. Anat.)*, **26,** 391

55. Anderman, F. (1976). Nicolaus Friedreich and degenerative atrophy of the posterior columns of the spinal cord. *Can. J. Neurol. Sci.*, **3,** 275

56. Greenfield, J. G. (1954). *The Spinocerebellar Degenerations.* (Springfield, Illinois: Charles C. Thomas)

57. Sjögren, T. (1943). Klinische und erbbiologische untersuchungen über die heredoataxien. *Acta. Psychiatr. Neurol.*, **27,** 1

58. Adams, R. D. and Victor, M. (1977). *Principles of Neurology,* p. 836. (New York: McGraw-Hill)

59. Brain, W. R. and Walton, J. N. (1969). *Diseases of the Nervous System,* p. 589. (Oxford: Oxford University Press)

60. Kark, R. A. P., Rosenberg, R. and Schut, L. (1978). *The Ataxias. Advances in Neurology,* p. 21. (New York: Raven Press)

61. Scott, C. R. and Farrell, D. F. (Personal communication)

62. Stumpf, D. A. and Parks, J. D. (1978). Friedreich's ataxia. I. Normal pyruvate dehydrogenase complex activity in platelets. *Ann. Neurol.*, **4,** 366

63. Barbeau, A., Butterworth, R. F., Ngo, T., Breton, G., Melancon, S., Shapcott, D., Geoffroy, G. and Lemieux, B. (1976). Pyruvate metabolism in Friedreich's ataxia. *Can. J. Neurol. Sci.*, **3,** 379

64. Barbeau, A. (1978). Friedreich's ataxia 1978 – an overview. *Can. J. Neurol. Sci.*, **5,** 161

65. Dunn, H. G. and Dolman, C. L. (1969). Necrotizing encephalomyelopathy: report of a case with relapsing polyneuropathy and hyperalaninemia and with

manifestations resembling Friedreich's ataxia. *Neurology*, **19,** 536

66. Exss, R., Gulotta, F., Kallfelz, H. C. and Völpel, M. (1974). Wernicke's encephalopathy and Friedreich's ataxia. *Neuropaediatrie*, **5,** 162

67. Guggenheim, M. A. and Stumpf, D. A. (1977). Familial metabolic disease with clinicopathological findings of both Leigh's Disease and adult-type spinocerebellar degeneration. *Ann. Neurol.*, **2,** 264

68. DeVivo, D. (Personal communication)

69. Kark, R. A. P., Blass, J. P. and Spence, A. (1975). Physostigmine in patients with familial ataxias. *Neurology*, **27,** 70

70. Rodriguez-Budelli, M. M., Kark, R. A. P., Blass, J. P., Spence, M. A. (1978). Action of physostigmine on inherited ataxias. *Adv. Neurol.*, **21,** 195

71. Barbeau, A. (1978). Emerging treatments: replacement therapy with choline or lecithin in neurological diseases. *Can. J. Neurol. Sci.*, **5,** 157

72. Barbeau, A. (1978). Phosphatidylcholine (Lecithin) in neurologic disorders. *Proc. Am. Acad. Neurol.*, **30,** 81

73. Whitehouse, S., Cooper, R. H. and Randle, P. J. (1974). Mechanism of activation of pyruvate dehydrogenase by dichloroacetate and other halogenated carboxylic acids. *Biochem. J.*, **141,** 761

74. Stacpoole, P. W., Moore, G. W. and Kornhauser, C. M. (1978). Metabolic effects of dichloroacetate in patients with diabetes mellitus and hyperlipoproteinemia. *N. Engl. J. Med.*, **298,** 526

75. Saudubray, J. M. (Personal communication)

76. McKhan, G. (Personal communication)

77. Evans, O. B., Kilroy, A. W. and Fenichel, G. M. (1978). Acetazolamide in the treatment of pyruvate dysmetabolism syndromes. *Arch. Neurol.*, **35,** 302

78. DiPalma, J. R. and Ritchie, D. M. (1977). Vitamin toxicity. *Annu. Rev. Pharmacol. Toxicol.*, **17,** 133

79. Nahas, G. G. (1959). Use of an organic carbon dioxide buffer *in vivo*. *Science*, **26,** 782

80. Blass, J. P. and Lewis, C. A. (1973). Kinetic properties of the partially purified pyruvate dehydrogenase complex of ox brain. *Biochem. J.*, **130,** 31

81. Butler, J. R., Pettit, F. H., Davis, P. F. and Reed, L. J. (1977). Binding of thiamin thiazolone pyrophosphate to mammalian pyruvate dehydrogenase and its effect on kinase and phosphatase activities. *Biochem. Biophys. Res. Commun.*, **74,** 1667

82. Pincus, J. H., Solitare, G. B. and Cooper, J. R. (1976). Thiamine triphosphate levels and histopathology. Correlation in Leigh's disease. *Arch. Neurol.*, **33,** 759

83. Rosenberg, L. E. (1974). Vitamin-responsive inherited diseases affecting the nervous system. In F. Plum (ed.). *Brain Dysfunction in Metabolic Disorders*, p. 271. (New York: Raven Press)

84. Taylor, W. M. and Halperin, M. L. (1973). Regulation of pyruvate dehydrogenase in muscle. Inhibition by citrate. *J. Biol. Chem.*, **248,** 6080

85. Holtzman, D. (Personal communication)

86. Shapira, Y., Cederbaum, S. D., Cancilla, P. A., Nielsen, D. and Lippe, B. M. Familial poliodystrophy, mitochondrial myopathy, and lactate acidemia. *Neurology*, **25,** 614

87. Gibson, G. E., Jope, R. and Blass, J. P. (1975). Reduced synthesis of acetylcholine accompanying impaired oxidation of pyruvic acid in rat brain

minces. *Biochem. J.*, **148**, 17

88. Blass, J. P. and Gibson, G. E. (1977). Cholinergic systems and disorders of carbohydrate catabolism. In D. Jenden (ed.). *Cholinergic Mechanisms and Psychopharmacology*, pp. 791–803. (New York: Plenum Press)

89. Wurtman, R. J., Hirsch, M. J. and Growdon, J. H. (1977). Lecithin consumption raises serum-free-choline levels. *Lancet*, **2**, 68

90. Evans, O. B. (Personal communication)

91. Manfredi, F., Sicker, H. O., Spoto, A. P. and Saltzman, H. A. (1960). Severe carbon dioxide intoxication. Treatment with organic buffer (Trishydroxy-methylaminomethane). *J. Am. Med. Assoc.*, **173**, 999

92. Gibson, G. E., Shimada, M. and Blass, J. P. (1979). Protection by THAM against behavioral and neurochemical effects of hypoxia. *Biochem. Pharm.*, **28**, 747

93. Blass, J. P., Cederbaum, S. D. and Kark, R. A. P. (1976). Rapid diagnosis of pyruvate and ketoglutarate dehydrogenase deficiencies in platelet-enriched preparations from blood. *Clin. Chim. Acta.*, **75**, 21

94. Silverstein, E. and Boyer, P. D. (1964). Instability of pyruvate-C^{14} in aqueous solutions as detected by enzymic assay. *Anal. Biochem.*, **8**, 470

95. Clark, A. F., Farrell, D. F., Burke, W. and Scott, C. R. (1976). The effect of mycoplasma contamination on the *in vitro* assay of pyruvate dehydrogenase activity in cultured fibroblasts. *Clin. Res.*, **24**, 147

96. Chen, T. R. (1977). *In situ* detection of mycoplasma contamination in cell culture by fluorescent Hoechst 33258 stain. *Exp. Cell. Res.*, **104**, 255

97. Schneider, E. L., Stanbridge, E. J. and Epstein, C. J. (1974). Incorporation of ^{3}H-Uridine and ^{14}C-Uracil into RNA. A simple technique for the detection of mycoplasma contamination of cultured cells. *Exp. Cell. Res.*, **84**, 311

98. Mårdh, P. A. (1975). Elimination of mycoplasmas from cell cultures with sodium polyanethol sulphonate. *Nature*, **254**, 515

99. Gibson, G. E. and Vasil, A. (Personal communication)

100. Stansbie, D. (1976). Regulation of the human pyruvate dehydrogenase complex. *Clin. Sci. Mol. Med.*, **51**, 445

101. Johnson, W. G. and Chutorian, A. M. (1977). Inheritance of a new form of hexosaminidase deficiency. *Ann. Neurol.*, **2**, 266

14

Pyruvate carboxylase deficiency, studies on patients and on an animal model system

F. A. Hommes, J. Schrijver and Th. Dias

Pyruvate carboxylase plays a central role in the regulation of the flux of carbon in metabolism[1], not only in liver and kidney tissues with a high activity of pyruvate carboxylase but in other tissues as well, particularly in the developing brain[2]. A deficiency of this enzyme may therefore give rise to a variety of biochemical abnormalities and clinical symptoms. A further complication is the possible relationship with subacute necrotizing encephalomyelopathy (Leigh) or SNE[3]. However, this histopathologically defined disease may be associated with more than one biochemical abnormality[4], such as disorders in thiamine triphosphate metabolism[5], pyruvate dehydrogenase deficiency[6] and pyruvate carboxylase deficiency[7].

In the following discussion a review will be given of the clinical abnormalities, the identification of the enzyme defect, treatment, studies on an animal model of pyruvate carboxylase deficiency, and some of the implications of these studies.

CLINICAL STUDIES

Fourteen patients have been described in whom there is substantial evidence for altered pyruvate carboxylase activity (Table 14.1). The most prominent clinical findings include retarded development, seizures, hypotonia and acidosis. The age of onset of symptoms varies considerably. In four patients symptoms became apparent at birth and in the remaining ten patients within 2 years. The number of patients is too small to draw any conclusions about unequal expression of the deficiency in males or females, although nine of the 14 patients were females. Cases 9 and 10 were siblings, one male and one female.

TABLE 14.1   Patients with pyruvate carboxylase deficiency

Case	Reference	Sex	Siblings affected	Prominent clinical findings	Onset	Blood lactate (mmol/l)	Lactate/ pyruvate ratio	Fasting glucose (mmol/l)	Alanine loading test	Residual pyruvate carboxylase activity
1	7	m.	yes	vomiting, diarrhoea, seizures, retarded development, aminoaciduria	4 months	3.2	normal	3.6	NA	low
2	59, 60	f.	yes	retarded development, hypotonia, rolling eye movements	1 year	0.9–4.0	normal	5.0	normal	20%
3	27	f.	NA	seizures, retarded development, acidosis	birth	3.5	normal	0.8	NA	low
4	25	f.	NA	apathy, spasticity	4 months	8.7	increased	NA	NA	low
5	18	m.	yes	seizures, retarded development, acidosis	8 months	3.5	NA	NA	abnormal	100%; 10%
6	24	f.	no	ataxia, hypotonia	16 months	40	increased	4.4	NA	30%
7	61	NA	NA	NA	NA	high	NA	NA	NA	low
8	62	f.	no	seizures, retarded development, hypotonia	10 weeks	3.2	normal	4.8	abnormal	low
9	23	m.	yes	hypotonia, acidosis	birth	9.4	increased	normal	NA	2%
10	23	f.	yes	hypertonia, acidosis	birth	7.1	increased	normal	NA	10%
11	20, 63	f.	yes	retarded development, acidosis, hypotonia, rolling eye movements	10 months	4.2	increased	4.3	normal	20%
12	64	f.	NA	retarded development, acidosis, hypotonia, strabismus	birth	8.1	increased	1.1	NA	low
13	35	f.	NA	seizures, retarded development, acidosis	3 months	11.2	increased	4.6	NA	6%
14	63	m.	no	vomiting, seizures, hypotonia, ataxia, retarded development, nystagmus	29 months	10.0	increased	normal	NA	45%

NA = no information available

The clinical symptoms are certainly not specific for pyruvate carboxylase deficiency. They may be observed in a large variety of inborn errors of metabolism. This necessitates special clinical and laboratory tests to ascertain the diagnosis. As a preliminary screening, determination of the urinary lactate concentration can be helpful since it is a good indicator of blood lactate concentration[8]. A recently developed rapid test makes this screening easy to perform[9]. All reported cases of pyruvate carboxylase deficiency showed increased blood lactate levels with normal to increased lactate/pyruvate ratios. An increased blood lactate concentration is not specific for pyruvate carboxylase deficiency and is expected with all disturbances in pyruvate utilization.

It is surprising in this defect of gluconeogenesis, that severe fasting hypoglycaemia has only been reported in two cases. This is in sharp contrast to other defects of gluconeogenesis, i.e. glucose-6-phosphatase deficiency[10], fructose-1,6-diphosphatase deficiency[11] and phosphoenol pyruvate carboxykinase deficiency[12], which are invariably associated with severe hypoglycaemia.

An *in vivo* test for defects of gluconeogenesis is given by the alanine loading test, described by Fernandes and Blom[13]. Only limited information on such tests carried out on pyruvate carboxylase deficient patients is available. A normal alanine clearance from the blood after an oral alanine load was found in case 2, but blood lactate and blood glucose levels were not reported. Case 5 showed an abnormal increase in blood lactate after an oral alanine load but no blood glucose values were reported. An oral alanine loading test in case 11 did not cause an increase in the blood lactate level but blood glucose values are lacking. Case 8 is the only one where no increase of blood glucose could be demonstrated after an oral intake of alanine. No information is available on the other cases.

ENZYME STUDIES

Pyruvate carboxylase is a notoriously difficult enzyme to assay. It is highly dependent for its activity on the presence of the allosteric activator, acetyl coenzyme A. In the absence of this activator, the activity is only 20% of that of the fully activated enzyme, but high, unphysiological concentrations of K^+, pyruvate, ATP and HCO_3^- are required to obtain this full activity[14]. Half maximal activation by acetyl coenzyme A with the purified human enzyme is obtained at a concentration of 15 μmol/l[14]. In whole homogenates a considerably higher concentration of the activator is needed[15]. Several investigators have reported inactivation of human liver pyruvate carboxylase at lower temperatures[14-16]. Since pyruvate carboxylase is a mitochondrial enzyme[17], extraction of the tissue poses another pitfall. It is therefore not surprising that a wide range of activities of pyruvate carboxylase in normal human liver has been reported, namely from 0.2–14.6 (μmol/min)/g wet weight[7, 18-25].

In order to clarify some of these discrepancies, optimal conditions for storage and extraction of the tissue and assay of the enzyme were determined. The results are shown in Table 14.2. The human enzyme proved to be rather unstable at temperatures below 20 °C. Similar results were obtained with the enzyme from rat liver. Part of the large variation reported for the activity of pyruvate carboxylase in control human liver can certainly be explained by this instability of the enzyme. The nutritional status of the patient at the time the liver sample was taken may furthermore contribute to this variability[26].

TABLE 14.2 Inactivation of human liver pyruvate carboxylase at low temperatures

Storage	Temperature of homogenization medium	Pyruvate carboxylase activity (mean ± SEM)		n
		μmol/min/g wet weight	μmol/min/mg protein	
Fresh	room temp.	4.9 ± 1.4	26.4 ± 4.4	4
Fresh	0 °C	0.1	0.9	1
Dry at −60 °C	room temp.	0.1; 0.2	0.5; 1.7	2
Dry at −60 °C	0 °C	0.2	1.1	1
At −60 °C in medium	room temp.	5.1 ± 0.7	16.2 ± 2.7	7
At −60 °C in medium	0 °C	0.1	0.3	1

Liver tissue (20 mg/ml) was homogenized in a Potter-Elvehjem homogenizer in 10 mmol/l tris–HCl (pH 7.4), 1 mmol/l EDTA, 2 mmol/l dithiothreitol (DTT) and 0.1% Triton X-100. Pyruvate carboxylase was assayed according to Utter and Keech[65] at 30 °C in a medium containing 175 mmol/l tris–HCl, 35 mmol/l $NaH^{14}CO_3$ (specific activity 600 dpm/nmol), 10 mmol/l $MgCl_2$, 2 mmol/l DTT, 0.5 g/l bovine serum albumin, 4 mmol/l ATP, 10 mmol/l acetyl phosphate, 1 mmol/l CoA-SH, 10 mmol/l pyruvate, 10 U/ml phosphotransacetylase and 4.4 U/ml citrate synthase. After preincubation for 10 min, the reaction was started by the addition of homogenate to a final concentration of 2 mg/ml. The reaction was terminated by the addition of 0.1 ml 25% $HClO_4$. After gassing with carbon dioxide for 45 s and centrifugation, the supernatant was counted. Tissue samples were stored for at least 2 weeks. The storage medium for pyruvate carboxylase consisted of 2 mol/l sucrose, 1 mmol/l EDTA, and 50 mmol/l potassium phosphate, pH 7.4[22]

Grover et al.[18, 19] reported a normal pyruvate carboxylase activity in a liver biopsy of their patient (case 5) but a decreased activity at autopsy. It has been suggested that this decreased activity is not the primary cause of the disease but results from the disease process itself. The specificity of this decrease remains unexplained.

Brunette et al.[27] and Delvin et al.[28] observed two forms of pyruvate carboxylase activity in human liver, differing in their K_m for pyruvate. The low K_m component was supposed to be missing in their patient (case 3). The interpretation of the kinetic data has however been criticized by Scrutton and White[14]. A biphasic response to the pyruvate concentration in Lineweaver–Burk plots can easily be explained in control human liver by the specific kinetics of pyruvate carboxylase[14, 15].

It is difficult to deduce from the data in the literature whether or not all necessary precautions have been taken for the assay of pyruvate carboxylase activity in liver biopsies of the patients summarized in Table 14.1. How far control biopsies have been assayed on the same day, using the same solutions and presumably under the same conditions, cannot be evaluated. However this is essential to obtain reliable data. One patient formerly diagnosed as pyruvate carboxylase deficient[29], proved to have a normal activity when assayed under better conditions for storage and homogenization of the tissue[15], although the acetyl coenzyme A dependency has not been tested as yet. This patient has been under thiamine therapy for a number of years, which may have influenced his gluconeogenic capacity (see below).

TREATMENT

Early attempts at treatment of pyruvate carboxylase deficiency have been focussed on decreasing the blood lactate levels. Following reports by Clayton et al.[30] and Crome and Stern[31], it was demonstrated that lipoic acid administration effectively decreased the blood lactic acid concentration[7, 18, 20]. Some clinical improvement was observed as well but the treatment was ineffective in that it did not stop further deterioration of the patient. The use of high doses of lipoic acid for a prolonged period of time is not without danger because of possible liver damage.

A more rational approach has been proposed by Tang and coworkers[25]. Since pyruvate carboxylase is not only of importance for gluconeogenesis but for effective operation of the Krebs cycle as well, Tang et al.[25] hypothesized that oxaloacetate deficiency may play an important role in the pathogenesis of the symptoms. If so, the 4-carbon dicarboxylic acid pool should be increased. This has been accomplished by supplementation of the diet with L-glutamine. Large doses of vitamin B_6 were also given, to ensure adequate rates of transamination. A similar approach has been reported, using aspartic acid[32]. Substantial decreases of blood lactate have been observed as well as an improvement of the clinical condition. This does not seem to be a general finding as case 10 did not respond at all. The synthesis of oxaloacetate via the pyruvate carboxylase catalysed reaction is important not only in liver, but in brain as well[2]. There is a limitation to the use of glutamate and aspartate owing to the restricted permeability of these amino acids in several tissues. This has been demonstrated for liver[33] and brain[34]. The non-essential amino acids, especially those involved in neurotransmission, are kept out of the brain very effectively. It is therefore doubtful whether the glutamate or aspartate therapy can ever be effective in correcting the biochemical abnormalities in the central nervous system. The theoretical basis of the glutamate/aspartate approach is nevertheless sound, particularly since De Vivo et al.[35] demonstrated a decreased concentration of oxaloacetate, citrate, α-ketoglutarate, malate and aspartate in a liver biopsy of their patient (case 11). The calculated oxaloacetate concentration was about 10% of that of a control liver biopsy, suggesting that the Krebs cycle activity was severely limited by the decreased availability of oxaloacetate. In support of this conclusion, an intravenous glucose tolerance test gave rise to the synthesis of ketone bodies.

Another attempt to combat the lactic acidaemia consists of the administration of high doses of thiamin, as originally suggested by Lonsdale et al.[36]. The absorption of thiamin from the intestinal tract is limited, however. This explains the use of thiamin propyldisulphide and thiamin tetrafurfuryldisulphide[37] which are absorbed more easily[38]. In some cases, with or without administration of glutamate or aspartate (cases 6 and 8), a decrease of blood lactate was observed but not in others (4, 7 and 10). Improvement of the clinical condition has not been reported and at best further deterioration of the patient has been halted.

Considerable controversy exists regarding the mechanism of action of such a treatment with pharmacological doses of thiamin. Cooper et al.[5] have suggested that the pathology in some patients can be explained by a deficiency of thiamin triphosphate in brain, due to the presence in body fluids of these patients of an inhibitor of ATP:thiamin pyrophosphate phosphotransferase, the enzyme responsible for the synthesis of thiamin triphosphate. It has recently been demonstrated that the methods currently in use to measure the activity of this enzyme are inadequate[39]. It has been suggested that only bound endogenous thiamin diphosphate is phosphorylated to thiamin triphosphate[40] but this is unlikely since the synthesis far exceeds the endogenous amount of total thiamin[41-43]. The nature of the inhibitor, if it exists, remains unclear. Any application as a diagnostic tool has to wait until a reliable assay system has been worked out in more detail. It cannot be decided at present whether thiamin exerts its effect via thiamin triphosphate.

A beneficial effect of thiamin in lowering the blood lactate concentration could be explained by an increased concentration of thiamin disphosphate in the mitochondria resulting in more of the active form of pyruvate dehydrogenase[44, 45]. The impressive and rapid improvement observed in one case (case 3) after thiamin administration seems to be rather unique. Nevertheless it should be tried in all cases of pyruvate carboxylase deficiency.

Conversion of the inactive, phosphorylated form of pyruvate dehydrogenase into the active, dephosphorylated, form of the enzyme can also be accomplished by dichloroacetate[46, 47]. It has been applied to patients with diabetes mellitus to lower blood lactate levels[48]. Although it is highly effective in combating lactacidaemia, the use in patients with pyruvate carboxylase deficiency is not without danger as it has been shown that dichloroacetate decreases the blood glucose level significantly, both in starved animals[49] and in diabetic humans[48]. It does not affect blood sugar levels in normally fed rats[50]. Inhibition of gluconeogenesis by dichloroacetate, presumably at the level of glyceraldehyde-3-phosphate dehydrogenase, has been demonstrated[51]. Since gluconeogenesis is decreased in patients with pyruvate carboxylase deficiency, extreme care should be taken in using this drug in such patients.

ANIMAL MODEL

In view of the conflicting reports on the effect of thiamin and of glutamate/aspartate therapy in patients with pyruvate carboxylase deficiency, it was considered worthwhile to develop an animal model to study the effect of these agents in more detail. Pyruvate carboxylase is a biotin containing enzyme. By making rats biotin depleted, they will become deficient in pyruvate carboxylase activity.

Biotin depletion can be induced in rats by feeding them a biotin deficient diet, supplemented with avidin to bind biotin synthesized by the intestinal flora. It proved difficult to induce sufficient biotin deficiency in rats by this method, as judged by the residual pyruvate carboxylase activity in liver and brain (25% and 60% respectively). More extreme deficiency could be induced in newborn rats by feeding pregnant rats the biotin deficient, avidin rich diet from the moment of conception. This procedure resulted in 10% and 30% residual pyruvate carboxylase activity in liver and brain respectively[52].

Biotin deficient rats show a normal distribution of thiamin and its phosphate esters in the brain (Table 14.3). Intraperitoneal treatment of rats with thiamin for 3 consecutive days at a dose of 100 mg per kg body weight per 24 h increased the level of thiamin and its phosphate esters in certain

TABLE 14.3 Thiamin and its phosphate esters in brain of control biotin deficient rats. Amounts are given in $\mu g/g$ wet weight (mean $\pm$ SEM) or as percentage of total thiamin

	Control rats	Biotin deficient rats
Whole brain ($\mu g/g$ wet weight)	5.12 ± 0.21 ($n = 9$)	4.80 ± 0.44 ($n = 12$)
Thiamin + thiamin monophosphate (%)	17.2 ± 1.0	17.9 ± 1.7
Thiamin diphosphate (%)	78.0 ± 2.5	76.7 ± 2.2
Thiamin triphosphate (%)	4.8 ± 0.8	5.4 ± 0.3
Cerebrum ($\mu g/g$ wet weight)	5.05 ± 0.28 ($n = 5$)	5.02; 5.07
Cerebellum ($\mu g/g$ wet weight)	3.26 ± 0.48 ($n = 5$)	4.04; 3.15
Stem ($\mu g/g$ wet weight)	3.27 ± 0.32 ($n = 5$)	3.85; 2.82

tissues, although 75% of the thiamin injected can be recovered from the urine within 24 h. The total thiamin content of liver increased from $0.124 \pm 0.004 \mu g$ per mg protein ($n = 14$) to $0.278 \pm 0.049 \mu g$ per mg protein ($n = 10$). The distribution of thiamin and its phosphate esters in liver mitochondria is shown in Table 14.4. Treatment did not, however, increase the total thiamin content of the brain [$5.22 \pm 0.21 \mu g$ per gramme wet weight ($n = 9$) and $4.96 \mu g$ per gramme wet weight ($n = 2$) for normal rat brain and brain of thiamin-treated rats respectively].

To explain the effect of thiamin on lowering the blood lactate and pyruvate levels, three possibilities were considered:

(1) Stimulation of lactate excretion in urine.
(2) Stimulation of gluconeogenesis from lactate.

TABLE 14.4 The distribution of thiamin and its phosphate esters in liver mitochondria of control and thiamin treated rats. Amounts are given in μg per mg protein $\pm$ SEM

Rats	Thiamin + Thiamin monophosphate	Thiamin disphosphate	Thiamin triphosphate
Control ($n = 3$)	0.010 ± 0.001	0.100 ± 0.010	0.008 ± 0.001
Thiamin treated ($n = 7$)	0.039 ± 0.002	0.182 ± 0.019	0.013 ± 0.001

Thiamin was given intraperitoneally (100 mg/kg body weight) for 3 consecutive days prior to sacrifice. Liver mitochondria, suspended in 0.25 mol/l sucrose and 0.1 mmol/l EDTA were extracted at 0 °C with 4 ml 18% $HClO_4$ per ml mitochondrial suspension. After neutralization to pH 5.0, the sample was centrifuged and the supernatant applied to a Dowex 1 x 4 column for separation of thiamin and its phosphates according to Koike and Yusa[66]. Thiamin and its phosphate esters were determined fluorimetrically according to Cooper et al.[5]

(3) Stimulation of pyruvate oxidation at the level of pyruvate dehydrogenase.

Tables 14.5 and 14.6 show the blood and urine lactate concentrations in control and biotin deficient rats and the effect of thiamin administration. A significant decrease of blood lactate concentration was found after fed, normal rats had been treated with thiamin ($p < 0.0005$). This effect of thiamin could not be observed in fasted normal rats. The opposite was found in the biotin deficient rats. Administration of thiamin did not result in a decrease of the blood lactate level in fed, biotin deficient rats, but was significantly lower ($p < 0.0005$) in the fasting state. An increased excretion of lactate in the urine could be observed in normal fed rats treated with thiamin ($p < 0.025$), but not in the biotin deficient rats.

Thiamin can therefore, under certain conditions at least, lower the blood lactate level. Increased excretion in the urine seems to be partly responsible for this phenomenon. In view of the low concentration of lactate in the urine, it is doubtful whether this can fully explain the decreased blood lactate level.

Ketone bodies in the fed and fasting state are considerably higher in the biotin deficient rats than in normal rats (Table 14.7). This is to be expected because of the limited availability of oxaloacetate in pyruvate carboxylase deficiency.

An increased intake of aspartate was supplied with the drinking-water (1 g/l). The rats received in this way 135 ± 15 (μmol/24 h)/100 g body weight of aspartate. A change in blood glucose was not observed, a further indication that oxaloacetate is not limiting gluconeogenesis (c.f. De Vivo et al.[35]). In the rat about 90% of phosphoenolpyruvate carboxykinase is localized in

TABLE 14.5 The effect of thiamin on blood glucose, lactate and pyruvate of normal and biotin deficient rats. Concentrations are given in mmol/l ± SEM

Treatment	Fed rats				Fasted rats			
	Glucose	Lactate (L)	Pyruvate (P)	L/P ratio	Glucose	Lactate (L)	Pyruvate (P)	L/P ratio
None	6.98 ± 0.13	1.90 ± 0.34	0.13 ± 0.01	12.8 ± 0.8	5.45 ± 0.07	1.09 ± 0.07	0.09 ± 0.01	12.3 ± 0.6
n	15	26	18	18	7	9	9	9
Thiamin	7.03 ± 0.03	1.23 ± 0.12	0.13 ± 0.01	10.6 ± 1.0	5.56 ± 0.34	1.19 ± 0.15	0.19 ± 0.01	8.6 ± 1.0
n	4	11	6	6	6	9	6	6
Biotin deficient	4.27 ± 0.51	4.70 ± 1.03	0.19 ± 1.0	21.3 ± 3.0	2.98 ± 0.29	3.31 ± 0.49	0.16 ± 0.02	21.1 ± 2.3
n	14	23	14	14	10	14	13	12
Biotin deficient + thiamin	4.59 ± 0.25	4.09 ± 0.59	0.20 ± 0.20	19.2 ± 1.5	2.68 ± 0.46	1.19 ± 0.14	0.07 ± 0.03	18.4 ± 2.3
n	6	12	6	6	8	6	6	6

Rats were fasted for at least 12 h. Thiamin was administered as described in Table 3

TABLE 14.6 The effect of thiamin on the lactate concentration in the urine of normal and biotin deficient fed rats. Concentrations are given in (μmol/24 h)/100 g body weight. Thiamin was administered as described in Table 14.3

Treatment	Lactate (L)	Creatinine (C)	L/C ratio	n
Control	0.89 ± 0.07	28.3 ± 3.1	0.034 ± 0.003	12
Thiamin	1.39 ± 0.22	28.9 ± 3.0	0.046 ± 0.005	10
Biotin deficient	40.0 ± 13.9	5.6 ± 1.8	9.16 ± 1.74	4
Biotin deficient + thiamin	28.8 ± 8.0	5.8 ± 1.4	5.11 ± 1.02	4

the cytoplasm[17], with apparently sufficient oxaloacetate or its precursors present to maintain gluconeogenesis. In the mitochondrial compartment, however, oxaloacetate seems to be deficient because blood β-hydroxybutyrate dropped from 4.17 ± 0.55 mmol/l ($n = 13$) to 2.19 ± 0.17 mmol/l ($n = 5$) when aspartate was supplied in the drinking water.

When normal rats were injected with thiamin an increase of about 40% was observed in the rate of gluconeogenesis in the isolated liver cells (Table 14.8). Hardly any glucose production could be demonstrated in hepatocytes isolated from biotin deficient rats, but there was a significant increase in gluconeogenesis after the biotin deficient rats had been pretreated with thiamin. These results, and the data obtained on blood in the intact animal, are consistent with the hypothesis that thiamin stimulates gluconeogenesis. The mechanism of this activation remains unknown.

It has previously been suggested that the beneficial effects of high doses of thiamin are at least in part due to maintenance of the pyruvate dehydrogenase complex in its active form, thus facilitating the oxidation of pyruvate[45].

CONCLUSIONS

Although a prenatal diagnosis of pyruvate carboxylase deficiency has not yet been reported, the recent demonstration of the presence of this enzyme in cultured fibroblasts opens up this possibility[53-55]. Detailed further studies are required because some strains showed virtually no activity, while the activity of other strains of cells was variable, possibly due to genetic polymorphism[55].

Diagnosis at the enzymatic level remains essential for this disease, as the clinical symptoms and autopsy findings resemble those of pyruvate dehydrogenase deficiency[4, 6]. This is perhaps not surprising since the activity

TABLE 14.7 Effect of thiamin on blood ketone bodies of control and biotin deficient rats. Concentrations are given in mmol/l ± SEM. Thiamin was administered as described in Table 14.3

	Fed rats			Fasted rats		
	β-Hydroxybutyrate	Acetoacetate	βOH/Acac	β-Hydroxybutyrate	Acetoacetate	βOH/Acac
None	0.08 ± 0.01	0.03 ± 0.01	2.7 ± 0.52	1.31 ± 0.19	0.44 ± 0.07	3.16 ± 0.26
n	12	12	12	8	7	7
Thiamin	0.09 ± 0.02	0.04 ± 0.01	2.7 ± 0.32	0.75 ± 0.13	0.24 ± 0.03	2.87 ± 0.51
n	4	4	4	5	3	3
Biotin deficient	1.09 ± 0.25	1.16 ± 0.32	1.22 ± 0.37	4.17 ± 0.55	1.54 ± 0.15	3.48 ± 0.49
n	8	8	8	13	13	13
Biotin deficient + thiamin	0.60 ± 0.10	0.58 ± 0.10	1.19 ± 2.9	4.39 ± 2.07	1.56 ± 0.38	3.19 ± 1.26
n	6	6	6	3	3	3

TABLE 14.8 The effect of thiamin on gluconeogenesis by isolated liver cells of fasted control and biotin deficient rats. The rates are given in (nmol glucose/h)/mg protein

Treatment	Substrate	
	Endogenous	Lactate
None	—	172.7
	80.9	208.6
	—	207.5
Thiamin	58.5	337.7
		234.8
Biotin deficient	10	10
Biotin deficient + thiamin	10	47.6

Liver hepatocytes were prepared from 24 h fasted rats according to the method of Berry and Friend[67]. Cells (15–30 mg protein) were incubated for 60 min at 37 °C in 5 ml of Krebs–Ringer solution after gassing with 95% O_2/5% CO_2 in the presence of 10 mmol/l lactate and 1 mmol/l pyruvate. The reaction was terminated by the addition of 1 ml 18% $HClO_4$. After neutralization and centrifugation, glucose was determined in the supernatant. Thiamin was administered as described in Table 14.3

of pyruvate carboxylase shows regional variation in brain[52] similar to pyruvate dehydrogenase deficiency[56]. Rigorous care should be taken to standardize and optimize the conditions of storage and homogenization of the tissue, as well as the assay procedure. As with the enzymatic diagnosis of other inborn errors of metabolism, the assay of the enzyme should not be limited to a determination of the overall activity, usually determined under optimal conditions, but should include a determination of the K_m values of the substrates. An additional source of aberrant kinetic behaviour of pyruvate carboxylase activity is given by the allosteric activator acetyl coenzyme A. This aspect has not been explored at all in any of the reported cases of pyruvate carboxylase deficiency and could be responsible for the variation in residual pyruvate carboxylase activity.

Studies on the animal model have suggested that administration of high doses of thiamin may be beneficial to patients with pyruvate carboxylase deficiency. First by decreasing the blood lactate level via interaction at the level of pyruvate dehydrogenase, and second by stimulating gluconeogenesis via an unknown mechanism. It should be noted that thiamin only penetrates the brain very slowly. The thiamin content of the brain did not increase after treatment of rats with thiamin for 3 consecutive days. Similar observations were made by Itokawa on rabbits[57]. This casts some doubt on the efficiency of thiamin administration in improving cerebral thiamin triphosphate deficiency[5, 37]. None of the patients summarized in Table 14.1 showed neurological improvement after thiamin therapy.

The case of glutamate/aspartate deserves further discussion. It suffers from the same disadvantage as thiamin since these amino acids reach the brain only slowly. They do have a profound effect on the mitochondrial oxaloacetate pool, as exemplified by the decrease in blood ketone bodies in the biotin deficient rats after aspartate supplementation. It should be noted that in man, 80% of phosphoenol pyruvate carboxykinase is localized in the mitochondrion[17, 58]. In man, glutamate/aspartate may therefore have a greater effect on gluconeogenesis.

Acknowledgement

The investigations reported here were supported in part by the Foundation for Medical Research (FUNGO) by grants from the Netherlands Organization for the Advancement of Pure Research (ZWO).

References

1. Denton, R. M. (1979). Pathways and regulation of pyruvate metabolism. This volume, p. 209
2. Land, J. M. and Clark, J. B. (1975). The changing pattern of brain mitochondrial substrate utilization during development. In F. A. Hommes and C. J. van den Berg (eds.). *Normal and Pathological Development of Energy Metabolism*, pp. 155–167. (London: Academic Press)
3. Leigh, D. (1951). Subacute necrotizing encephalomyelopathy in an infant. *J. Neurol. Neurosurg. Psychiatry*, **14**, 216
4. Blass, J. P., Cederbaum, S. D. and Dunn, H. G. (1976). Biochemical abnormalities in Leigh's disease. *Lancet*, **1**, 1237
5. Cooper, J. R., Itokawa, Y. and Pincus, J. H. (1969). Thiamin triphosphate deficiency in subacute necrotizing encephalomyelopathy. *Science*, **164**, 72
6. Farmer, F. W., Veath, L., Miller, A. L., O'Brien, J. S. and Rosenberg, R. M. (1973). Pyruvate decarboxylase deficiency in familial intermittent cerebellar ataxia. *Neurology*, **23**, 429
7. Hommes, F. A., Polman, H. A. and Reerink, J. D. (1968). Leigh's encephalomyelopathy: an inborn error of gluconeogenesis. *Arch. Dis. Child.*, **43**, 423
8. Daalmans-De Lange, M. M. and Hommes, F. A. (1974). The urinary lactate excretion in children. *Helv. Paediatr. Acta*, **29**, 599
9. Daalmans-De Lange, M. M. and Hommes, F. A. (1978). A rapid screening test for lactaciduria. *J. Clin. Chem. Clin. Biochem.*, **16**, 349
10. Brown, B. I. and Brown, D. H. (1968). Glycogen-storage diseases: Types I, III, IV, V, VII and unclassified glycogenoses. In *Carbohydrate Metabolism and its Disorders*, **Vol. II**, p. 23 (New York: Academic Press)
11. Pagliara, A. S., Karl, I. E., Keating, J. P., Brown, B. I. and Kipnis, D. M.

(1972). Hepatic fructose-1,6-diphosphatase deficiency. A cause of lactic acidosis and hypoglycemia in infancy. *J. Clin. Invest.*, **51**, 2115

12. Hommes, F. A., Bendien, K., Elema, J. D., Bremer, H. J. and Lombeck, I. (1976). Two cases of phosphoenolpyruvate carboxykinase deficiency. *Acta Paediatr. Scand.*, **65**, 233

13. Fernandes, J. and Blom, W. (1974). The intravenous L-alanine tolerance test as a means for investigating gluconeogenesis. *Metabolism*, **23**, 1149

14. Scrutton, M. C. and White, M. D. (1974). Purification and properties of human liver pyruvate carboxylase. *Biochem. Med.*, **9**, 271

15. Schrijver, J. (1978). Thesis, University of Groningen

16. Marsac, C., Saudubray, J. M., Moncion, A. and Leroux, J. P. (1976). Development of gluconeogenic enzymes in the liver of human newborns. *Biol. Neonate*, **28**, 317

17. Wieland, O., Evertz-Prüsse, E. and Stukowski, B. (1968). Distribution of pyruvate carboxylase and phosphoenolpyruvate carboxykinase in human liver. *FEBS Lett.*, **2**, 26

18. Grover, W. D., Auerbach, V. H. and Patel, M. S. (1972). Biochemical studies and therapy in subacute necrotizing encephalomyopathy (Leigh). *J. Pediatr.*, **81**, 39

19. Gruskin, A. B., Patel, M. S., Linshaw, M., Ettenger, R., Huff, D. and Grover, W. (1973). Renal function studies and kidney pyruvate carboxylase in subacute necrotizing encephalomyelopathy (Leigh's Syndrome). *Pediatr. Res.*, **7**, 832

20. Maesaka, H., Kaniga, K., Misugi, K. and Tada, K. (1976). Hyperalaninemia, hyperpyruvicemia and lactic acidosis due to pyruvate carboxylase deficiency of the liver, treatment with thiamin and lipoic acid. *Eur. J. Pediatr.*, **122**, 159

21. Murphy, J. V. (1974). Efficacy of recommended therapeutic regimes in Leigh's disease. *Dev. Med. Child. Neurol.*, **16**, 362

22. Robinson, B. H., Gall, D. G. and Cutz, E. (1977). Deficient activity of hepatic pyruvate dehydrogenase and pyruvate carboxylase in Reye's syndrome. *Pediatr. Res.*, **11**, 279

23. Saudubray, J. M., Marsac, C., Charpentier, C., Cathelineau, L., Besson Leaud, M. and Leroux, J. P. (1976). Neonatal congenital lactic acidosis with pyruvate carboxylase deficiency in two siblings. *Acta Paediatr. Scand.*, **65**, 717

24. Tada, K., Sugita, K., Fujikawi, K., Kesaki, T., Takada, G. and Omura, K. (1973). Hyperalaninemia with pyruvicemia in a patient suggestive of Leigh's encephalomyelopathy. *Tohoku. K. Exp. Med.*, **109**, 13

25. Tang, T. T., Good, Th. A., Dyken, P. R., Johnson, S. D., McCready, S. R., Sy, S. T., Lardy, H. A. and Rudolph, F. B. (1972). Pathogenesis of Leigh's encephalomyelopathy. *J. Pediatr.*, **81**, 189

26. Störmer, B. and Staib, B. (1971). Activities of pyruvate carboxylase, phosphoenolpyruvate carboxykinase and pyruvate kinase of New Zealand obese mice liver during different phases of diabetes after starvation, cortisol and insulin treatment. In H. D. Söling and B. Willms (eds.). *Regulation of Gluconeogenesis*, pp. 63–65 (Stuttgart: Thieme Verlag)

27. Brunette, M. G., Delvin, E., Hazel, B. and Scriver, C. R. (1972). Thiamin responsive lactic acidosis in a patient with deficient low K_m pyruvate carboxylase activity in liver. *Pediatrics*, **50**, 702

28. Delvin, E., Scriver, C. R. and Neal, J. C. (1974). Pyruvate carboxylase in human liver. Apparent loss of a component of catalytic activity in a form of lactic acidosis with hypoglycemia. *Biochem. Med.*, **10**, 97

29. De Groot, C. J., Jonxis, J. H. P. and Hommes, F. A. (1972). Further studies on Leigh's encephalomyelopathy. In J. Stern and C. Toothill (eds). *Organic Acidurias*, pp. 40–45. (London: J. F. Churchill and Livingstone)

30. Clayton, B. E., Dobbs, R. H. and Patrick, A. D. (1967). Leigh's subacute necrotizing encephalopathy: clinical and biochemical study, with special reference to therapy with lipoate. *Arch. Dis. Child.*, **42**, 467

31. Crome, L. and Stern, J. (1967). *The Pathology of Mental Retardation*, p. 314. (London: J. and A. Churchill)

32. De Groot, C. J. and Hommes, F. A. (1973). Further speculation on the pathogenesis of Leigh's encephalomyelopathy. *J. Pediatr.*, **82**, 541

33. Hems, R., Stubbs, M. and Krebs, H. A. (1968). Restricted permeability of rat liver for glutamate and succinate. *Biochem. J.*, **107**, 807

34. Oldendorf, W. H. (1971). Brain uptake of radiolabelled amino acids, amines and hexoses after arterial injection. *Am. J. Physiol.*, **221**, 1629

35. De Vivo, D. C., Haymond, M. W., Leckie, M. P., Bursmann, Y. L., McDougal, D. B. and Pagliara, A. S. (1977). The clinical and biochemical implications of pyruvate carboxylase deficiency. *J. Clin. Exp. Med.*, **45**, 1281

36. Lonsdale, D., Faulkner, W. R., Price, J. W. and Smelby, R. R. (1969). Intermittent cerebellar ataxia associated with hyperpyruvic acidemia, hyperalaninemia and hyperalaninuria. *Pediatrics*, **43**, 1025

37. Pincus, J. H., Cooper, J. R., Murphy, J. V., Robe, E. F., Lonsdale, D. and Dunn, H. G. (1973). Thiamine derivatives in subacute necrotizing encephalomyelopathy. *Pediatrics*, **51**, 716

38. Thompson, A. D., Frank, O., Baker, H. and Leevy, C. M. (1971). Thiamin propyldisulphide: absorption and utilization. *Ann. Intern. Med.*, **74**, 529

39. Schrijver, J., Dias, Th. and Hommes, F. A. (1978). Studies on ATP-thiamin diphosphate phosphotransferase activity in rat brain. *Neurochem. Res.*, **3**, 699

40. Ruenwongsa, T. P. and Cooper, J. R. (1977). The role of bound thiamin pyrophosphate in the synthesis of thiamin triphosphate in rat liver. *Biochim. Biophys. Acta*, **482**, 64

41. Hoekstra, D., Berger, R. and Hommes, F. A. (1974). The thiamin diphosphate content of liver mitochondria of the pregnant and developing rat. *Nutr. Metab.*, **16**, 317

42. Itokawa, Y. (1976). Assay method and some properties of thiamin diphosphate-adenosine triphosphate phosphoryl transferase in rat brain. In C. J. Gubler, M. Fujiwara and P. M. Dreyfus (eds). *Thiamin*, pp. 361–368 (New York: John Wiley and Sons)

43. Rindi, G. and de Giuseppe, L. (1961). A new chromatographic method for the determination of thiamin and its mono-, di and tri-phosphates in animal tissues. *Biochem. J.*, **78**, 602

44. Hoekstra, D., Berger, R. and Hommes, F. A. (1974). Control of pyruvate oxidation in fetal and maternal tissue by the thiamin level. *Pediatr. Res.*, **8**, 132

45. Hommes, F. A., Berger, R. and Luit-De Haan, G. (1973). The effect of thiamin treatment on the activity of pyruvate dehydrogenase: relation to the

treatment of Leigh's encephalomyelopathy. *Pediatr. Res.*, **7**, 616
46. Whitehouse, S., Cooper, R. H. and Randle, P. J. (1974). Mechanism of activation of pyruvate dehydrogenase by dichloroacetate and other halogenated carboxylic acids. *Biochem. J.*, **141**, 761
47. Whitehouse, S. and Randle, P. J. (1973). Activation of pyruvate dehydrogenase in perfused rat heart by dichloroacetate. *Biochem. J.*, **134**, 651
48. Stacpoole, P. W., Moore, G. W. and Kornhauser, D. M. (1978). Metabolic effects of dichloroacetate in patients with diabetes mellitus and hyperlipoproteinemia. *N. Engl. J. Med.*, **298**, 526
49. Blackshear, P. J., Holloway, P. A. H. and Alberti, K. G. M. M. (1974). The metabolic effects of sodium dichloroacetate in the starved rat. *Biochem. J.*, **142**, 279
50. Stacpoole, P. W. and Felts, J. M. (1970). Di-isopropylammonium dichloroacetate (DIPA) and sodium dichloroacetate (DCA): Effect on glucose and fat metabolism in normal and diabetic tissue. *Metabolism*, **19**, 71
51. Stacpoole, P. W. (1977). Effect of dichloroacetate on gluconeogenesis in isolated rat hepatocytes. *Metabolism*, **26**, 107
52. Schrijver, J., Dias, Th. and Hommes, F. A. (1979). Some biochemical observations on biotin deficiency in the rat as a model for human pyruvate carboxylase deficiency. *Nutr. Metab.*, **23**, 179
53. Atkin, B., Utter, M. F., Winberg, M. B. and Buist, N. R. M. (1977). Detection of pyruvate carboxylase deficiency in leucocytes and fibroblasts. *Pediatr. Res.*, **11**, 452
54. Hanson, T. L. Christensen, C. and Brandt, N. J. (1977). Pyruvate carboxylase activity in cultured human fibroblasts and amniotic fluid cells. *Proc. 11th FEBS Meeting*, Copenhagen, AI-8.052
55. Raghunathen, R., Russell, J. D. and Arinze, J. J. (1977) Pyruvate carboxylase and phosphoenolpyruvate carboxykinase in cultured human fibroblasts. *J. Cell Physiol.*, **92**, 285
56. Blass, J. P., Cederbaum, S. D. and Gibson, G. E. (1975). Clinical and metabolic abnormalities accompanying deficiencies in pyruvate oxidation. In F. A. Hommes and C. J. van den Berg (eds). *Normal and Pathological Development of Energy Metabolism*, pp. 193–210 (London: Academic Press)
57. Itokawa, Y. (1977). (Personal communication)
58. Söling, H. D., Willms, B. and Kleineke, J. (1971). Regulation of gluconeogenesis in rat and guinea pig. In H. D. Söling and B. W. Willms (eds). *Regulation of Gluconeogenesis*, pp. 210–229 (Stuttgart: Thieme Verlag)
59. Yoshida, T., Tada, K., Konno, T. and Arakawa, T. (1969). Hyperalaninemia with pyruvicemia due to pyruvate carboxylase deficiency. *Tohoku J. Exp. Med.*, **99**, 121
60. Yoshida, T., Tada, K. and Arakawa, T. (1970). Abnormally high levels of lactate and pyruvate in cerebrospinal fluid of hyperalaninemia with hyperpyruvicemia. *Tohoku J. Exp. Med.*, **101**, 375
61. Moosa, A. and Hughes, E. A. (1974). L-glutamine therapy in Leigh's encephalomyelopathy. *Arch. Dis. Child.* **43**, 246
62. Gröbe, H., von Bassewitz, D. B., Donenick, H. C. and Pfeiffer, R. A. (1975). Subacute necrotizing encephalomyelopathy. Clinical, ultrastructural, biochemical and therapeutic studies in an infant. *Acta. Paediatr. Scand.*, **64**, 755

63. Tada, K., Takada, G., Omura, K. and Itokawa, Y. (1978). Congenital lactic acidosis due to pyruvate carboxylase deficiency: absence of an inhibitor of TPP-ATP phosphoryl transferase. *Eur. J. Pediatr.*, **127,** 141

64. van Biervliet, J. P. G. M., Bruinvis, L., van der Heiden, C., Ketting, D., Wadman, S. K., Willemse, J. L. and Monnens, L. A. H. (1977). Report of a patient with severe, chronic lactic acidaemia and pyruvate carboxylase deficiency. *Dev. Med. Child. Neurol.*, **19,** 392

65. Utter, M. F. and Keech, D. B. (1963). Pyruvate carboxylase. I. Nature of the reaction. *J. Biol. Chem.*, **283,** 2603

66. Koike, H. and Yusa, T. (1970). Thiamin and its phosphoric esters: estimation by an ion exchange method. In D. B. McCormick and L. D. Wright (eds). *Methods of Enzymology.* **Vol. 18A,** pp. 105–108 (New York: Academic Press)

67. Berry, M. M. and Friens, D. S. (1969). High yield preparation of isolated rat liver parenchymal cells: a biochemical and fine structural study. *J. Cell Biol.*, **43,** 506

SECTION SIX

Glycogen Storage Diseases

15

Recent advances and problems in the glycogen storage diseases

Brenda E. Ryman

The first description of a glycogen storage disease is attributable to von Gierke in 1929[1]. Since this time our knowledge has advanced quickly and these diseases now form an area of inborn errors of metabolism in which the basic enzyme defects are understood (Table 15.1) and the clinical symptoms and the differential diagnosis based on simple tests and biopsy examination, are well documented and clearly defined. Several recent reviews have been published[2-4] but there has probably been none better used than the early one by Hers[5], who has contributed so much to our understanding of this group of diseases.

Why then is it necessary to have extensive discussions during this symposium on the glycogen storage diseases, when there seems to be more order and understanding than is found in many other groups of genetic disorders? The reason is, without doubt, to examine and note progress, to attempt to clarify areas which are still somewhat hazy and, hopefully, to integrate observations which hitherto have been difficult to accommodate into our present state of knowledge. The following sections are a brief contribution to this objective, particularly considering some areas not covered by other speakers and citing literature not included in recent reviews.

TABLE 15.1   **The glycogen storage diseases**

Type	Disease	Principal site of glycogen storage	Enzymic lesion
I	von Gierke's	Liver, kidney, intestine	Glucose 6-phosphatase
II	Pompe's	Liver, heart, muscle	Lysosomal α-glucosidase
III	Cori's limit dextrinosis	(A) Liver and muscle	Amylo-1,6-glucosidase
		(B) Liver	(debranching enzyme) and/or 4-α-glucanotransferase
IV	Andersen's amylopectinosis	Liver	1,4-α-glucan branching enzyme
V	McArdle's	Muscle	Phosphorylase
VI	Hers'	(A) Liver, muscle	Phosphorylase kinase (sex linked)
		(B) Liver	Phosphorylase or phosphorylase kinase (autosomal)
VII	Tarui's	Muscle	Phosphofructokinase

THE BIOCHEMICAL DISORDER AND ENZYME DIAGNOSIS

The glycogen storage diseases have one biochemical feature in common, that is abnormal storage of glycogen. This is more often an increase, but sometimes a decrease, and the glycogen may have normal or abnormal structure. Many other secondary biochemical changes may occur, e.g. hypoglycaemia, changes in blood lipid components and lactate levels, to name but a few. These are considered in detail in recent reviews[2,3]. Some of these secondary changes may be used to make a provisional diagnosis[3], but the final diagnosis must rest on a direct enzyme assay of suitable tissue.

The most suitable tissues for enzymological examination are usually liver or muscle, but in some disorders leucocytes, erythrocytes or fibroblasts can be used. The type of tissue preferred for each disease and the methodology of the enzyme assays have been discussed in detail[3-6]. An innovation in respect of Type II disease is the reported use of tears and conjunctival biopsy to make a successful diagnosis[7]. Amniotic fluid cells have been useful in assessing fetuses at risk for the lethal Types II and IV glycogen storage diseases. The sensitive fluorimetric assay of α-glucosidase described by Fujimoto et al.[8] is applicable to amniotic fluid cells and has facilitated the prenatal diagnosis of two pregnancies at risk of Pompe's disease.

INCIDENCE AND INHERITANCE

The glycogen storage diseases show an overall frequency of approximately 1 in 60 000 live births and are almost all autosomally inherited. However, there are some exceptions to this pattern. Autosomal recessive and sex linked forms of Type VI (liver phosphorylase deficiency) have been described[9, 10], which obviously represent different enzyme defects. Whilst McArdle's disease (Type V) is usually believed to be inherited as an autosomal recessive condition, Chui and Munsat[11] have documented some evidence which suggests that the inheritance is of a dominant nature.

CLINICAL PRESENTATION AND TREATMENT

Within the group of glycogen storage diseases, varying degrees of clinical severity exist. For example, Types II and IV are almost invariably lethal within the first 3–12 months of life, whereas Type III is often relatively mild. More surprisingly, varying degrees of severity exist even within the same enzyme defect. This is particularly marked in Type I (glucose-6-phosphatase deficiency), in which symptoms may vary from severe (particularly the hypoglycaemia) to relatively mild. We have no idea why this is so and it would certainly be useful if we understood the adaptive mechanisms which result in a mild form of Type I, despite a total lack of glucose-6-phosphatase. If such understanding could be achieved, treatment designed to stabilize Type I patients might be improved.

A later paper in the symposium describes the strides forward which have already been made in the treatment of children with Type I disease, by counteracting the effects of persistent hypoglycaemia using continuous nasogastric glucose administration[12]. From my own laboratory there has been a report of an attempt to treat a child with Type II glycogen storage disease by the use of liposomes (phospholipid vesicles), containing amyloglucosidase, with encouraging results[13].

Type I

The observation that the hydrolysis of glucose 6-phosphate may involve both a transport protein and glucose 6-phosphatase[15] may explain the results obtained on a patient with *in vivo* evidence of Type I glycogenosis and normal enzyme activity *in vitro*[14].

Earlier reports that von Gierke's disease (Type 1) may be associated with the development of hepatomas has led Miller *et al.*[16] to investigate scintigraphic abnormalities in 15 patients. They recommend careful scanning of all such patients as a routine.

There has also been a very recent report of the excretion of 2-oxoglutaric acid in the urine of Type I patients[14].

Type II

Pompe's disease   There are still some mysteries associated with Pompe's disease (lysosomal α-glucosidase deficiency). In this condition glycogen accumulates in every tissue of the body which has been examined. There is some evidence that metachromatic staining material also accumulates, but the underlying reason for this is not obvious. A recent report showed preferential localisation of large glycogen molecules in the lysosomes with smaller ones in the cytoplasm[17]. This observation may indicate some specialised selectivity of lysosomes based on physical parameters of molecules and this specificity may be related to the accumulation of other macromolecules than glycogen.

Adult variant   There is an adult form of Type II which has some puzzling features. It is necessary to explain why the clinical disorder is widespread in Pompe's disease, whereas there appears to be no cardiac involvement in the adult variant of α-glucosidase deficiency. In the severe form (Pompe's) the enzyme is equally deficient in liver, skeletal muscle and cardiac muscle and, in support of common genetic control of α-glucosidase, Koster et al.[18] have failed to find any difference in the physico-chemical and immunological properties of the enzyme from the three tissues. A recent publication has reported an absence of α-glucosidase in heart muscle of a patient with the adult form of Type II[19]. The reason why no functional abnormality occurs in the cardiac muscle remains obscure.

It is not always easy to distinguish the adult variant of Type II from patients with secondary deficiencies of α-glucosidase. The enzyme has rather low levels in muscle and it seems possible that other factors may reduce its activity still further. During our biopsy work, we have observed a patient with hypothyroidism and marked muscle weakness who also showed a very low level of α-glucosidase; but he was clearly not a case of adult variant Type II glycogen storage disease.

Type IV

Since the published reviews[2-5], a further case of Type IV glycogen storage disease (1,4-α-glucan branching enzyme) has been reported in a Latin American girl by Bannayan et al.[20]

Type V

McArdle's disease (muscle phosphorylase deficiency) has been investigated further, and the mysterious reappearance of phosphorylase activity in regenerating and cultured muscle cells from a patient with this disorder reported by Roelofs et al.[21], has now been explained. Sato et al.[22] have shown by electrophoretic and immunochemical techniques that the phosphorylase activity observed in these circumstances corresponded to the fetal and liver enzyme, and that no adult skeletal muscle phosphorylase could be detected.

Nolte and Schollmeyer[23] have shown that the level of phosphoenolpyruvate carboxykinase is increased in McArdle's disease. They believe that this reflects an adaptive mechanism which provides phosphorylated intermediates for energy supply to the muscle.

Type VI

Type IV glycogen storage disease has been a somewhat unsatisfactory group for a long time. As was mentioned previously it has accommodated both sex linked and autosomal recessive defects associated with the phosphorylase system[9]. The situation has been clarified by Lederer et al.[10] by investigations of phosphorylase and its interconverting enzymes using haemolysates from normal and Type VI patients. It is questionable whether defects of the activating system associated with rather unique clinical manifestations, not normally seen in Type VIA or B, should be called Types VIII or IX, as has been suggested[24-30]. Hopefully this matter will be discussed and might be resolved during this symposium.

References

1. von Gierke, E. (1929). Hepato-nephromegalis-glykogenica (glykogen-speicherkrankheit der Riber und nieren). *Beitr. pathol. Anat.*, **82,** 497
2. Ryman, B. E. (1974). The glycogen storage diseases. *J. clin. Pathol.*, **27,** *Suppl. (Roy. Coll. Path.)*, **8,** 106
3. Ryman, B. E. (1976). The glycogen storage diseases. In J. H. Wilkinson (ed.). *The Principles and Practice of Diagnostic Enzymology*, pp. 503–517 (London: Edward Arnold)
4. Huijing, F. (1975). Glycogen metabolism and glycogen-storage diseases. *Physiol. Rev.*, **55,** 609
5. Hers, H. G. (1964). Glycogen storage disease. In R. Levine and R. Luft (eds). *Advances in Metabolic Regulation*. **Vol. 1,** pp. 1–44 (New York: Academic Press)
6. Hers, H. G. and van Hoof, F. (1966). Enzymes of glycogen degradation in biopsy material. In E. F. Neufeld and V. Ginsberg (eds). *Methods in Enzymology*. **Vol. VIII,** pp. 525–532
7. van Hoof, F., Libert, J., Aubert-Tulkens, G. and Serra, M. V. (1976). The assay of lacrymal enzymes and the ultra-structural analysis of conjunctival

biopsies: New Techniques for the study of inborn lysosomal diseases. *Metab. Ophthalmol.*, **1**, 165

8. Fujimoto, A., Fluharty, A. L., Stevens, R. L., Kihara, H. and Wilson, M. G. (1976). Two alpha-glucosidases in cultured amniotic fluid cells and their differentiation in the prenatal diagnosis of Pompe's disease. *Clin. Chim. Acta.*, **68**, 177

9. Huijing, F. and Fernandes, J. (1969). X-chromosomal inheritance of liver glycogenosis with phosphorylase kinase-deficiency. *Am. J. Hum. Genet.*, **21**, 275

10. Lederer, B., van Hoof, F., van den Berghe, G. and Hers, H. G. (1975). Glycogen phosphorylase and its converter enzymes in haemolysates of normal human subjects and of patients with Type VI glycogen storage disease. *Biochem. J.*, **147**, 23

11. Chui, L. A. and Munsat, T. L. (1976). Dominant inheritance of McArdle syndrome. *Arch. Neurol.*, **33**, 636

12. Stacey, T. E., Macnab, A., and Strang, L. B. (1979). Recent work on treatment of Type I glycogen storage disease. ibid.

13. Tyrrell, D. A., Ryman, B. E., Keeton, B. R. and Dubowitz, V. (1976). Use of liposomes in treating Type II glycogenosis. *Br. Med. J.*, 88

14. Chalmers, R. A., Ryman, B. E. and Watts, R. W. E. (1978). Studies on a patient with *in vivo* evidence of Type I glycogenosis and normal enzyme activities *in vitro*. *Acta. Paediatr. Scand.*, **67**, 201

15. Nilsson, O. S., Arion, W. J., DePierre, J. W., Dallner, G. and Ernster, L. (1978). Evidence for the involvement of a glucose-6-phosphate carrier in microsomal glucose-6-phosphatase activity. *Eur. J. Biochem.*, **82**, 627

16. Miller, J. H., Gates, G. F., Landing, B. H., Kogut, M. D. and Roe, T. F. (1978). Scintigraphic abnormalities in glycogen storage disease. *J. Nucl. Med. Allied Sci.*, **19**, 354

17. Geddes, R. and Stratton, G. C. (1977). The influence of lysosomes on glycogen metabolism. *Biochem. J.*, **163**, 193

18. Koster, J. F., Slee, R. G., van der Klei-Van Moorsel, J. M., Rietra, P. J. G. M. and Lucas, C. J. (1976). Physico-chemical and immunological properties of acid α-glucosidase from various human tissues in relation to glycogenosis Type II (Pompe's disease). *Clin. Chim. Acta.*, **68**, 49

19. Soyama, K., Ono, E., Shimada, N., Tanaka, K. and Kusunoki, T. (1977). Urinary α-glucosidase analysis for the detection of the adult form of Pompe's disease. *Clin. Chim. Acta*, **77**, 61

20. Bannayan, G. A., Dean, W. J. and Howell, R. R. (1976). Type IV glycogen-storage disease. Light-microscopic, electron-microscopic and enzymatic study. *Am. J. Clin. Pathol.*, **66**, 702

21. Roelofs, R. I., Engel, W. K. and Chauvin, P. B. (1972). Histochemical phosphorylase activity in regenerating muscle fibers from myophosphorylase-deficient patients. *Science*, **177**, 795

22. Sato, K., Imai, F., Hatayama, I. and Roelofs, R. I. (1977). Characterization of glycogen phosphorylase isoenzymes present in cultured skeletal muscle from patients with McArdle's disease. *Biochem. Biophys. Res. Commun.*, **78**, 663

23. Nolte, J. and Schollmeyer, P. (1973). Metabolic adaptation in muscle of phosphorylase deficiency (McArdle's disease)? *Klin. Wochenschr.*, **51**, 250

24. Hug, G., Garancis, J. C., Schubert, W. K. and Kaplan, S. (1966). Glycogen storage disease, Types II, III, VIII and IX. *Am. J. Dis. Child.*, **3,** 457

25. Ludwig, M., Wolfson, S. and Rennart, O. (1972). Glycogen storage disease type VIII. *Arch. Dis. Child.*, **47,** 830

26. Hug, G., Schubert, W. K. and Chuck, G. (1966). Phosphorylase kinase of the liver: deficiency in a girl with increased hepatic glycogen. *Science*, **153,** 1534

27. Hug, G., Schubert, W. K. and Chuck, G. (1969). Deficient activity of dephosphophosphorylase kinase and accumulation of glycogen in the liver. *J. Clin. Invest.*, **48,** 704

28. Morishita, Y., Nishiyama, K., Yamamura, H., Kodama, S., Negishi, H., Matsuo, M., Matsuo, T. and Nishizuka, Y. (1973). Glycogen phosphorylase kinase deficiency. *Biochem. Biophys. Res. Commun.*, **54,** 833

29. Hug, G., Sper, M. R. and Schubert, W. K. (1973). Adult versus infantile glycogenosis in type II. *Pediatr. Res.*, **7,** 389

30. Hug, G., Schubert, W. K. and Chuck, G. (1970). Loss of cyclic 3′5′-AMP dependent kinase and reduction of phosphorylase kinase in skeletal muscle of a girl with deactivated phosphorylase and glycogenosis of liver and muscle. *Biochem. Biophys. Res. Commun.*, **40,** 982

THE F. P. HUDSON MEMORIAL LECTURE

Introduction by G. Komrower

I am delighted to have been given the honour of introducing the first F. P. Hudson lecturer. The idea for this Annual Memorial Lecture came from Gordon Jones, the Managing Director of Scientific Hospital Supplies, friend and admirer of Freddie Hudson, and we are indebted for this generous action.

I think I was asked because Freddie and I were both proud Lancastrians and old friends, who had added the study of biochemical genetics to our routine clinical work. Neither of us were biochemists, but learnt our biochemistry by a process of osmosis.

Freddie was a founder member and president of this society. As I have said, he was a general physician who was attracted to inherited disease and, early on, he undertook to run the PKU Register for the Medical Research Council. This was a great success, largely because he was a good physician, kind and a great catalyst. He was able to communicate well with the general paediatricians around the country and advise them about any clinical problems relating to their cases of PKU. Unfortunately he died before the result of this work became available for publication, but there is no doubt that as a result of his groundwork we will be afforded considerable information about the early progress of PKU children diagnosed in the newborn period and treated immediately.

May I welcome his widow Marjorie Hudson to our presence this morning. She was always extremely interested in Freddie's work and very proud of his achievements. We are delighted to see her here today.

Who better than Dr Fernandes to be the first Freddie Hudson lecturer. Dr Fernandes, who has just been appointed to the Chair of Paediatrics in Groningen, is an excellent doctor, kind and friendly, who has made a real contribution to the paediatric literature with articles that have a very good clinical content. In addition, he is an excellent investigator and a good speaker and we are greatly looking forward to hearing him today. Ladies and gentlemen, I would like to present to you Dr Fernandes as the first F. P. Hudson Memorial lecturer who will address us on the subject of 'Metabolic abnormalities in various types of hepatic Glycogen Storage Disease and their management'.

16

Hepatic glycogenosis: diagnosis and management

J. Fernandes

I would like to thank the Society for inviting me to give the first lecture to commemorate the late Dr Hudson. It is a great honour for me to participate in this new tradition. It means a recognition of the oldest way of research in medicine, namely research directly related to the patient. It is with this approach in mind that I present my studies of children with different types of glycogenosis.

Ninety-one children with glycogen storage disease have been seen. The majority of them were distributed between three types of enzyme defect: glucose-1-phosphatase, Type 1 (18 patients); debranching enzyme system, Type III (13 patients); phosphorylase system, Type VI (42 patients). In addition, there were 9 patients with lysosomal 1,4-glucosidase deficiency (Type II) and 2 with an abnormality in the branching enzyme (Type IV). Only the more common types will be discussed in this paper.

The physical symptoms are very similar: all three types are characterised by an enlarged liver and the large protruding abdomen contrasts sharply with the thin extremities. Often the children show retarded motor development during the first years of life. They are usually later in sitting, standing and walking than normal children. Moreover, there is distinct growth retardation which is especially striking in children with glucose-1-phosphatase deficiency. Children deficient in debranching enzyme usually follow the lower percentile zones of the Tanner charts, but phosphorylase deficient children have a normal growth pattern.

The most prominent features of the metabolic disturbance are hypoglycaemia, acidosis with elevated blood lactate levels, fasting ketosis, hyperlipaemia and hyperuricaemia. In contrast with the similarity of the physical symptoms, the metabolic abnormalities are highly dependent on the underlying type of enzyme defect[1] (Table 16.1). This means that early diagnosis is very important for appropriate treatment.

TABLE 16.1   **Main metabolic abnormalities associated with the three most frequently occurring types of glycogenosis**[1]

Metabolic characteristic	Enzyme deficiency		
	Glucose-6-phosphatase	Amylo-1,6-glucosidase	Phosphorylase
Hypoglycaemia	+ +	+	±
Acidosis	+	—	—
Ketosis	—	+	±
Hyperlipaemia	+ +	+	±
Hyperuricaemia	+	—	—

The most direct approach to making a correct diagnosis is by enzyme assay of a liver biopsy or a leukocyte preparation. This is a complicated and laborious procedure performed in only a few specialized centres. It is therefore of great importance to have a screening procedure available to limit the number of specialised tests.

SCREENING PROCEDURE

Figure 16.1 shows a diagram of the diagnostic procedure that has been developed[2]. It is very useful as a preliminary screen when the diagnosis of glycogenosis seems probable and prior to the enzymic examination. Firstly, a glucose tolerance test is performed. The possible results of this are shown in the three upper diagrams of Figure 16.1. The fall of an initially raised lactate level is quite characteristic for glucose-6-phosphatase deficiency and no further tests are needed. An abnormally large rise of an initially normal lactate level indicates either a debranching enzyme or phosphorylase deficiency, but does not differentiate between the two. A borderline normal lactate curve suggests either a deficiency of debranching enzyme, or of the phosphorylase complex. Further differentiation between these two

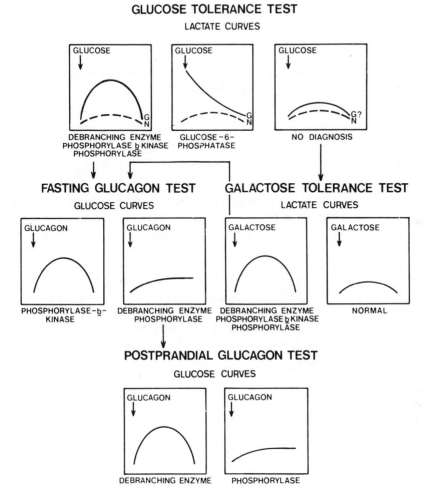

Figure 16.1 A diagnostic screening procedure for patients with suspected glycogen storage disease[2]. Enzyme deficiencies suggested by the curves shown are listed below the boxes. For the glucose tolerance tests; G = results suggesting a glycogenosis, N = normal

possibilities is achieved by a glucagon test after an overnight fast: a normal glucose peak points to a phosphorylase kinase deficiency, whilst a flat glucose curve points to a deficiency of debranching enzyme or of phosphorylase proper. These two can be differentiated further by a postprandial glucagon test. The glucose response remains flat in phosphorylase deficiency and is normal in debranching enzyme deficiency.

The procedure outlined above leads to an early tentative diagnosis which may be confirmed afterwards by enzyme assay. As already indicated, early differentiation is of practical importance for the management of the patients, as this differs for each type of enzyme deficiency. The management of the metabolic complications of the disorders will be considered in some detail.

CLINICAL MANAGEMENT

Hypoglycaemia

Hypoglycaemic attacks are most common and severe in children with Type I glycogenosis. There is almost complete dependence on exogenous glucose as glucose production from glycogenolysis and gluconeogenesis is blocked. Frequent feeds with an ample supply of glucose are needed. It may be difficult to maintain the frequency of the feeds necessary to sustain the blood sugar at normal levels but the situation may be improved in the various ways suggested in Figure 16.2. The glucose tolerance curve was studied following the administration of glucose in water and the same amount of glucose in curd[1]. The slope of the glucose curve was very steep after glucose in water, but its course was more gradual after a mixed feed. Presumably the effect of curd is twofold: it causes delayed emptying of the stomach and

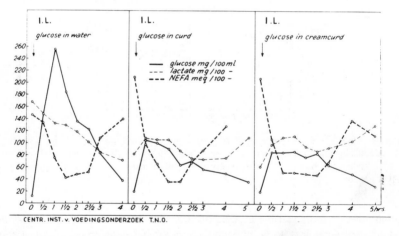

CENTR. INST. v. VOEDINGSONDERZOEK T.N.O.

Figure 16.2 The differing effect of oral glucose administration in water, curd or cream curd on blood glucose, lactate and free fatty acids, in a patient with glucose-6-phosphatase deficiency[1]. For glucose, mg/100 ml × 0.06 = mmol/l. For lactate, mg/100 ml × 0.11 = mmol/l

serves as an extra source of fuel, thus saving glucose. Giving starch instead of glucose also improved the ensuing glucose curve. During the starch test the glucose rise was less abrupt and its decrease more gradual. This means that the intervals between feeds can be longer with the ingestion of starch in porridge, rather than glucose in water, tea or fruit juices.

In children with debranching enzyme deficiency, prevention of hypoglycaemia does not depend exclusively on an adequate and timely supply of starch and glucose. They can utilize all kinds of sugars, since they can easily convert galactose and fructose into glucose[1]. Yet children with this type of enzyme deficiency do need frequent feeds, high in carbohydrate, especially in the first year of life. Moreover, they have an active, or even enhanced rate of gluconeogenesis from protein[3] (Figure 16.3). The nature of

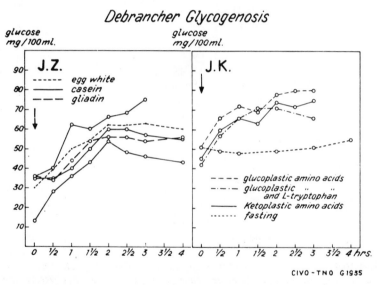

Figure 16.3 Oral tolerance tests with different proteins and amino acid mixtures in a patient with debranching enzyme deficiency[3]. For glucose, mg/100 ml × 0.06 = mmol/l

the protein or amino acid mixture given makes no perceptible difference to the ensuing glucose increase. These patients benefit from extra protein, particularly a high protein feed at bedtime.

Phosphorylase deficient patients have only mild symptoms of hypoglycaemia and do not need special dietary measures.

Acidosis and ketosis

Of the three types of glycogenosis under consideration, severe acidosis occurs only in glucose-6-phosphatase deficiency. On the other hand, fasting ketosis is most pronounced in debranching enzyme and virtually absent in glucose-6-phosphatase deficiency. This is in contrast to former assumptions. Only during severe metabolic acidosis were slightly elevated ketone body levels observed in patients with glucose-6-phosphatase deficiency. Thus, abnormally high lactate levels are the main cause of the acidosis.

The effect of oral glucose administration on blood lactate levels in Type I patients is shown in Figure 16.4. Thus, the prevention of hyperlactacidaemia

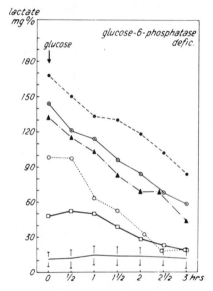

Figure 16.4 Blood lactate concentrations during oral glucose tolerance tests in five patients with glucose-6-phosphatase deficiency (symbols) and in controls (lowest line showing mean ± s.d.)[4]. For lactate, mg/100 ml × 0.11 = mmol/l

as well as hypoglycaemia depends mainly on frequent feeds high in starch or glucose. Sucrose and lactose are undesirable nutrients compared with maltose[5]. This is because galactose from lactose, and fructose from sucrose, cannot be converted to glucose, and their degradation enhances lactate production. Therefore lactose and particularly sucrose are restricted in the diet, which then consists largely of glucose and starch as sources of carbohydrate.

Figure 16.5 summarizes the data collected on fasting ketosis. Surprisingly, the total ketone bodies in the blood of glucose-6-phosphatase deficient patients were all within the range of control subjects, but practically all debranching enzyme deficient children had a striking fasting ketosis. The results in phosphorylase deficient children were more variable, some had a marked ketosis, others did not. This diversity appears to be related to age[6].

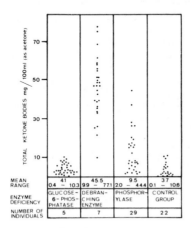

Figure 16.5   Fasting ketone bodies in patients with the three most frequently occurring glycogenoses[6]. For ketone bodies (as acetone), mg/100 ml × 0.17 = mmol/l

The tendency to fasting ketosis is greatest in the very young and it decreases with age until it disappears at 7 years. This change with age could be accounted for by improved adaptation in the older patients.

Dietary management to prevent excessive ketosis is essentially the same as for hypoglycaemia and, therefore, separate dietary measures are not indicated.

Hyperlipidaemia

It is not known whether the hyperlipidaemia in these conditions involves an increased risk of atherosclerosis in adult life. However, in view of the early atherosclerosis of diabetics it is desirable to attempt to reduce the hyperlipidaemia. Dietary measures had little effect on the hyperlipidaemia of children with glucose-6-phosphatase deficiency. In debranching enzyme and phosphorylase deficient children, on the other hand, there was a reduction. This was achieved by the combination of a low carbohydrate content in the diet and the use of dietary fats high in polyunsaturated fatty acids, such as corn oil.

The effect of diet on blood total fatty acids and cholesterol in a child with phosphorylase kinase deficiency is shown in Figure 16.1. The total fatty acid levels were very high on a high carbohydrate diet, fell significantly on substitution of corn oil for an equivalent amount of carbohydrate and rose again on the reintroduction of the original diet. The patient has maintained normal lipid levels, at home now, on a diet with extra corn oil. In some

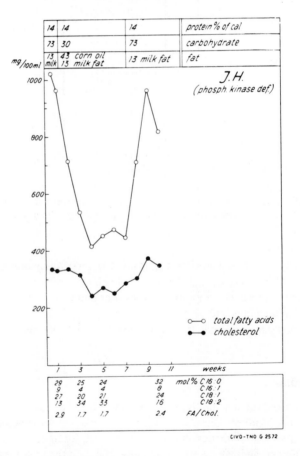

Figure 16.6 Serum lipid concentrations of a patient with phosphorylase kinase deficiency during iso-caloric diets with varying carbohydrate and fat content[7]. For cholesterol, mg/100 ml × 0.026 = mmol/l. For fatty acids, mg/100 ml × 0.035 = mmol/l (mean mol. wt. of 277 assumed)

patients with phosphorylase or debranching enzyme deficiency the corn oil diet has had little effect, but the majority respond to these dietary measures.

Hyperuricaemia

Hyperuricaemia is a serious complication which is seen more often as more patients with glucose-6-phosphatase deficiency survive the precarious first years of life. Because of long standing high blood uric acid levels they run the risk of developing gout. Besides this, renal damage due to hyperuricaemia may be even more serious. Therefore, the tendency towards hyperuricaemia is suppressed at an early age. We have had no success with Probenicid, which acts by stimulating the renal excretion of uric acid; but Allopurinol, the xanthine oxidase inhibitor, which prevents the conversion of precursors into uric acid, produced a distinct decrease of uric acid levels in the blood[1]. Figure 16.7 shows the hands, with tophi, of a patient, now 32 years old, before and after treatment.

NOCTURNAL GASTRIC FEEDS

Finally I would like to show briefly some results of nocturnal gastric drip feeding in six patients with glucose-6-phosphatase deficiency.

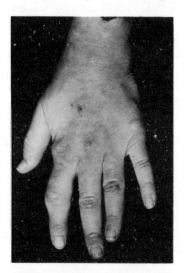 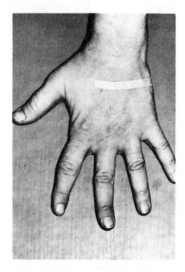

Figure 16.7   The effect of treatment with Allopurinol on the tophi of a patient with glucose-6-phosphatase deficiency. To the left, before treatment; to the right, after treatment

The idea of this treatment came after referral to us of a remarkable patient. His paediatrician had introduced a gastric drip with glucose every night from the age of 11 months because the usual night feeds had not prevented hypoglycaemic symptoms. The patient was in very good condition and, surprisingly, had normal growth, whereas most of our patients had severe growth retardation. After this observation nocturnal gastric feeding was introduced in five other patients, with some modifications to the method. A complete soy milk feed was used without lactose or sucrose but with added glucose or maltose. The gastric drip feed at night provides approximately 30–35% of total energy.

We were especially interested in the effect on lactic acidosis, hyperlipidaemia and clinical symptoms. As far as possible the blood glucose concentration was kept between 4 and 6 mmol/l during the 12 hours of night drip feeding. This steady glucose homeostasis might diminish lactate production. Lactate production is reflected by the urinary lactate excretion more accurately than by blood lactate level, which often varies considerably over short periods. Figure 16.8 shows the data on the first patient. The high initial lactate excretion fell after hospitalization and before starting treatment. There was a further slight decrease during the experimental drip period and a scatter of data during the last control period. Rather low values were maintained during the ensuing 3 years' treatment. Some other patients with pronounced hyperlactic aciduria improved markedly[8], but in others the

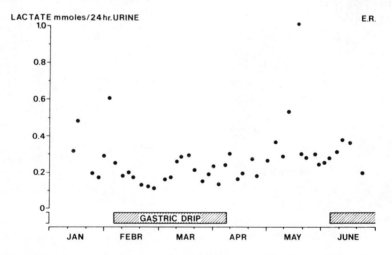

Figure 16.8 Urinary lactate excretion of patient 1, with glucose-6-phosphatase deficiency, during periods of nocturnal gastric drip feeding and at other times with frequent meals around the clock[8]

results were variable.

The effect of the dietary regime on acid–base equilibrium is shown in Figure 16.9. The degree of acidaemia is reflected by the base excess and the number of observations, the means and standard deviations are shown during basal and gastric drip feeding periods, in the morning and evening. Base excess was significantly lower during the two basal periods as compared with the drip period. Thus the tendency for acidaemia was less during the experimental feeding.

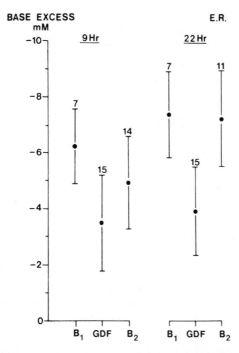

Figure 16.9 Blood base excess data of patient 1, with glucose-6-phosphatase deficiency, during basal periods (B) and periods of gastric drip feeds (GDF)[8]

Regarding the effect of gastric drip on serum lipids, Figure 16.10 shows the serum triglyceride and cholesterol concentration of one patient during three dietary periods. Serum lipid levels were extremely high initially. They decreased significantly during the first control period but were lowest during the drip feeding. Subsequently a gradual increase occurred and, during 3 years nocturnal treatment at home, her serum triglyceride increased further but the serum cholesterol remained in the normal range.

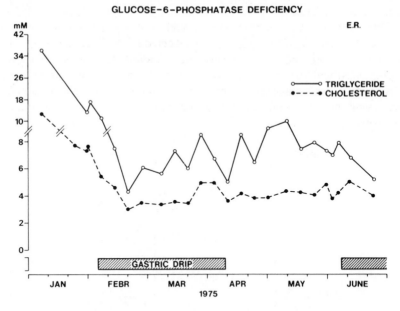

Figure 16.10 Serum triglyceride and cholesterol concentrations (mmol/l) in patient 1, with glucose-6-phosphate deficiency, during basal periods and periods of gastric drip feeds

The hypertriglyceridaemia may be related to increased production or decreased elimination. The clearance of triglycerides from the blood is affected by the enzyme lipoprotein lipase, which consists of two main components, extrahepatic and hepatic lipase. Table 16.2 shows the activity of hepatic and extrahepatic lipase in three patients. Extrahepatic lipase is situated at the vascular endothelium of adipose and muscle tissue. It is released into the blood by intravenous administration of heparin. The 5 min sample represents the component immediately available which hydrolyses triglycerides from chylomicrons and Very Low Density Lipoproteins. The 40 min sample represents the reserve pool in the cells. Normal lipase activities are between 100 and 200 (μmol free fatty acids/ml plasma)/min. The activity of the 40 min sample is normally higher than the 5 min sample. From the table it appears that all pre-treatment lipase activities were abnormally low. After 2 weeks nocturnal drip treatment the 5 min post heparin lipase activities tended to normal, but the 40 min activities were lower than those at 5 min. This unusual finding might reflect a low lipoprotein lipase pool. This is in keeping with the fact that the serum triglyceride levels

TABLE 16.2 Serum triglyceride cholesterol and phospholipid concentration, and hepatic triglyceride lipase and extrahepatic lipoprotein lipase activity in three patients before and after gastric drip feeding (GDF)[8]

Patient and treatment	Triglyceride (mmol/l)	Cholesterol (mmol/l)	Phospholipid (mmol/l)	Lipase			
				Hepatic		Extrahepatic	
				5 min	40 min	5 min	40 min
2. Before GDF	11.2	8.2	7.3	59	92	42	74
After GDF (17 days)	10.1	6.5	6.3	112	95	94	66
3. Before GDF	4.3	3.4	3.9	80	71	66	28
After GDF (14 days)	3.8	4.4	3.1	163	148	104	37
5. Before GDF	5.3	3.8	3.8	249	147	73	15
After GDF (15 days)	11.3	2.9	5.3	266	242	31	15

The 5 min and 40 min post-heparin activity is expressed as μmol free fatty acid released from an artificial triglyceride emulsion per min per litre plasma. Normal 5 min post-heparin activity in young adults is 166 to 896 for hepatic triglyceride lipase and 123 to 382 for extrahepatic lipoprotein lipase[9]

remained elevated in all patients, though improvement was observed in some.

With regard to hepatic lipase activities of the same three patients, there is much speculation about the role of this component in the process of lipid clearing. It appears that hepatic lipase activity, though decreased in two patients before treatment, was normal in all three patients after treatment. It is not apparent whether the improvement has any significance for fat clearing. Thus the hyperlipidaemia appears to be related to both increased liponeogenesis and decreased fat elimination.

In contrast with the moderate changes in the metabolic disorder, the clinical improvement of most patients during prolonged gastric drip feeding was striking. The patients' vitality increased, the bleeding tendency disappeared, the sleep became less superficial, the tendency for excessive sweating diminished and the liver size decreased in five of the six patients. A catch-up growth of patients with retarded growth was observed (Figure 16.11).

CONCLUSIONS

The treatment of glycogenosis patients is summarized in Table 16.3. The

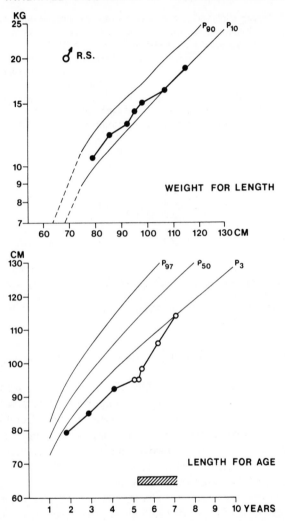

Figure 16.11   Growth before and during a period of gastric drip feeding (hatched period) in a patient with glucose-6-phosphatase deficiency

benefits of drip feeding should be weighed against the risks of this artificial procedure. Among the risks is the fact that, at a certain age, the treatment has to be abandoned. So the ultimate outcome is yet uncertain.

Here we should keep in mind the words of Dr Hudson[10], to whose memory my lecture is dedicated: I quote, 'Whatever regimen is adopted, the

TABLE 16.3 Diets for children with liver glycogen storage disease

Diet component	Type of enzyme deficiency		
	Glucose-6-phosphatase	Debranching enzyme system	Phosphorylase system
Carbohydrate (% of energy)	50–70, as starch and glucose (lactose and sucrose restricted)	40–50, preferably as starch	
Fat (% of energy)	15–35, as polyunsaturated fat e.g. corn oil	30–40 polyunsaturated fat (corn oil)	
Protein (% of energy)	15	20	
Remarks	frequent meals (glucose drip feeds). 1–2 g NaHCO₃ daily to counteract acidosis	protein rich supper recommended	dietary measures not very stringent

therapist must not forget that the subject being treated is, or should usually be, a normal growing child in a normal home environment; he is not an experimental subject in a metabolic unit. Administration of the diet must be within the competence of the average mother who has many daily duties in addition to food preparation.'

References

1. Fernandes, J. (1975). Hepatic glycogen storage diseases. In D. N. Raine (ed.). *The Treatment of Inherited Metabolic Disease*, pp. 115–149 (Lancaster: Medical and Technical Publishing Co.)
2. Fernandes, J., Koster, J. F., Grose, W. F. A. and Sorgedrager, N. (1974). Hepatic phosphorylase deficiency: Its differentiation from other hepatic glycogenoses. *Arch. Dis. Child.*, **49,** 186
3. Fernandes, J. and van de Kamer, J. H. (1968). Hexose and protein tolerance tests in children with liver glycogenosis caused by a deficiency of the debranching enzyme system. *Pediatrics*, **41,** 935
4. Fernandes, J., Huijing, F. and van de Kamer, J. H. (1969). A screening method for liver glycogen disease. *Arch. Dis Child.*, **44,** 311
5. Fernandes, J. (1974). The effect of disaccharides on the hyperlactic-acidaemia of glucose-6-phosphatase deficient children. *Acta. Paediatr. Scand.*, **63,** 695

6. Fernandes, J. and Pikaar, N. A. (1972). Ketosis in hepatic glycogenosis. *Arch. Dis. Child.*, **47,** 41

7. Fernandes, J. and Pikaar, N. A. (1969). Hyperlipemia in children with glycogen disease. *Am. J. Clin. Nutr.*, **22,** 617

8. Fernandes, J., Jansen, H. and Jansen, T. C. (1979). Nocturnal gastric drip feeding in glucose-6-phosphatase deficient children. *Pediatr. Res.*, **13** (In press)

9. Huttunen, J. K., Ehnholm, C., Kinnunen, P. K. J., Nikkila, E. A. (1975). An immunochemical method for the selective measurement of two triglyceride lipases in human post heparin plasma. *Clin. Chim. Acta*, **63,** 335

10. Hudson, F. P. (1971). General introduction to the dietary treatment of phenylketonuria. In H. Bickel, F. P. Hudson and L. I. Woolf (eds). *Phenylketonuria and Some Other Inborn Errors of Amino Acid Metabolism*, p. 158

17

Recent work on treatment of Type I glycogen storage disease

T. E. Stacey, A. Macnab and L. B. Strang

This paper concerns the clinical and biochemical course in two siblings with glucose-6-phosphatase deficiency, who have been treated with supplementary glucose according to a variety of regimes.

PATIENT 1

This girl is now 16 years old, and is the second child of healthy, unrelated parents of above average intelligence. Her elder brother was already known to have absent hepatic glucose-6-phosphatase. She was born at term, weighing 3.88 kg, after an unremarkable pregnancy. A plasma glucose of 1 mmol/l was recorded on the first day of life, and marked hyperlipaemia was present from the ninth day. Episodes of sweating and pallor occurred, but symptoms of more severe hypoglycaemia were pre-empted by frequent feeding. By age 5 months, hepatomegaly was marked and hyperlipaemia was persistent. Formal oral glucose tolerance test showed a 3 hour plasma glucose of only 0.6 mmol/l and a diagnosis of glycogen storage disease Type I was considered to be warranted without a liver biopsy. A regime of high carbohydrate meals was continued, 3 hourly day and night.

In early childhood the patient had many hospital admissions with severe acidosis, associated with infective illnesses. Acidosis always responded rapidly to intravenous infusion of dextrose and sodium bicarbonate. Excessive bleeding occurred from a laceration of the frenulum at age 18 months and from a scalp wound at $3\frac{1}{2}$ years. Haematuria and rectal bleeding occurred at $9\frac{1}{2}$ years. Her developmental milestones were within normal limits, although motor performance was influenced by muscle weakness and her large abdomen.

Growth was poor. Her height fell progressively below the 3rd percentile from about 4 years of age. At age $6\frac{1}{2}$ years she was given growth hormone (10 mg twice weekly) for one year, to explore the possibility that her growth might increase in response to very high plasma levels of growth hormone. No effect in growth was seen, but a rapid increase in bone age was noted; she developed genu valgum and radiological evidence of rickets, along with a low plasma phosphate and high alkaline phosphatase. This was treated by adding 4–6 g sodium bicarbonate per day to her diet. She improved clinically, her rickets healed over the next few months, the alkaline phosphatase level fell and her plasma phosphate eventually increased to normal. There was no increase in her height velocity, then down to 1.5 cm/year compared to the 3rd percentile for height velocity of 4 cm/year, in spite of regular 3 hourly glucose supplements.

Treatment regimes

Her glucose supplementation regime has been changed several times: the details are summarized in Table 17.1. From shortly after birth, her parents had given her supplementary oral glucose, at a dose of approximately 0.3 g/kg . h. The frequency was 3 hourly at night, and usually 3 hourly or occasionally 2 hourly during the day. Frequency was increased during acidotic episodes. At the age of 10 years $8\frac{1}{2}$ months a period of 140 days of continuous intravenous glucose was started, via a silicone rubber catheter of outside diameter 0.6 mm. The sterile dextrose infusate passed from an air free plastic bag via a bacterial filter, a silastic pump chamber with PTFE rollers and a second bacterial filter attached to the indwelling catheter. The pump was a modified lightweight, battery operated, peristaltic pump[1] which could be worn in a small harness around the chest. It allowed the child to be fully ambulant. Treatment was maintained at home by medically qualified members of the family and for some of this period she returned to normal school.

Initially the catheter tip was placed at the entrance to the right atrium, and 25% dextrose solution was used. After 30 days, an episode of fever and chest pain occurred. There was no clinical, X-ray or ECG evidence of a

TABLE 17.1 Glucose supplementation regimes in patient 1

Treatment period	Age	Glucose regime	Dose rate (g/kg . h)	Growth rate (cm/year)
A	Birth to 10 y 8½ m	Oral 3 hourly	0.3	1.5
B	10 y 8½ m to 11 y 1 m	Intravenous	0.44	16.5
C	11 y 1 m to 11 y 8 m	Oral 2 hourly	0.44	1.5
D	11 y 8 m to 13 y 10 m	Continuous nasogastric	0.44	6.0
E	13 y 10 m to 16 y 4 m	Nocturnal nasogastric + 1 hourly oral	0.36	2.5–5.8

pulmonary embolus, and a parainfluenza virus was subsequently isolated, but it was felt that an embolus could not be excluded. Thereafter a peripheral venous site was used for the silastic catheter, along with 10% dextrose solution. Following several episodes of thrombophlebitis, an arteriovenous anastomosis was created surgically at the wrist for future use.

Intravenous infusions were discontinued after 140 days, and for the next 7 months (period C), glucose supplementation was given at the same total daily dose, but 2 hourly, orally, day and night. The fourth regime was started at the age of 11 years 8 months (period D). This was continuous (24 hour) infusion of supplementary dextrose by the same pump, but via a fine nasogastric silicone rubber catheter. This continued at home, and at school, for a total of 2 years 2 months. Again, the glucose dose was the same. The patient passed her own nasogastric tube when necessary. The final, and current, treatment regime (E) consists of continuous nasogastric infusion at night, but with hourly oral supplements during the day.

Biochemical data

The biochemical changes observed are summarized in Table 17.2. The most striking finding was the effect on lipid metabolism, as reflected by plasma cholesterol and glyceride glycerol concentrations. For both parameters, the levels during continuous glucose supply (B, D, E) are considerably lower than the intermittent oral supplementation periods (A, C) ($p < 0.01$). Similar results are seen for serum glutamateoxaloacetate transaminase ($p < 0.05$) although the levels did not revert completely to normal. The apparently wide variation in period C is due to a progressive rise in SGOT throughout the 2

TABLE 17.2   Biochemical data obtained in patient 1 during different treatment periods, as shown in Table 17.1 (Where multiple observations were made figures shown are the mean ± 1 SEM with number of observations in brackets)

Treatment period	Cholesterol (mmol/l)	Glyceride glycerol (mmol/l)	SGOT (u/l)	uric acid (μmol/l)	Lactate (mmol/l)	Pyruvate (μmol/l)
A	13.9 ± 1.0 (6)	29.0	69	513 ± 15 (5)	5.6	200
B	6.7 ± 0.3 (15)	7.4 ± 0.7 (13)	21.4 ± 1.7 (16)	399 ± 33 (10)	2.5 ± 0.2 (9)	156 ± 18 (10)
C	11.8 ± 0.8 (5)	26.5 ± 3.6 (4)	41.0 ± 8.7 (6)	524 ± 24 (5)	4.3 ± 0.7 (16)	344 ± 57 (3)
D	8.7 ± 0.4 (2)	8.8 ± 0.8 (18)	20.6 ± 1.5 (17)	482 ± 18 (20)	4.4 ± 0.3 (19)	301 ± 23 (13)
E	9.13 ± 0.4 (8)	9.0 ± 1.0 (11)	23.4 ± 3.7 (9)	481 ± 28 (5)	5.3 ± 0.3 (11)	280 ± 18 (10)

hourly glucose regime; by the end of this time, levels were again above 60 u/l.

In this patient uric acid levels have always been near the upper limit of normal, but the intravenous therapy (B) resulted in significantly lower levels than the bracketing periods (A and C) ($p < 0.01$). Plasma lactate ($p < 0.01$) and pyruvate ($p < 0.05$) levels were also lowest during intravenous therapy, but were unaffected by nasogastric supplementation.

The mean random blood glucose levels were similar in all the treatment regimes, but the range is markedly different. Figure 17.1 shows plasma glucose sampled every half hour for 4 hours during continuous nasogastric supplementation, contrasted with the same dose given orally by 2 hourly boluses. The mean level is identical, at around 5 mmol/l, but the variation of glucose levels in intermittent oral supplementation is more marked; the recurrent hypoglycaemia in 2 hourly oral supplementation is particularly obvious.

As expected, the plasma insulin levels also vary. Figure 17.2 shows data from the same two modified tolerance tests as Figure 17.1 and the difference in variation in peripheral insulin concentration is clear. During continuous intravenous infusion of glucose, plasma glucose levels were similar to those for nasogastric infusion as shown in Figure 17.1, but mean plasma insulin levels were some 30% lower than those for nasogastric infusion. Continuous

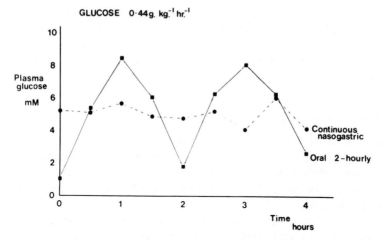

Figure 17.1   Peripheral venous plasma glucose concentration in patient 1 during continuous nasogastric glucose (●– – – –●), or oral glucose boluses at 0 and 2 hours (■———■). Total dose of glucose was the same in each case, at a mean rate of 0.44 g/kg.h

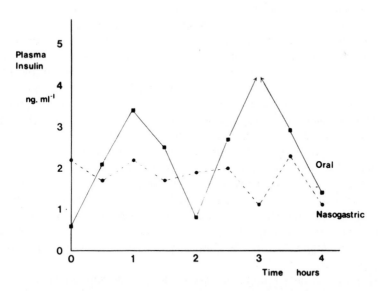

Figure 17.2   Data from the same tests as Figure 1, showing peripheral venous plasma insulin concentration. Symbols as in Figure 1. Value at 3 hours in oral test was greater than 4 ng/ml

intravenous or nasogastric infusion did not suppress the growth hormone secretion seen during spontaneous sleep.

The typical quantitative defect seen in platelet aggregation studies[2] was also reversed by continuous supplementation, associated with an increase in platelet nucleotide levels.

Clinical course

As far as the patient was concerned, the greatest change from the pretreatment period (A) was that she felt better. Within hours of starting the intravenous infusion, her respiratory rate had decreased and she was able to maintain a reasonable plasma pH without much respiratory compensation. Her spontaneous activity increased and her appetite improved. During the intravenous supplementation period (B) her total energy intake doubled, although the supplementary glucose accounted for less than half the carbohydrate intake. Perhaps of greatest importance was the fact that catch-up growth occurred[3, 4].

Figure 17.3 shows her growth chart since the age of 8, based on measurements made independently. The height velocity data are summarized in Table 17.1. In 140 days of intravenous supplementation (B), she grew more than she had grown in the previous 2 years (A). She continued to grow at this rate for a short time when supplementation was changed to 2 hourly, but the rate then decreased again to unsatisfactory levels (C). During the 140 days free of hypoglycaemia (B), she became more sensitive to fasting. A week after discontinuing continuous intravenous therapy, while nominally on 2 hourly supplements, she was half an hour late with one dose. Symptoms of hypoglycaemia were rapidly followed by a hypoglycaemic convulsion, her first ever. An intentional delay of the same dose the following day again resulted in symptomatic hypoglycaemia, which was rapidly treated. The plasma glucose level was shown subsequently to be 1 mmol/l, a level which had been well tolerated previously.

Adequate growth occurred during continuous nasogastric supplementation (D) but when this was replaced by hourly oral glucose by day, height velocity initially decreased; this coincided with a period of low morale and poor compliance, and, in retrospect, the frequency of daytime glucose was less than suggested. In the last year, there has been considerable improvement.

Obesity became a problem during intravenous supplementation. Her weight percentile changed from below the 3rd to above the 50th between $10\frac{1}{2}$ and $11\frac{1}{2}$ years of age, by which time she was 100% overweight. By careful energy control, there has been little weight gain for the last 3 years

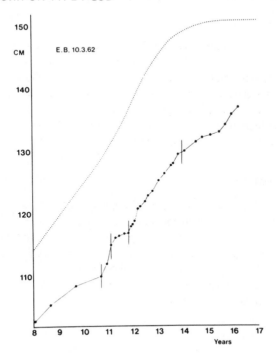

Figure 17.3 Growth in height of patient 1 compared to the 3rd percentile of Tanner. The five consecutive treatment periods are separated by the vertical lines

and her weight is just above the 3rd percentile.

At a chronological age of 16 years 3 months her bone age was 13 years. It has always been delayed, but there has been no episodic rapid increase similar to that in height velocity, although before intensive treatment started the discrepancy was much greater.

Puberty is also late. Menarche has not yet occurred, but first signs of puberty are appearing, and FSH and LH levels are increasing. If growth can be maintained at the current rate, the prognosis for final adult height should be good.

The hepatomegaly decreased by about 40% as estimated clinically during intravenous infusion, and has remained of similar size since then. She remains generally well in herself, goes to a normal school, and will shortly take 'O level' examinations.

PATIENT 2

The elder brother of patient 1 was diagnosed at the age of 5 months as glycogen storage disease, Type I. Liver biopsy showed no glucose-6-phosphatase activity, and a glycogen content of 8.5%. Muscle biopsy was normal. He was given a course of growth hormone, at the age of 9 years, similar to that given to his sister. His iatrogenic rickets was effectively treated with added bicarbonate and later vitamin D. He was less growth retarded than his sister, although always below the 3rd percentile.

Treatment regimes

Until the age of $13\frac{1}{2}$ years, oral glucose supplementation was given 3 hourly, day and night, at a rate of approximately 0.3 g/kg . h (Table 17.3). This was followed by 15 months of 2 hourly supplementation, day and night. For the next 15 months, supplementation was increased to hourly during the day, but again at the same overall rate of about 0.33 g/kg . h. For the last 3 years, he has had a continuous nasogastric infusion of glucose at night, with hourly oral glucose during the day.

Results

The progress in amelioration of biochemical parameters is obvious from Table 17.3, but we do not have data as extensive as that on his sister.

Since starting nocturnal nasogastric supplementation, he has shown considerable catch-up growth (Figure 17.4), more than can be attributed simply

TABLE 17.3 Growth and biochemical findings in patient 2 during different dietary regimes (Where shown, figures represent the mean $\pm$ 1 SEM, with number of observations in brackets.)

Age	Regime (glucose 0.33 g/kg . h) Day	Night	Cholesterol (mmol/l)	Glyceride glycerol (mmol/l)	SGOT (u/l)	growth (cm/year)
Birth to 13 y 6 m	3 hourly		10.8 ± 0.6 (9)	—	75	3.9
13 y 6 m to 14 y 9 m	2 hourly		10.2 ± 0.9 (4)	18.2 ± 3.1 (4)	48 ± 8 (3)	7.6
14 y 9 m to 16 y	1 hourly + 2 hourly		7.7 ± 0.5 (5)	8.6 ± 0.6 (6)	34 ± 4 (5)	9.1
16 y to 19 y	1 hourly α nasogastric		6.1 ± 0.4 (8)	4.5 ± 0.6 (7)	17 ± 2 (8)	11.2

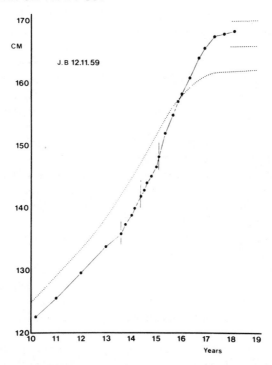

Figure 17.4 Growth in height of patient 2, compared to the 3rd percentile and finally the 10th and 25th percentiles of Tanner. The four treatment regimes are separated by the vertical lines

to puberty which in his case was not delayed and is now almost complete. He has crossed the 3rd and 10th percentiles, and final adult height is therefore quite satisfactory. He is doing well at a school with a high academic standard and is generally well adjusted to his problems, although limitation of sustained vigorous exercise, because of failure to mobilize glucose, is obviously a handicap for an otherwise apparently normal young man.

SUMMARY

Both these siblings were able to maintain a normal growth rate by increasing the frequency of their glucose supplementation and catch up growth has been possible in each child. The intravenous route seems best, but is least practical. It has advantages pre-operatively[5], in terms of decreasing the liver size, and correcting coagulation defects. Folkman *et al.*[6] described the effect of a short period of intravenous hyperalimentation in two young children prior to portacaval shunt procedure; their infusion contained amino acids, electrolytes and trace elements as well as glucose, but the period of time was too short to document changes in growth rate resulting from infusion. Greene *et al.*[7] demonstrated increased linear growth in three older children treated with nocturnal nasogastric supplementation containing glucose, oligosaccharides and aminoacids, but with 3 hourly diurnal feeding. They demonstrated a lowering of previously elevated glucagon levels in two of their patients. Burr[8] gives an account of 3 weeks each of intravenous and continuous nasogastric feeding, prior to portacaval surgery in a 16 year old.

The mechanism of action of glucose supplementation is unclear, but in our patients supplementation with glucose alone seems to be sufficient. Correction of lactic acidosis by intravenous infusion was associated with the best growth, but good growth was obtained during nasogastric supplementation in spite of high plasma lactates. It is probable that avoidance of recurrent hypoglycaemia is a major factor in promoting growth, but it is important that the apparent loss of ability to cope with hypoglycaemia should be remembered in any child on such a regime. Differences between patients may well represent heterogeneity in efficiency of metabolism or its control, especially in regard to use of alternative substrates. In any event, it seems that improvement can be obtained in both growth and plasma biochemistry. The aim must be to find the method which is best suited to the individual, by balancing his requirements against the difficulties, and the risks, of the treatment.

Acknowledgements

The liver biopsy data was provided by Professor Hers. The insulin levels were measured by Dr Richard Himsworth. Growth data was obtained from Professor Tanner. The data could not have been collected without the outstanding co-operation, goodwill and encouragement of the patients and their family.

References

1. Ball, G., Chenery, L., Hemsley, D. and Macnab, A. J. (1974). A miniature peristaltic pump with electronic rate control: technical adaption to a clinical need. *Biomedical Engineering*, **9**, 563
2. Hutton, R. A., Macnab, A. J. and Rivers, R. P. A. (1976). Defect of platelet function associated with chronic hypoglycemia. *Arch. Dis. Child.*, **51**, 49

3. Macnab, A. J. (1974). Type 1 glycogenosis: effects of prolonged intravenous dextrose infusion on growth and plasma biochemistry. *Pediatr. Res.*, **8**, 136

4. Macnab, A. J. (1974). Increased growth velocity in type 1 glycogen storage disease during reversal of metabolic abnormalities by two periods of prolonged dextrose infusion. *Pediatrica XIV: Proceedings of 14th International Congress of Paediatrics*, **10** (Metabolism), p. 195

5. Starzl, T. E., Putnam, C. W., Porter, K. A., Halgrimson, C. G., Corman, J., Brown, B. I., Gotlin, R. W., Rodgerson, D. D. and Green, H. L. (1973). Portal diversion for the treatment of glycogen storage disease in humans. *Ann. Surg.*, **178**, 525

6. Folkman, J., Philippart, A., Tze, W-J and Crigler, J. (1972). Portacaval shunt for glycogen storage disease: value of prolonged intravenous hyperalimentation before surgery. *Surgery*, **72**, 306

7. Greene, H. L., Slonim, A. E., O'Neill, J. A. and Burr, I. M. (1976). Continuous nasogastric feeding for management of type 1 glycogen storage disease. *N. Engl. J. Med.*, **294**, 423

8. Burr, I. M., O'Neill, J. A., Karzon, D. T., Howard, L. J. and Green, H. L. (1974). Comparison of the effects of total parenteral nutrition, continuous intragastric feeding, and portacaval shunt on a patient with type 1 glycogen storage disease. *J. Pediatr.*, **85**, 792

18

Pre- and postnatal diagnosis of glycogen storage disease

G. Hug

DEFINITION OF GLYCOGENOSIS

Glycogen storage disease (GSD) exists when the concentration or structure of glycogen is abnormal in any tissue of the body due to an inherited disease. Hepatic glycogen concentration is often decreased during starvation, haemodynamic shock, in Reye's syndrome, or at autopsy, and increased in hypoglycaemia or diabetes. Abnormal glycogen concentration in these situations is not accepted as evidence for GSD since it is either an artifact (autopsy), is acquired and not inherited (Reye's syndrome) or is secondary to a different disease (diabetes). The syndrome of GSD can be divided further following the rule first suggested by Gerti T. Cori[1] that each newly recognized enzymatic defect be assigned a new type. If the defective enzyme is not known, typing should still be done if it is based on distinct clinical and biochemical features. Indeed, in Dr Cori's original classification of four types, generalized glycogenosis was listed as GSD II although the associated defect of acid α-glucosidase had not yet been described[1]. The resulting focus on the unique clinical features of GSD II facilitated the diagnosis of the disease in additional patients.

Our classification of GSD is listed in Table 18.1 (see p. 360) and contains the diagnostic features of each type. Figure 1 depicts the associated metabolic pathways. Table 18.2 presents glycogen concentration and en-

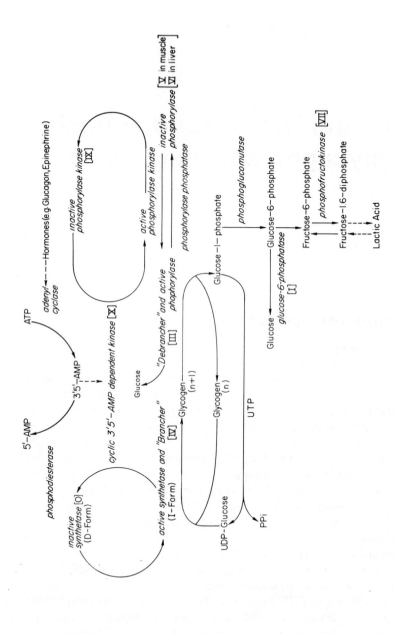

Figure 18.1 System of phosphorylase activation and anaerobic glycolysis. Roman numerals in brackets indicate the type of GSD that is associated with the deficiency of the respective enzyme activity (see also Table 18.1)

TABLE 18.2 Biochemical analysis of tissue from glycogenosis

Cases	Glycogen concentration (% of wet tissue)	Phosphorylase (μmoles phosphate/g.min) Total	Active	Phosphorylase kinase (nmoles of added crystalline phosphorylase b converted to a/g.min)	Acid α-glucosidase (μmoles glucose/g.min)	Amylo-1,6-glucosidase*	Glucose-6-phosphatase (μmoles phosphate/g.min)
Normal							
Liver	2.5–6.0	44.3 ± 9.6	25.1 ± 6.5	28.2 ± 8.3	0.258 ± 0.093	3750 ± 490	4.7 ± 1.9
Muscle	0.1–1.5	78.0 ± 21.1	47.7 ± 13.2	147.7 ± 46.0	0.035 ± 0.011	7113 ± 553	
Type I							
Liver	8.9	42	23	normal	0.242	normal	0
Muscle	0.6	59	38	normal	0.041	normal	
Pseudo-Type I							
Liver	7.4	53	46	normal	0.261	normal	3.9
Muscle	1.1	77	28	normal	0.037	normal	
Type IIa							
Liver	8.8	47	26	normal	0	normal	3.2
Muscle	7.5	64	42	normal	0	normal	
Type IIb							
Liver	11.5	45	29	normal	0.026	normal	5.4
Muscle	1.6	80	31	normal	0	normal	
Type III							
Liver	9.3	40	19	normal	0.210	45	2.9
Muscle	6.0	72	45	normal	0.030	43	
Type V							
Liver	4.5	48	26	normal	0.260	normal	3.8
Muscle	3.8	0	0	normal or increased up to seven times	0.028	normal	

TABLE 18.2 (cont.)

| Cases | Glycogen concentration (% of wet tissue) | Phosphorylase (μmoles phosphate/g.min) | | Phosphorylase kinase (nmoles of added crystalline phosphorylase b converted to a/g.min) | Acid α-glucosidase (μmoles glucose/g.min) | Amylo-1,6-glucosidase* | Glucose-6-phosphatase (μmoles phosphate/g.min) |
		Total	Active				
Type VI							
Liver	7.6	2	1.8	normal	0.176	normal	3.4
Muscle	0.3	61	46	normal	0.025	normal	
Type VIII							
Liver	12.0	43	6	normal	0.312	normal	5.1
Muscle	0.4	58	35	normal	0.040	normal	
Type IXa							
Liver	9.9	46	2.3	7.9‡	0.155	normal	3.7
Muscle	0.3	70	58	normal	0.026	normal	
Type IXb							
Liver	10.5	44	0.8	8.4‡	0.318	normal	2.6
Muscle	.1.4	100	72	normal	0.029	normal	
Type X							
Liver	10.5	39	0.1	normal	0.292	normal	6.8
Muscle	2.9	54	0	81.7§	0.025	normal	
Type XI							
Liver	10.8	53	37	normal	0.243	normal	5.1
Muscle	0.7	69	42	normal	0.029	normal	

* Glucose-^{14}C incorporated into -1,6- branch points expressed as cpm/((mg glycogen)(g tissue)(hour)

† Mean value ± 1 SD

‡ Values obtained with crystalline muscle phosphorylase b as substrate; if endogenous liver phosphorylase is the substrate, the rate of activation is less than 5% of normal

§ Enzyme is demonstrable at physiological pH in GSD X only if I-strain mouse muscle and 3',5'-AMP (i.e. 'activated' cyclic 3'5'-AMP dependent kinase) have been added to homogenate of patient's muscle; in other types of GSD or in normal muscle, the addition of mouse muscle is not needed

zymatic activities in liver and skeletal muscle of normal individuals and of one patient for each type of glycogenosis that we have encountered.

BENEFITS OF DIAGNOSIS

Diagnosis of any disease is important for the following three reasons: (1) it forms the basis for treatment, (2) it excludes other conditions that require different modes of treatment, (3) it is the basis for counselling the patient and his family.

Treatment

Table 18.3 summarizes therapeutic needs of patients with GSD. Therapy may be needed intermittently to relieve symptoms as in some children with GSD 0, I, V, and VII. In an individual patient with GSD I it may be a matter of judgment whether treatment should be instituted. In such a situation an important requirement is that treatment must not be harmful. For this reason therapy with drugs such as Dilantin, or surgical treatment with portacaval shunt, does not have a place in the management of GSD. Dilantin is not effective despite contrary statements in the literature[2]. Regarding portacaval shunt, the published success stories indicate that there may be

TABLE 18.3   The therapy of glycogen storage disease

A. *Treatment not needed*
GSD III, VI, IX, X and many cases of GSD I, V, VII

B. *Treatment needed and available*
GSD 0 and I for hypoglycaemia and acidosis;
GSD I for gout and hyperlipidaemia;
GSD III for recurrent pneumonia;
'Combined' defects (e.g. GSD III/IX) for ? hypoglycaemia;
GSD I may be improved by continuous feeding via intragastric drip to maintain normoglycaemia.

C. *Treatment needed but not available*
GSD II, IV, VIII are fatal despite therapy. Rational therapeutic attempts (e.g. enzyme replacement) may be indicated.
GSD V, VII may present with chronic muscle pain that can be difficult to relieve.
In GSD XI the markedly retarded growth does not respond to available therapy (such as Vitamin D, phosphate supplementation, etc.).

D. *Treatment to be avoided*
Dilantin, phenobarbital, portacaval shunt operation.

the occasional patient who not only escapes the side effects of the procedure but perhaps is helped by it[3]. However, in many patients any kind of treatment may be unnecessary. Patients with GSD VI and IX do well if left alone but such patients have been shunted inadvertently, because typing was not done in sufficient detail prior to the operation, or despite the demonstration of a totally benign type of GSD[4]. As a rule, GSD I is not a malignant disease. If such patients are shunted, good results may occur because of the natural course of the disease and not on account of the operation[4]. It can make matters worse, as indeed it often does[5]. Portacaval shunt is never good therapy in GSD if one also considers the unpublished cases where the operation was followed by death, cirrhosis, closure of the anastomosis or encephalopathy rather than just the published success stories. With the advent of continuous intragastric feeding in patients with GSD I[6], consideration of portacaval shunt operation should no longer be necessary.

There remains the group of GSD where therapy is not available either to relieve an annoying or serious symptom (such as intermittent muscle cramps in GSD V or retarded growth in GSD XI) or to prevent death such as in GSD II, IV and VIII. In these instances, rational therapeutic experimentation should continue provided it does not cause the patient additional problems or pain. Such experimentation may provide insight into the pathophysiological process of these diseases. This understanding is the prerequisite for future effective therapy.

Differential diagnosis

The cardinal symptoms of GSD are hepatomegaly, cardiac enlargement, muscular dysfunction such as cramps or hypotonia, progressive degenerative brain disease, metabolic acidosis and/or hypoglycaemic convulsions. These symptoms may also be indicative of other childhood diseases some of which can be treated successfully. Hence, the correct diagnosis of GSD is important to exclude other treatable diseases.

Genetic counselling

As a rule, genetic advice is requested by the family and the patient with GSD. These conditions are inherited as autosomal recessives except for GSD IXb which follows a sex linked recessive pattern. On average one in four children of an affected family will have the disorder and one of two boys in GSD IXb. Almost without exception the question of prenatal diagnosis is then raised by the family. This procedure engages the public's emotions because of the erroneous belief that it is the first step in a chain of events leading to abortion. In fact, more children are alive because of prenatal diagnosis than would exist without the procedure. This is because couples at risk only want healthy future babies and will avoid pregnancy, or if it occurs will resort to abortion unless they can be assured that the fetus is normal. Since on average the fetus is normal three out of four times, prenatal diagnosis is actually a life saving procedure. In my experience, it is also a procedure that the woman might request to satisfy her 'need to know'. It gives her a chance to prepare herself for the arrival of a sick baby whom she wants.

Table 18.4 indicates the feasibility of prenatal diagnosis of the various types of GSD. It is usually accomplished by the assay of the respective en-

TABLE 18.4   Prenatal diagnosis of glycogenosis

A. *Can be done and is needed*
GSD II (by electronmicroscopy of uncultured amniotic fluid cells)
GSD II, IV (by enzymatic analysis of cultured amniotic fluid cells)

B. *Can be done but is not needed*
GSD III (if the enzymatic defect is generalized, involving skin fibroblasts and cultured amniotic fluid cells)

C. *Cannot be done but is needed*
GSD VIII (brain and liver are the only organs that are involved)

D. *Cannot be done and is not needed*
GSD 0, I, VI, VII, IX, X, XI
GSD III (if the defect is limited to liver and/or muscle and does not involve skin fibroblasts or cultured amniotic fluid cells)

zymatic activities in cultured amniotic fluid cells. The culture of these cells lengthens the time between the earliest date in pregnancy (i.e. the 15th–16th week) when amniocentesis can safely be done and when a diagnosis is available. The need to save time has led to the introduction of enzymatic microassays on short-term microcultures[7]. In short-term cultures, however, types of cells may be prevalent that are different from those predominant in long-term cultures[8]. Enzyme assays on uncultured amniotic fluid cells are fraught with danger and should not be done since 90% of these cells may be non-viable. Biochemical assays on amniotic fluid can be useful but only in combination with proper controls, as illustrated by the fact that acid alpha-glucosidase activity is present in amniotic fluid even if the fetus has GSD II. For success of any method of prenatal diagnosis, optimal collection at amniocentesis and subsequent careful preparation of the specimen are absolutely crucial[9]. All these caveats, only lightly touched upon here, lead to the conclusion that prenatal diagnosis should not be undertaken frivolously. As summarized in Table 18.4, there is no need for prenatal diagnosis in GSD I, III, V, VI, VII, IX, X and XI since these disorders are usually compatible with a reasonably normal life. Thus the risk of losing a normal fetus by mis-diagnosis is not acceptable.

PROCEDURES FOR DIAGNOSIS

There are numerous tests for the diagnosis of GSD and their non-selective use would be prohibitively expensive in effort, time, and money spent and in discomfort to the patient. In Table 18.5 I present a summary of our selective approach. Other diagnostic routes can be taken and might be as effective.

TABLE 18.5   Methods used for the diagnosis of glycogenosis

Obligatory 'hard data'	Facultative 'soft data'
History of patient and family	Tolerance tests:
Physical examination	glucagon, epinephrine
Note: Enlargement of heart, liver, kidney and/or spleen; hypotonia; cerebral malfunction; convulsion	galactose, fructose (potentially dangerous since acute acidosis may be precipitated)
Blood chemistry: uric acid, glucose, lipids, trans-aminases, pH, lactic acid	Biochemical and morphologic analysis of blood cells, cultured skin fibroblasts and urine
Urine analysis	
Biopsy of affected organ(s) (if by 'open' technique, always take muscle)	
Tissue specimens for (a) biochemical analysis (b) morphologic analysis by light microscopy electron microscopy	

Obligatory 'hard data' are derived from procedures that we consider essential. 'Soft data' are the result of ancillary procedures.

Patient history and physical examination

As usual the history of family and patient is of paramount importance as are clinical observations and physical examination. Twitching after overnight fasting and skipped breakfast does suggest hypoglycaemia. In such a situation, affixing the label 'ketotic hypoglycaemia' is not an acceptable alter-native to making a diagnosis, even in the presence of ketosis. Ketotic hypoglycaemia is a biochemical symptom that is associated with disorders such as deficient activity of glycogen synthetase (GSD 0) and fructose-1,6-diphosphatase, or defective secretion of catecholamines. A child who was sent home with the label ketotic hypoglycaemia died during an episode of viral gastroenteritis, when food intake was decreased. After a cousin died under similar circumstances and a sibling had hypoglycaemic convulsions, deficient activity of fructose-1,6-diphosphatase was finally demonstrated in a hepatic biopsy specimen. 'Ketotic hypoglycaemia' is both an intellectually unsatisfactory label and a dangerous one.

Testing procedures

The selection of suitable tests is a matter of judgment although it is easy to list the tests that are available. Non-invasive tests are those done on urine, ECG, X-ray for rickets or size of heart. In our experience, a plain abdominal X-ray has always separated the slightly enlarged kidneys of GSD I from those of GSD III that are of normal size. Examination of liver size by ultrasound is of sufficient precision for the evaluation of therapeutic attempts. In our estimate, ultrasound is superior to isotope liver scan. Blood cells and serum are usually not difficult to obtain, although blood volumes that can safely be withdrawn are limited. Electromyography is useful in differentiating primary myopathy from primary nerve disease with secondary muscle involvement. Glucagon tolerance test is the most useful tolerance test in GSD but is seldom conclusive. It produces a blood sugar curve that is flat in GSD I, VI and XI but is normal in GSD IX. It is flat in GSD III after fasting, but normal if glucagon is given soon after a meal.

Need for biopsy

The decisive procedures are the biochemical and morphologic analyses done on affected tissues. Biopsies are not considered often enough, and not soon enough. Biopsy must not be done casually[10]. There ought to be a discussion as to whether to do a biopsy and if so, of which organs and finally whether to do it with the needle or via an open operation.

My position is that biopsy should be done (in the absence of contraindications such as a tendency for bleeding, etc.) if the examination of tissue is required not only to make the diagnosis of GSD but to exclude the presence of other potentially treatable diseases. For example, one must avoid finding a choledochal cyst at autopsy in a child who was treated for a genetic disease which had not been confirmed by hepatic biopsy.

In general, the organ to be biopsied is the one manifesting the clinical symptoms. There are exceptions to this rule. In a patient suspected on clinical grounds of having GSD II, a small superficial skin biopsy specimen size 1 mm × 2 mm, obtained without bleeding in a one second procedure with sharp curved scissors, will show the diagnostic glycogen accumulations surrounded by a membrane, on electron microscopy. No further diagnostic tests are then required.

Needle biopsy is a convenient approach but that is the least convincing reason for its use. It may not deliver sufficent tissue. One can expect about 50 mg of liver from the Menghini needle. Repeated needle liver biopsies are useful to follow the progress of a disease at intervals for evaluation of treatment. It may be adequate for the initial biopsy, either to solve the problem or to establish the need for an open operation. Needle biopsy of muscle is painful but carries little risk. Needle biopsy of cerebral cortex is dangerous. Needle biopsies of kidney or liver are not painful but they must be considered operations. They are not outpatient procedures. The pre- and postoperative handling of the patient has to follow a precise protocol[11]. Complications must be recognized and treated promptly. With this formalized approach our record of many thousands of needle biopsies has been good.

Liver biopsy at laparotomy

If an open liver biopsy is performed, the patient's physician should be present in the operating room to receive the specimens from the surgeon and deal with them precisely as required. If the indications are good enough for a biopsy, it is essential that the physician personally ensures the success of the procedure. Muscle tissue, also, is diagnostically valuable and should be obtained from the incised abdominal wall. It should be taken on the way in, when it will be fresh and viable. The biopsy specimens should be divided immediately into the various pieces needed. For example, just enough (three to four cubes of 1 mm) should be taken for electron microscopy into glutaraldehyde (3% in 0.1 mol/l phosphate buffer, pH 7.2 to 7.4), but the lion's share must go for biochemistry. If the amount of tissue is too small the surgeon should be told immediately, so that he may be able to take a second biopsy.

Failure of the operation is more often due to lack of detailed planning than to technical difficulties in the surgical procedure. Prior arrangements for the necessary investigations should be made so that the specimens can be sent immediately to the co-operating laboratory. The tissue for the biochemical tests must be transported in dry ice, but it is equally important that the electron-microscopy specimen is kept unfrozen. It should go without saying that a clinical summary of the patient should accompany these specimens, but this is very frequently forgotten.

SUMMARY OF FINDINGS INDICATIVE OF GSD

The work up for GSD is one of the less complex exercises in paediatrics. Hepatomegaly, cardiomyopathy, stunted growth and muscular hypotonia, either isolated or combined, should trigger at least a fleeting thought of GSD. Symptoms more specific to one type of GSD are detailed in Table 18.1.

It should be remembered that, although convulsions may occur in Type 1, blood glucose concentrations of 1.2 mmol/l, or less, may be well tolerated. However, a child who has been maintained for some time with a normal blood glucose by continuous feeding, is then likely to react with severe hypoglycaemic convulsions if the blood sugar is allowed to fall[12].

LIMITATIONS OF PROCEDURES

As Table 18.5 indicates, we do not rely much on indirect tests such as tolerance tests that work through layers of uncontrollable metabolic happenings, interposed between the administration of the test substance and its measured effect. This complexity makes it difficult to define the body's normal response and also the pathological results. The glucagon tolerance test is certainly a useful adjunct for making a diagnosis, particularly if the response of urinary cyclic 3′,5′-AMP is also determined. If cyclic 3′,5′-AMP is increased in the urine after glucagon but the blood glucose remains unchanged, the metabolic response is intact as far as and including the activation of adenyl cyclase (Figure 18.1). This is the case in GSD VI and XI.

Assays of enzymes are generally not reliable if they are made on tissues that have gone through complex sequences of extracorporeal manipulations such as culturing of fibroblasts, or isolation of white cells. Repeated assay on aliquots of the pooled homogenate of different fibroblast cultures may give nearly identical results, while the same assay technique on separate homogenates made of fibroblast cultures grown in different flasks but derived from the same skin biopsy may give results that differ from each other by 100%. Culture conditions vary greatly between the different flasks although all are maintained in the same incubator. Consequently, we have been unable to confirm experiments with fibroblast cultures reported from other laboratories, demonstrating, for example, the sex linked recessive inheritance of GSD IXb[13]. Similar considerations pertain to white blood cells as indicated in Tables 18.6 and 18.7 which show representative results of rather extensive studies on white cell phosphorylase activity. Standard deviations are much too large to instill any degree of confidence with respect to the significance of the means. Again, other workers have reported reliable results on isolated white cell phosphorylase activity[14].

TABLE 18.6 **The effect of the method of cell isolation and assay conditions on white blood cell phosphorylase activity in 11 normal volunteers. The activities are expressed as mean ($\pm$ SD) in (μmol P/mmol N_2)/min**

	Method of cell isolation	
Assay conditions	in the presence of NaF	in the absence of NaF
In the presence of 5'AMP	1.76 $\pm$ 0.7	1.14 $\pm$ 0.9
In the absence of 5'AMP	0.82 $\pm$ 0.3	0.59 $\pm$ 0.5

Regardless of the fact that in our hands the assay of white cell phosphorylase and its activation system is not a reliable diagnostic procedure, I also believe that it is in the patient's best interest if one examines his liver tissue in order to determine why his liver is enlarged. It is

TABLE 18.7 **Phosphorylase activity in white cells (mean $\pm$ SD) of five different blood specimens obtained in the presence of NaF, from three normal volunteers activities are expressed as (μmol P/mmol N_2)/min**

	In the presence of 5'-AMP	In the absence of 5'-AMP
R.C.	3.9 $\pm$ 2.6	2.6 $\pm$ 1.2
A.W.	1.3 $\pm$ 0.6	0.9 $\pm$ 0.4
G.H.	2.9 $\pm$ 0.8	1.6 $\pm$ 1.1

dangerous to explain hepatomegaly by white cell assays even if they worked well. For example in the course of the study of a family with GSD VI, low leucocyte phosphorylase activity has been reported in a child with normal sized liver[14]. If this child's liver had been enlarged because of other hepatic disease, such as neuroblastoma, the diagnosis would have been missed, since the hepatomegaly would have been interpreted as a consequence of GSD VI. Hepatomegaly requires liver biopsy, not because of GSD but for the diagnosis of other conditions that may kill the patient.

PRACTICAL ASPECTS OF THE GLYCOGEN STORAGE DISEASES

GSD 0

Glycogen synthetase deficiency has been demonstrated in twins and an unrelated 9-year-old girl. Enzyme activity was defective in liver but normal in muscle and blood cells. Hypoglycaemia, hyperketonaemia, non-responsiveness to glucagon, and convulsions occur after fasting and can all be corrected by regular food intake. The latter prevents mental retardation[15].

GSD I

Lipid droplets within hepatocytes may be of enormous size as shown in Figure 18.2. The specimen is from a boy who at 2 years of age had a large liver, stunted growth, episodes of hypoglycaemia and acidosis, as well as all the other biochemical and clinical characteristics of the disease. He was conventionally treated with frequent feeding. He is now in his twenties, leads a normal life and has a healthy child. He has gout which is being treated. His liver is moderately enlarged on palpation, but the previous marked abdominal protuberance has disappeared. Such histories indicate the good prognosis of the condition without surgery and that prenatal diagnosis of GSD I is a low priority. Prenatal diagnosis using cultured amniotic fibroblasts is not possible since these cells normally do not contain glucose-6-phosphatase. Hepatoma seems to occur with increased frequency in some children with GSD I[16].

Pseudo GSD I

Clinical observations indicate GSD I with a certainty that makes it difficult for the physician to accept the finding of normal activity of hepatic glucose-6-phosphatase, and liver glycogen concentration is increased. Perhaps the glucose-6-phosphatase present is not active *in vivo*. In any case, the clinical course and symptoms are indistinguishable from those of GSD I[17].

GSD II

Dr Putschar, now of Massachusetts General Hospital, reported the first light microscopic analysis of the disease. His account is remarkable and

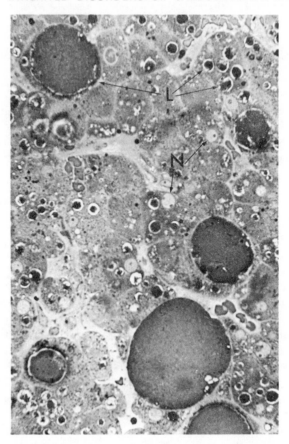

Figure 18.2 Liver biopsy specimen of GSD 1. There are numerous lipid droplets (L) of great variation in size. Nuclei (N) (× 490)

noteworthy not only for reasons of priority but also because of the clear and beautiful description of abundantly present intracellular vacuoles[18], now known to be abnormal lysosomes[19], which are the accepted morphological hallmark of the disease. In Figure 18.3, these abnormal lysosomes are visible in every hepatocyte of an infant with GSD IIa. The infant was then treated with daily infusions of glycogen degrading enzymes prepared from *Aspergillus niger*[20]. Three weeks later, we biopsied the child's liver again. The hepatic glycogen concentration had dropped from abnormally high pretreatment values (7.8%) to within normal range (2.9%) and concomitantly the abnormal lysosomes had disappeared from the patient's hepatocytes (Figure 18.4). This course of events can also be demonstrated by electron

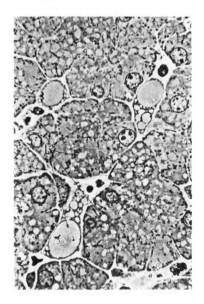
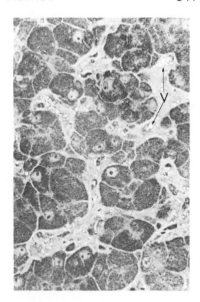

Figure 18.3 (*left*) Liver biopsy specimen of GSD IIa before enzyme infusion. Numerous 'abnormal lysosomes' filled with glycogen (Ly) are visible in every hepatocyte (× 500) **Figure 18.4** (*right*) Liver biopsy specimen from the same child with GSD IIa as in Figure 18.3 but obtained after 3 weeks of daily infusion of glycogen degrading enzymes. The abnormal lysosomes that were visible within hepatocytes prior to the enzyme administration have now disappeared. Kupffer cells are hypertrophic and contain clear vacuoles (V) (× 350)

microscopy[20, 21]. Unfortunately, success in the treatment of the hepatic morphology was not translated into clinical improvement. The disease took its usual relentless course and the child died of GSD IIa despite continuous enzyme administration.

If one considers the havoc caused by GSD II in muscle and heart (Figures 18.5 and 18.6) it is understandable that these children are hypotonic and die of respiratory and cardiac failure. It is less clear why the increased amount of cytoplasmic glycogen outside the abnormal lysosomes, is not degraded by the enzymes of the phosphorylase pathway with which it is presumably in contact[9, 21, 22]. During the continuous daily administration of fungal enzymes, hepatic glycogen, which was now deposited solely in the cytoplasm, increased again steadily after the initial fall, although abnormal lysosomes did not reappear. This observation may indicate the formation in these hepatocytes of a type of glycogen that cannot be degraded by the phosphorylase pathway analogous perhaps to that which occurs in muscle.

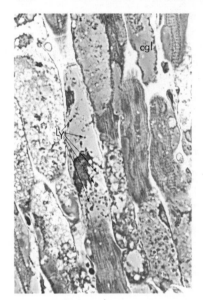 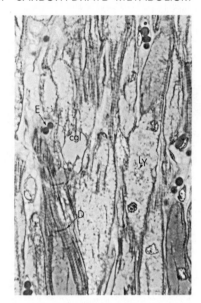

Figure 18.5 (*left*)   Muscle biopsy specimen of GSD IIa. Contractile elements are scarce and disrupted by large areas of cytoplasmic glycogen (cgl) that surrounds 'abnormal lysosomes' (Ly) (× 350)   **Figure 18.6** (*right*)   Heart autopsy specimen of GSD IIa. Contractile elements are replaced by extensive cytoplasmic glycogen (cgl) within which 'abnormal lysosomes' (Ly) are visible. (E), erythrocytes; (D), intercalated disk (× 350)

For its removal this glycogen would normally require segregation into lysosomes followed by acid alpha-glucosidase mediated intralysosomal degradation. In GSD II, because of defective alpha-glucosidase, the lysosomal degradation would not occur and the lysosomes would become engorged by glycogen. During treatment with fungal enzymes, abnormal lysosomes would be modified by a mechanism previously described[21]. As a consequence the type of glycogen usually deposited within lysosomes would remain in the cytoplasm where it would accumulate because the phosphorylase pathway could not degrade it.

Although we do not understand all aspects of the abnormal lysosomes, we find that they have great diagnostic potential. Their presence in cultured skin fibroblasts (Figure 18.7) implies that they may be useful for diagnosis in superficial skin biopsy specimens, as shown in Figure 18.8. In addition, we find that they can be used for the prenatal diagnosis of GSD II[9, 23]. It is, of course, possible to culture amniotic fluid cells and measure acid alpha-glucosidase activity in these cells. The activity is defective if the fetus has

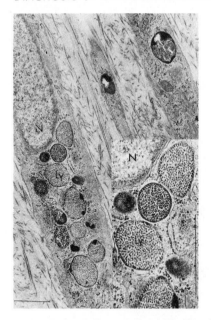
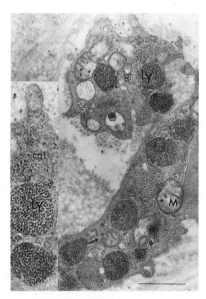

Figure 18.7 (*left*) Cultured skin fibroblasts of GSD IIa. There are numerous glycogen accumulations each surrounded by a membrane (Ly). (N), nucleus. Bar indicates 2 microns **Figure 18.8** (*right*) Skin biopsy specimen of GSD IIa. Diagnostic 'abnormal lysosomes' contain glycogen and are surrounded by a membrane (Ly). (M), mitochondrion; (cgl), cytoplasmic glycogen. Bar indicates 2 microns

GSD IIa. Additional enzymes should also be measured in the same cultures to demonstrate their viability. Alternatively, we found it useful to search, with the electron microscope, for abnormal lysosomes in the uncultured amniotic fluid cells. This prenatal diagnosis by ultrastructural analysis can be completed within one day after the amniocentesis[9, 23]. The collected cells, properly prepared and fixed as described[9], can be sent by airmail letter for analysis from anywhere in the world.

Figure 18.9 indicates the ultra-structural appearance of a normal uncultured amniotic fluid cell. Most of these cells are probably not viable. The nucleus is disintegrating and mitochondria are scarce and defective. Even if present in abundance, cytoplasmic glycogen is entirely normal. In Figure 18.10 an uncultured amniotic fluid cell is shown from a 16 week pregnancy at risk for GSD II. In addition to the aforementioned features, this cell contains several abnormal lysosomes that are characteristic for GSD IIa. These abnormal lysosomes illustrate well the stringent morphologic criteria that must be fulfilled for reliable diagnosis. A single, uninterrupted membrane

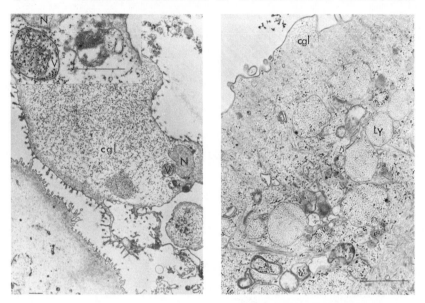

Figure 18.9 (*left*) Normal uncultured amniotic fluid cell. The nucleus (N) is disintegrating. The vacuolar structures (V) are not abnormal lysosomes but are probably disintegrating mitochondria. (cgl), cytoplasmic glycogen. Bar indicates 2 microns **Figure 18.10** (*right*) Uncultured amniotic fluid cell of GSD IIa. Cytoplasmic glycogen (cgl) is normal, but the membrane surrounding accumulations of glycogen (Ly) are diagnostic of the disease. Bar indicates 2 microns

must surround a tightly packed accumulation of glycogen particles among which no other intracellular constituents should be discernible. Between this membrane and the glycogen there should be no space, or rim of cytoplasm. The membrane must not be splintered or be discontinuous in any way. I have not found intracellular organelles of this description in any other uncultured amniotic fluid cells except those from pregnancies with a GSD IIa fetus. It is unlikely that they occur in a fetus who is a carrier of the disease since they are not found in muscle, liver or skin of obligatory carriers. They might occur in a fetus with GSD IIb, but this poses no problem since GSD IIa and IIb have not been encountered in members of the same family.

To date, 21 pregnancies at risk for GSD IIa have been examined. I found diagnostic inclusions in uncultured amniotic fluid cells of five of these pregnancies. The products of these five pregnancies had GSD IIa, as shown biochemically and morphologically at subsequent abortion or delivery. The remaining pregnancies produced healthy babies.

GSD IIa babies at birth are clinically healthy, although the diagnosis is already possible by the examination of muscle biopsy specimens in which the glycogen concentration is increased and alpha-glucosidase activity is defective. When examining fetal tissues for GSD II one should be aware that normal fetal heart and muscle may contain nearly as much glycogen as heart and muscle of GSD II. However, normal fetal liver does not contain abnormal lysosomes, in contrast to the latter's presence in fetal hepatocytes of GSD IIa (Figure 18.11).

GSD II of late onset, or GSD IIb, poses additional problems of comprehension that have been mentioned previously[9].

GSD III

This type of GSD is generally compatible with normal life though one of our patients, who also had GSD IX, died suddenly at home. Repeated episodes of pneumonia may cause problems in these children. Portacaval shunt has been performed, but there is no indication for this.

GSD IV

This disease is fatal in early childhood. It is the only glycogenosis associated with a degree of hepatic cirrhosis that leads to ascites, portal hypertension and splenomegaly. In most cases, tissue glycogen concentration is reduced due to a defect of glycogen synthesis[24].

GSD V

Muscle phosphorylase deficiency interferes with normal lactic acid production from the muscle's own glycogen. Serum lactic acid concentration should not increase during ischaemic exercise but this is not a practical diagnostic test. We prefer to rely on the clinical symptoms of ischaemia. The blood flow to the patient's arm, and thereby the supply of glucose and oxygen, are occluded by a blood pressure cuff inflated to above systolic pressure. The patient then pumps a rubber bulb with his doctor doing the same exercise simultaneously as control, and to show compassion. A patient with GSD will stop after less than 30 pumping movements because the fingers arrest in classical tetanic position and great pain, whereas the control pumps comfortably past 100. This test is reliable, dramatic, and possibly dangerous to the doctor since he might be hit by the patient because of the pain he is causing him.

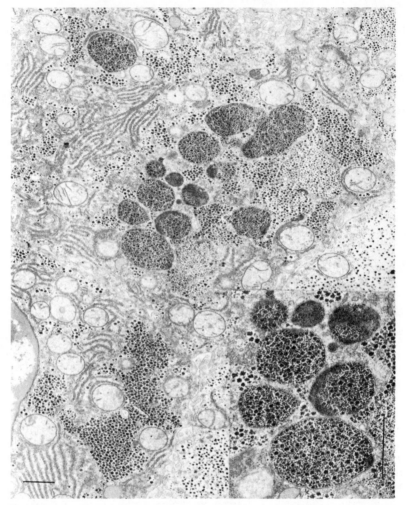

Figure 18.11 Hepatocytes of this 18 week old fetus with GSD IIa contain 'abnormal lysosomes'. Bar indicates 2 microns

Confusion regarding defects of the phosphorylase activation system

In the following section the arguments for the use of one type number for one defective enzyme are considered. GSD VI would be the exclusive designation for biochemically demonstrated liver phosphorylase deficiency.

This would resolve much of the confusion surrounding phosphorylase system defects.

The historical origin of this confusion is as follows. In 1959, reduced activity of liver phosphorylase was described by Hers in three human liver specimens[25]. Two of these specimens also had increased glycogen concentration. Normal glycogen (2.2%) in the third specimen was explained as the consequence of a missed breakfast in a patient with glycogenosis of the liver, We have not encountered any patient in whom hepatic glycogenosis was cured by missing breakfast! It seems more likely that the liver specimen with the normal glycogen concentration was not from a case of hepatic glycogenosis but had been processed suboptimally, producing a low liver phosphorylase as an artifact. This explanation is consistent with the fact that low liver phosphorylase activity occurs in any biopsy specimen that has been kept at room temperature for a few minutes[26].

Cognisant of the complex phosphorylase activating system in which any one of several different defects could result in low phosphorylase activity, Hers did not report the three initial specimens with this finding as representing phosphorylase deficiency[25]. This unwarranted label was attached to the condition of the same patients by their physicians the following year[27]. In fact, liver phosphorylase deficiency was only demonstrated biochemically in 1970 when we had the opportunity to do the necessary series of activation experiments in the defective liver homogenate of a patient[28]. These results were confirmed in a second patient[29]. In 1965 we reported the disease in a child with low liver phosphorylase activity that was reduced because of loss of control over the degree of normal phosphorylase activation[26]. This child had progressive degenerative brain disease, hepatomegaly, increased glycogen in the liver and cerebral cortex where it appeared as alpha-particles[9, 30], and this distinctive clinical picture was labelled GSD VIII[22].

In 1966, we described the first patient with liver phosphorylase kinase deficiency[31] and the defect was documented by biochemical analysis of liver tissue. This patient also had low liver phosphorylase activity, but since this was traced to yet another defect in the phosphorylase activation system, namely phosphorylase kinase, we called this entity GSD IX[22, 32]. The initial patient with GSD IX was a girl and additional patients demonstrating autosomal recessive inheritance have been described[32]. This condition was labelled GSD IXa after a sex linked recessive form of this condition was demonstrated[33], which we called GSD IXb. An earlier study suggested a sex linked inherited liver phosphorylase kinase deficiency but this was done on white blood cells exclusively[34]. Since the study did not contain any assays of liver phosphorylase kinase it is uncertain whether these patients had liver phosphorylase kinase deficiency, especially since muscle tissue was said to be defective also[35]. As a consequence the authors considered phosphorylase kinase deficiency to be a generalized disorder. Muscle tissue has been normal biochemically and morphologically in all of our patients with GSD IXa or IXb.

GSD IX is therefore not the counterpart in men of muscle phosphorylase kinase deficiency in mice. However, in 1970 we reported one patient with deactivated phosphorylase in liver and in muscle as well, and increased glycogen concentration in both tissues[36]. Phosphorylase deactivation in this patient was traced to the loss of cyclic $3',5'$-AMP dependent kinase activity, and the condition was labelled GSD X^{36}.

Although it has become apparent that several different defects might result in low phosphorylase activity, Hers had suggested that conditions of hepatic glycogenosis which were shown not to be GSD I, II or III, should be called GSD VI[37]. This diffuse concept of GSD VI is confusing, since it would include pseudo GSD I, cases of diabetes, different forms of hypoglycaemia, the benign hepatomegaly of GSD IXa and IXb, as well as the fatal GSD VIII, GSD X that also affects muscle, GSD XI with its distinct and different clinical appearance, as well as any as yet unrecognized form of liver glycogenosis. This use of GSD VI violates the rule of one type for one enzyme defect. The confusion is cleared instantly if we simply continue to assign a type with a roman numeral to each defect of a different enzyme or, this knowledge lacking, to a distinct clinical picture. For example, GSD VI is phosphorylase deficiency and only that. GSD IX is phosphorylase kinase deficiency and only that. If different modes were encountered by which the same enzymatic activity, e.g. that of phosphorylase kinase, became defective, then these would be classified as GSD IXa, IXb, etc., indicating that the same enzyme activity is defective but in different ways.

Biochemical diagnosis of phosphorylase system defects

The biochemical requirements for the demonstration of phosphorylase activation defects were described in 1966[31]. How does one diagnose biochemically GSD VI, VIII, IX or X, conditions that share the common symptom of low liver phosphorylase activity? The essential feature of a reliable assay is the correct handling of the biopsy. This must be frozen on dry ice or in liquid nitrogen immediately after its removal from the body. Any delay, such as that caused by transporting the specimen at room temperature by messenger from the operating room to the laboratory, renders the tissue useless for studies of phosphorylase, since it may introduce the artifactual reduction of phosphorylase activity[26]. In autopsy tissue, the enzyme activity is always markedly reduced even in liver known to be normal during life[26]. If artifact is excluded as the reason for low activity then the phosphorylase system must be evaluated by exposing the liver homogenate to conditions which normally lead to the complete activation of total phosphorylase[28-33]. This activation is best done enzymatically by adding ATP and Mg^{2+}, thus employing the endogenous activating system of the liver itself, although Appleman has shown that inactive liver phosphorylase may be demonstrated by the addition of sulphate ions to the homogenate[38]. We prefer the activation by endogenous enzymes since it is defects of these enzymes that we intend to study. In the absence of activation after the addition of ATP and Mg^{2+}, a defect in one of these enzymes may be suspected. The homogenate can then be split conveniently into two or three tubes. To tube 1 we add purified, crystalline rabbit muscle phosphorylase b (i.e. the inactive form of muscle phosphorylase); to the second tube we add purified phosphorylase kinase; and to the third tube, if available, we add muscle homogenate of GSD V.

The following observations can be made (Figure 18.12). If in tube 1 the liver homogenate activates rabbit muscle phosphorylase, and in tube 2 (and 3) endogenous phosphorylase activity does not appear even after kinase is added, we conclude that (1) the endogenous activation system is intact but (2) there is no liver phosphorylase to be activated. Consequently, we are dealing with GSD VI. If on the other hand, in tube 1 rabbit muscle phosphorylase is not converted into its active form, but in tube 2 (and 3) normal total activity of endogenous liver phosphorylase appears after kinase addition, we conclude that (1) liver phosphorylase is present but (2) its activating kinase is deficient. Consequently, we are dealing with GSD IX. There are, of course, nuances to this general outline. For example, muscle phosphorylase kinase regularly reveals about 25% more endogenous total liver phosphorylase than can be obtained using the liver's own activating system[32]. Similarly, although less than 5% of total kinase may be demonstrable in a liver of GSD IX using the rate of activation of the endogenous phosphorylase, the same liver homogenate will produce 30% of normal rate using rabbit muscle phosphorylase b as substrate[29]. There are degrees of reduction in enzyme activity both for phosphorylase and for phosphorylase kinase[29]. In principle, however, the proper biochemical workup requires testing of the adequacy of the liver phosphorylase activating system as summarized in Figure 18.12 in which it is shown also that the homogenate of GSD VIII behaves like that of normal liver (inasmuch as it is activated by ATP and Mg^{2+} alone) except that the initial phosphorylase activity is between 20 and 40% of normal.

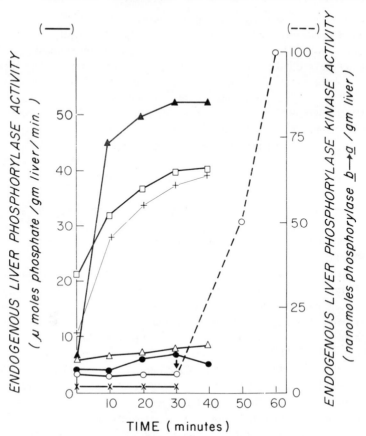

Figure 18.12 Biochemical demonstration of liver phosphorylase system defects. The 'left' ordinate indicates endogenous liver phosphorylase activity in the various homogenates. Activation of endogenous liver phosphorylase is depicted in solid lines. The 'right' ordinate indicates activity of rabbit muscle phosphorylase that was added in its inactive (*b*) form to the liver homogenate at 30 minutes (↓). All homogenates are fortified with ATP and MgCl₂. The 'normal' course of activation (□———□) is not different from that of GSD VIII (+———+) except that the latter starts well below normal. It is apparent that normal initial activity is > 50% of total phosphorylase activity whereas in GSD VIII it is < 30%, although total phosphorylase after 40 minutes of activation is seen to be the same in the control as in GSD VIII. In GSD VI there is no endogenous liver phosphorylase activity (●———●) but when the homogenate is fortified with crystalline phosphorylase (↓) the latter is activated by endogenous kinase (○———○----○) that is present in GSD VI homogenate. Hence GSD VI liver is deficient in phosphorylase. In GSD IX, initial activity is low and remains unchanged (△———△). However, if phosphorylase

GSD VI

Liver phosphorylase deficiency[28, 29] is clinically characterized by flat blood sugar curve after glucagon[29], although the urinary excretion of cyclic AMP increases normally. Liver enlargement with a long term tendency for moderate hepatic fibrosis[39], moderate elevation of serum transaminase and normoglycaemia also occur (Figures 18.2 and 18.13).

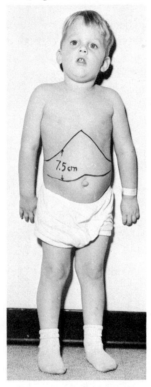

Figure 18.13 Patient with GSD VI. He is clinically not distinguishable from GSD IX or X

---

kinase * is added the latter activates the hepatic homogenate's endogenous phosphorylase (▲——▲). Hence, GSD IX liver is deficient in phosphorylase kinase. Total phosphorylase activity in the homogenate with the added kinase (▲——▲) is about 25% higher than that of normal control. This finding is consistent but unexplained.

  * The added kinase does not contain phosphorylase as impurity (×——×).

GSD VII

Phosphofructokinase deficiency[40] occurred in one of our patients who also was quite a good tennis player. At least in this young man, the defect was not incapacitating.

GSD VIII

In addition to the initial patient[22, 26, 30, 41] we may have seen one other child with this condition. However, no biopsy specimen of cerebral cortex for

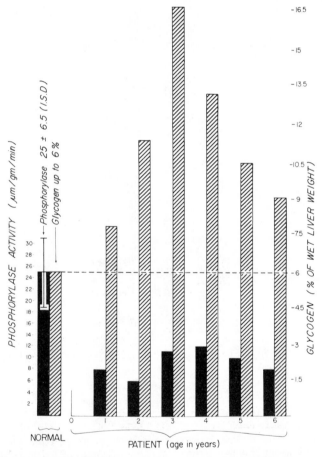

Figure 18.14 In GSD VIII liver specimens obtained by needle biopsy during a time span of 6 years the phosphorylase activity was reduced and glycogen concentration was increased

electron microscopic analysis was available from the second patient. Because of marked autolytic changes, brain autopsy specimens are not adequate for the ultrastructural diagnosis of GSD VIII. One other such patient with 7% of hepatic glycogen concentration and abnormal cerebral glycogen may have been published[42] but hepatic phosphorylase activity was not recorded. Cardinal features of GSD VIII are hepatomegaly, increased hepatic glycogen, low activity of liver phosphorylase (Figure 18.14) but an

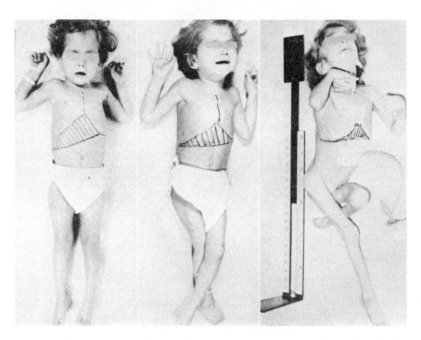

Figure 18.15   Child with GSD VIII. The pictures were taken in yearly intervals. They indicate progressive disease of the central nervous system

intact activation system for this enzyme (Figure 18.12), increased urinary catecholamine excretion in a child, with progressive degenerative brain disease beginning as hypotonia, ataxia, nystagmus, dancing eyes and ending in complete spasticity (Figure 18.15). Liver size and urinary catecholamine excretion may become normal during the end stage of the disease. In cerebral cortical biopsy specimens, there are increased numbers of glycogen particles of the alpha variety, which are not normally present in the brain (Figure 18.16).

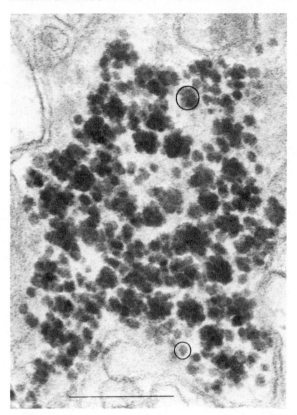

Figure 18.16 Biopsy specimen of cerebral cortex in GSD VIII. There are numerous glycogen particles of the alpha variety (large circle), usually present only in liver. Cerebral tissue normally contains small numbers of beta glycogen particles (small circle). Bar indicates 1 micron

GSD IX

Our initial patient with liver phosphorylase kinase deficiency was a girl[31] who now, thirteen years later, is a young lady without any symptoms except minimal hepatomegaly (Figure 18.17). A patient of ours with GSD IXb is a sailor in the Navy[33]. He is without any symptoms although hepatic activity of phosphorylase kinase remains defective and liver glycogen concentration is still increased. GSD IX may be the most frequent glycogenosis. For practical purposes, it is usually an example of benign hepatomegaly[31-33]. Liver enlargement of considerable proportion may be the only presenting symptom. Hepatocytes are large and engorged with glycogen, but fibrosis is not

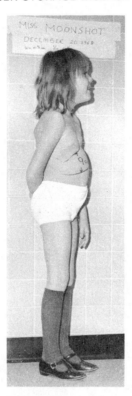

Figure 18.17   Initial patient with GSD IXa four years after she came to our attention. Her 'benign hepatomegaly' has since disappeared without treatment

prevalent (Figure 18.18). Serum transaminases may be elevated three to five times. Blood glucose concentration increases normally after glucagon administration, possibly because of the presence of a small amount of residual kinase activity[31-33]. The apparent K_m (as measured with rabbit muscle phosphorylase b as substrate) of the remaining kinase is normal. In GSD IXa and IXb, muscle tissue is normal in every respect (Figure 18.19). Liver phosphorylase activity is usually not as low as in GSD VI, though this finding is not sufficient to distinguish between the two conditions. It requires biochemical analysis of liver tissue, as detailed in Table 18.2. GSD IX may require no therapy. We had the opportunity to follow the disease in a girl who was treated with D-thyroxin[43]. After one year of such treatment, liver glycogen concentration, hepatic activity of phosphorylase and

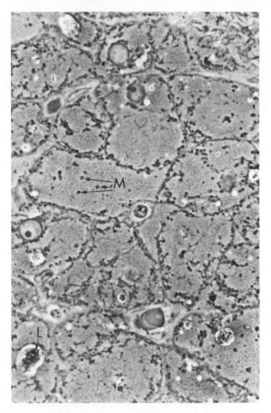

Figure 18.18   Liver biopsy specimen of GSD IX. The hepatocytes are large; some are confluent as if the plasma membranes had burst under the pressure of large areas of glycogen within which there are strings of mitochondria (M). There are some lipid inclusions (L) (× 490)

phosphorylase kinase, the morphological appearance of hepatocytes as well as liver size and function tests had reverted to normal[43]. However, in a boy and a girl of another family with GSD IX we found no such effect after similar treatment with D-thyroxin.

GSD X

To date one patient has been described with this condition[36]. Initially she presented with hepatomegaly. Now, eight years later, she also has minimal muscle symptoms, such as cramps on rare occasions. On liver biopsy,

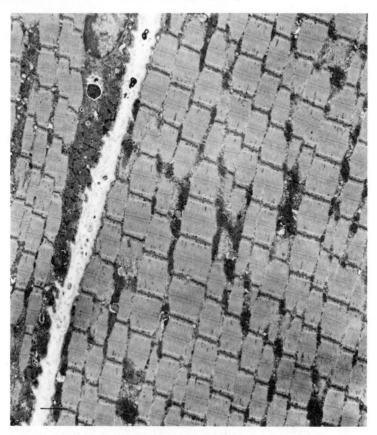

Figure 18.19 Muscle biopsy specimen of GSD IXa is indistinguishable from normal muscle. Occasional subsarcolemmal accumulations of mitochondria, especially paranuclear, are not unusual. Bar indicates 4 microns

glycogen was increased and phosphorylase activity was reduced to the level of GSD VI. In addition, a muscle specimen had increased glycogen biochemically and on electron microscopy[30,39] (Figure 18.20). Muscle phosphorylase existed entirely in the inactive form, i.e. as phosphorylase *b*. The activity of total phosphorylase was normal.

In biopsy specimens of normal muscle obtained as rapidly as possible, phosphorylase will be activated to between 50 and 80% of the total amount present, i.e. more than half of total human muscle phosphorylase is usually present as phosphorylase *a*, the active form, whereas the remainder exists as phosphorylase *b*, the inactive form. Phosphorylase *a* + *b* constitutes total phosphorylase. In GSD X, phosphorylase *b* was the only form demonstrable; its amount was equal to that normally present as *a* + *b*. Phosphorylase kinase was present since the child's own muscle was capable

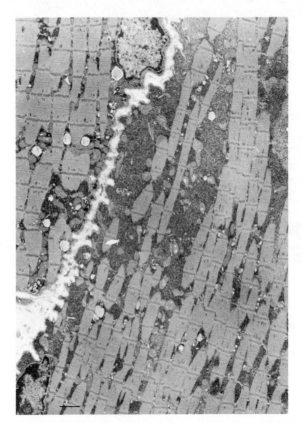

Figure 18.20   Muscle biopsy specimen of GSD X. There is a moderate increase of glycogen. The bar indicates 4 microns

of converting its phosphorylase into the *a*-form even in the absence of cyclic 3′,5′-AMP, provided the homogenate was adjusted to pH 8.6. She did not have a disease analogous to the I-strain mouse which is truly deficient in muscle phosphorylase *b* kinase and cannot activate phosphorylase under any condition. However, the girl's muscle homogenate, when adjusted to pH 6.8, could not activate its own phosphorylase even in the presence of cyclic 3',5'-AMP. Normally such activation would occur. This metabolic defect was corrected if her muscle homogenate had first been fortified by muscle obtained from a phosphorylase kinase deficient I-strain mouse. The girl's muscle homogenate at pH 6.8, and in the presence of cyclic 3',5'-AMP, became capable of activating muscle phosphorylase with the help of the I-strain mouse muscle. This had presumably supplied the cyclic 3',5'-AMP dependent kinase activity[36].

GSD XI

Children with this condition[9] are normal in their mental development but have gross growth retardation. They have marked hepatomegaly and show evidence of florid rickets, at least when they are actively growing. The glucagon tolerance test does not produce the expected increase in blood glucose but does produce the normal urinary increase of cyclic 3',5'-AMP. Nonetheless, all the enzyme activities that we have measured to date in the liver of such children have been within normal range. Liver glycogen concentration is increased markedly as is that of the kidney. The active rickets present during periods of growth and heal only when the patients receive up to 30 000 units of vitamin D daily and phosphate supplementation. There is excessive urinary excretion of phosphate, amino acids, and glucose. Tubular reabsorption of phosphate is markedly decreased. It is not difficult to identify these patients clinically and we have labelled their condition GSD XI. However, an understanding of the pathophysiologic mechanism responsible for the clinical picture is not yet possible.

TABLE 18.1 Glycogen storage diseases, Types 0–XI (GSD 0–XI)

Type, enzyme affected	Tissue distribution	Clinical symptoms	Alternative names and comments
Type 0 (GSD 0) Glycogen synthetase	Liver but not muscle; hepatic glycogen synthetase less than 2% of normal, but some hepatic glycogen (1%) demonstrable	Fasting hypoglycaemia; prolonged hyperglycaemia after glucose administration; mental retardation follows hypoglycaemic convulsions; when these are avoided by frequent protein-rich meals, psychomotor development can be normal	A glycogenosis; defect convincingly demonstrated in two unrelated families; early diagnosis and dietary treatment important for prevention of mental retardation; some children with 'ketotic hypoglycaemia' may have GSD 0
Type I (GSD I) Glucose-6-phosphatase	Liver, kidney, intestine; frequent intranuclear glycogen seen in these organs not diagnostic; continuous night-time feeding by tube and pump may alleviate clinical symptoms; portacaval shunt risky and clinically disappointing; treatment with phenytoin or phenobarbital ineffective	Enlarged liver and kidneys; 'doll face,' stunted growth, normal mental development; tendency to hypoglycaemia, lactic acidosis, hyperlipidaemia, hyperuricacidaemia, gout, bleeding; IV galactose or fructose not converted to glucose (caution: these tests may precipitate acidosis); abortive or no rise in blood glucose after IV glucagon; prognosis fair to good	von Gierke disease, hepato-renal glycogenosis; no involvement of skeletal or cardiac muscle, of leukocytes or cultured skin fibroblasts (glucose-6-phosphatase not normally present in these tissues)
Pseudo-Type I (pseudo-GSD I) (in vitro activity of glucose-6-phosphatase is normal)	Despite normal glucose-6-phosphatase activity, liver glycogen concentration is increased	Symptoms are as those of GSD I	Normal in vitro activity of glucose-6-phosphatase may not be operational in vivo.

TABLE 18.1 (continued)

Type, enzyme affected	Tissue distribution	Clinical symptoms	Alternative names and comments
Type IIa and IIb (GSD II) Lysosomal acid α-glucosidase (deficient activity of acid α-1,4- and of α-1,6,glucosidase; the latter could be considered 'lysosomal glycogen debrancher')	In the fatal, infantile, classic form (GSD IIa), glycogen concentration excessive in all organs examined; acid α-glucosidase deficiency was generalized in one patient; in others normal renal acid α-glucosidase; amniotic fluid (in contrast to cultured amniotic fluid cells) contains acid α-glucosidase activity even if the fetus has the disease. Cardiac muscle in GSD IIb normal clinically and morphologically, but deficient in α-glucosidase activity, although cardiac glycogen concentration is normal	Clinically normal at birth, though minimal cardiomegaly, abnormal ECG, increased tissue glycogen, abnormal lysosomes in liver and skin, and acid α-glucosidase deficiency demonstrable at birth; within a few months, marked hypotonia, severe cardiomegaly, moderate hepatomegaly; normal mental development; death usually in infancy (GSD IIa). Cases with involvement of muscle and liver but without cardiomegaly described in children and adults (GSD IIb). Normal blood glucose response to glucagon	Pompe's disease, generalized glycogenosis, cardiac glycogenosis; prenatal diagnosis within a few days after amniocentesis by the electron microscopic demonstration of abnormal lysosomes in uncultured amniotic fluid cells; for prenatal diagnosis by enzyme analysis, cultured amniotic fluid cells required, which also show the abnormal lysosomes GSD IIa: infantile fatal form GSD IIb: Late juvenile-adult form
Type III (GSD III) Amylo-1,6-glucosidase, 'debrancher enzyme'	Liver, muscle, heart, etc., in various combinations designated type IIIA to D; cultured amniotic fluid cells have diagnostic biochemical abnormality	Moderate to marked hepatomegaly; none to moderate hypotonia; none to moderate cardiomegaly; ECG rarely abnormal; no acidosis; no hypoglycaemia; no hyperlipaemia; glucagon produces a normal rise in blood glucose after a meal but not after fasting; normal mental development; prognosis fair to good	Limit dextrinosis, debrancher glycogenosis, Cori disease, Forbes disease; prenatal diagnosis by enzyme assay of cultured amniotic fluid cells feasible but perhaps unnecessary, owing to the usual benign course

TABLE 18.1 (continued)

Type, enzyme affected	Tissue distribution	Clinical symptoms	Alternative names and comments
Type IV (GSD IV) Amylo-1,4 → 1,6-trans-glucosidase, 'brancher enzyme'	Generalized (?); low to normal levels of abnormally structured glycogen (amylo-pectin-like molecules) with fewer branch points than in animal glycogen	Hepatosplenomegaly, ascites, cirrhosis, liver failure; normal mental development; death in early childhood	Amylopectinosis, brancher glycogenosis, Andersen disease; prenatal diagnosis of this incurable disease may be feasible and indicated by enzyme analysis of cultured amniotic fluid cells
Type V (GSD V) Muscle phosphorylase deficiency (congenital absence of skeletal muscle phosphorylase; phosphory-lase activating system intact)	Skeletal muscle; liver and myometrium normal	Temporary weakness and cramping of skeletal muscle after exercise; no rise in blood lactate during ischaemic exercise; symptoms like those of type VII glycogenosis; normal mental development; myoglobinuria in later life; fair to good prognosis	McArdle syndrome; liver and smooth muscle phosphorylase not affected; cardiac muscle phosphorylase not examined; prenatal diagnosis not feasible and not indicated
Type VI (GSD VI) Liver phosphorylase deficiency (phosphorylase-activating system intact)	Liver; skeletal muscle normal; leukocytes unsatisfactory for diagnosis	Marked hepatomegaly, no splenomegaly; no hypogly-caemia; no acidosis: no hyperlipaemia; no rise of blood glucose after IV glucagon; normal mental development; good prognosis	Lack of glucagon-induced hyperglycaemia distinguishes GSD VI from GSD IX; the latter shows a normal glucagon response; prenatal diagnosis not feasible and not indicated
Type VII (GSD VII) Phosphofructokinase	Skeletal muscle, erythrocytes (in initial report other tissues not examined); not known whether cultured amniotic fluid cells are affected but prenatal diagnosis not indicated	Temporary weakness and cramping of skeletal muscle after exercise; no rise in blood lactate during ischaemic exercise; normal mental development; symptoms identical to those of type V glycogenosis; good prognosis	Reduction of phosphofructo-kinase activity severe in skeletal muscle, mild in erythrocytes, not established in other tissues

TABLE 18.1 (*continued*)

Type, enzyme affected	Tissue distribution	Clinical symptoms	Alternative names and comments
Type VIII (GSD VIII) No enzymatic deficiency demonstrated. Total liver phosphorylase is normal but most of it is in the inactive form although the phosphorylase activating system is intact. This reflects loss of (? cerebral) control over the degree of hepatic phosphorylase activation	Liver, brain, skeletal muscle normal; cerebral glycogen increased; electron microscopy shows some cerebral glycogen in the form of giant α-particles within axon cylinders and synapses	Hepatomegaly; truncal ataxia, nystagmus, 'dancing eyes' may be present; neurologic deterioration progressing to spasticity, decerebration and death; urinary epinephrine and norepinephrine are increased during acute phase of disease, not in stationary end phase	Predominant clinical problem of the three patients with this presumptive diagnosis was progressive degenerative disease of brain. Addition of ATP and $MgCl_2$ to liver homogenate results in full activation of the endogenous (deactivated) phosphorylase
Type IXa and IXb (GSD IX) Liver phosphorylase kinase deficiency. Total liver phosphorylase is normal but most of it is in the inactive form because of deficient endogenous kinase	Liver, muscle tissue normal biochemically and microscopically; D-thyroxin induced liver phosphorylase kinase activity and corrected the other biochemical, clinical and morphological defects in one patient, but not in two others of a different family	Marked hepatomegaly; no splenomegaly; no hypoglycaemia or acidosis; normal rise in blood glucose after IV glucagon; prognosis good; treatment may not be necessary. 'Benign hepatomegaly' may disappear in early adulthood although the enzymatic defect persists	Liver phosphorylase can be activated *in vitro* by addition of exogenous kinase to the homogenate; not the human counterpart of muscle phosphorylase kinase deficiency in mice; normal glucagon response is a distinguishing feature *vs* GSD VI; GSD IXa: autosomal recessive; GSD IXb: X-linked recessive; prenatal diagnosis not demonstrated, not indicated

TABLE 18.1 *(continued)*

Type, enzyme affected	Tissue distribution	Clinical symptoms	Alternative names and comments
Type X (GSD X) Loss of activity of cyclic 3',5'-AMP dependent kinase in muscle and presumably liver. (Total phosphory-lase content of liver and skeletal muscle normal, but the enzyme completely deactivated in both organs; phosphorylase kinase activity 50% of normal, possibly owing to the loss of 3',5'-AMP dependent kinase activity)	Liver and muscle (other organs not tested); identical biochemical findings in muscle biopsy specimens obtained 6 years apart	Marked hepatomegaly; patient otherwise clinically healthy initially, but 6 years after diagnosis mild recurrent muscle pain; no cardiomegaly or hypoglycaemia; no rise in blood glucose after IV glucagon; the only individual known to have this condition not incapacitated at 12 years of age	*In vitro* activation of the patient's phosphorylase occurs (1) under assay conditions not requiring 3',5'-AMP dependent kinase; or (2) after the patient's muscle homogenate has been fortified with phosphorylase, kinase deficient mouse muscle that supplied 3',5'-AMP dependent kinase; postulated defect restricted to the activity of the cyclic 3',5'-AMP dependent kinase that phosphorylates phosphorylase kinase; other cyclic 3',5'-AMP dependent phosphorylations are intact
Type XI (GSD XI) All enzymatic activities measured to date are normal (adenyl cyclase, 3',5'-AMP dependent kinase, phosphorylase kinase, phosphorylase, debrancher, brancher, glucose-6-phosphatase)	Liver, or liver and kidney	Tendency for acidosis; markedly stunted growth; vitamin D resistant rickets (that may be cured with high doses of vitamin D and oral supplementation of phosphate); hyperlipidaemia, generalized aminoaciduria, galactosuria, glucosuria, phosphaturia; normal renal size; no rise in blood glucose after IV glucagon	Muscle usually not affected; GSD XI may include patients with glycogenoses of different enzymatic defects

References

1. Cori, G. T. (1958). Biochemical aspect of glycogen deposition disease. *Mod. Probl. Paediatr.*, **3**, 344

2. Jubiz, W. and Rallison, M. L. (1974). Diphenylhydantoin treatment of glycogen storage diseases. *Arch. In. Med.*, **134**, 418

3. Riddell, A. G., Davies, R. P. and Clark, A. D. (1966). Portacaval transposition in the treatment of glycogen-storage disease. *Lancet*, **2**, 1146

4. Starzl, T. E., Putman, C. W., Porter, K. A., Halgrimson, C. G., Corman, J., Brown, B. I., Gotlin, R. W., Rodgerson, D. O. and Green, H. L. (1973). Portal diversion for the treatment of glycogen storage disease in humans. *Ann. Surg.*, **178**, 525

5. Starzl, T. E., Brown, B. I., Blanchard, H. and Brettschneider, L. (1969). Portal diversion in glycogen storage disease. *Surgery*, **65**, 504

6. Burr, I. M., O'Neill, J. A., Karzon, D. T., Howard, L. J. and Green, H. L. (1974). Comparison of the effects of total parenteral nutrition, continuous intragastric feeding and portacaval shunt on a patient with type I glycogen storage disease. *J. Pediatr.*, **85**, 792

7. Fensom, A. H., Benson, P. F., Blunt, S., Brown, S. P. and Coltart, T. M. (1976). Amniotic cell 4-methylumbelliferyl-α-glucosidase activity for prenatal diagnosis of Pompe's disease. *J. Med. Genet.*, **13**, 148

8. Priest, R. E., Marimuthu, K. M. and Priest, J. H. (1978). Origin of cells in human amniotic fluid cultures. *Lab. Invest.*, **39**, 106

9. Hug, G. (1976). Glycogen storage disease. *Birth Defects*, **12**, 145

10. Symmers, W. S. C. (1974). *Curiosa.* (Chapter 50) (Baltimore: The Williams and Wilkins Company)

11. Hong, R. and Schubert, W. K. (1960). Menghini needle biopsy of the liver. *Am. J. Dis. Child.*, **100**, 42

12. Ehrlich, R. M. (1976). Nocturnal feeding for glycogen-storage disease. *N. Engl. J. Med.*, **294**, 1125

13. Migeon, B. R. and Huijing, F. (1974). Glycogen-storage disease associated with phosphorylase kinase deficiency: Evidence for X inactivation. *Am. J. Hum. Genet.*, **26**, 360

14. Guibaud, P. and Mathieu, M. (1972). Hétérogénéité de la glycogénose Type VI: Etude de l'activité de la phosphorylase leucocytaire dans deux familles. *Arch. Fr. Ped.*, **29**, 1043

15. Aynsley-Green, A., Williamson, D. H. and Gitzelmann, R. (1977). Hepatic glycogen synthetase deficiency: Definition of the syndrome from metabolic and enzyme studies on a nine year old girl. *Arch. Dis. Ch.*, **52**, 573

16. Howell, R. R., Stevenson, R. E., Ben-Menachem, Y., Phyliky, R. L. and Berry, D. H. (1976). Hepatic adenomata with type I glycogen storage disease. *J. Am. Med. Assoc.*, **236**, 1481

17. Chalmers, R. A., Ryman, B. E. and Watts, R. W. E. (1978). Studies on a patient with *in vivo* evidence of type I glycogenosis and normal enzyme activities *in vitro. Acta Paediatr. Scand.*, **67**, 201

18. Putschar, W. (1932). Uber angeborene glykogenspeicherkrankheit des herzens. *Beitr. Pathol. Anat.*, **90**, 222

19. Baudhuin, P., Hers, H. G. and Loeb, H. (1964). An electron microscopic and biochemical study of type II glycogenosis. *Lab. Invest.*, **13**, 1139

20. Hug, G. and Schubert, W. K. (1967). Lysosomes in type II glycogenosis; changes during administration of extract from *Aspergillus niger. J. Cell Biol.*, **35**, C1

21. Hug, G., Schubert, W. K. and Soukup, S. (1973). Treatment related observations in solid tissues, fibroblast cultures and amniotic fluid cells of type II glycogenosis, Hurler's disease and metachromatic leucodystrophy. *Birth Defects*, **9**, 160

22. Hug, G., Garancis, J. C., Schubert, W. K. and Kaplan, S. (1966). Glycogen storage diseases, types II, III, VIII, and IX. *Am. J. Dis. Child.*, **111**, 457

23. Hug, G., Schubert, W. K. and Soukup, S. (1970). Prenatal diagnosis of type II glycogenosis. *Lancet*, **1**, 1002

24. Bannayan, G. A., Dean, W. J. and Howell, R. R. (1976). Type IV glycogen storage disease: Light-microscopic, electron-microscopic, and enzymatic study. *Am. J. Clin. Pathol.*, **66**, 702

25. Hers, H. G. (1959). Etudes enzymatiques sur fragments hépatiques; application à la classification des glycogénoses. *Rev. Int. Hepatol.*, **9**, 35

26. Hug, G., Schubert, W. K. and Shwachman, H. (1965). Imbalance of liver phosphorylase and accummulation of hepatic glycogen in a girl with progressive disease of the brain. *J. Pediatr.*, **67**, 741

27. Lamy, M., Dubois, R., Rossier, A., Frezal, J., Loeb, H. and Blancher, G. (1960). La glycogénose par déficience en phosphorylase hépatique. *Arch. Fr. Pediatr.*, **17**, 14

28. Hug, G. and Schubert, W. K. (1970). Type VI glycogenosis; biochemical demonstration of liver phosphorylase deficiency. *Biochem. Biophys. Res. Commun.*, **41**, 1178

29. Hug, G., Chuck, G., Walling, L. and Schubert, W. K. (1974). Liver phosphorylase deficiency in glycogenosis type VI: Documentation by biochemical analysis of hepatic biopsy specimens. *J. Lab. Clin. Med.*, **84**, 26

30. Hug, G. (1972). Non-bilirubin genetic disorders of the liver. In *The Liver. International Academy of Pathology, Monograph* **No. 13** (Baltimore: The Williams and Wilkins Co.)

31. Hug, G., Schubert, W. K. and Chuck, G. (1966). Phosphorylase kinase of the liver; deficiency in a girl with increased hepatic glycogen. *Science*, **153**, 1534

32. Hug, G., Schubert, W. K. and Chuck, G. (1969). Deficient activity of dephosphophosphorylase kinase and accummulation of glycogen in the liver. *J. Clin. Invest.*, **48**, 704

33. Schimke, R. N., Zakheim, R. M., Corder, R. C. and Hug, G. (1973). Glycogen storage disease type IX: Benign glycogenosis of liver and hepatic phosphorylase kinase deficiency. *J. Pediatr.*, **83**, 1031

34. Huijing, F. and Fernandes, J. (1969). X-Chromosomal inheritance of liver glycogenosis with phosphorylase kinase deficiency. *Am. J. Hum. Genet.*, **21**, 275

35. Huijing, F. and Fernandes, J. (1970). Liver glycogenosis and phosphorylase kinase deficiency. *Am. J. Hum. Genet.*, **22**, 484

36. Hug, G., Schubert, W. K. and Chuck, G. (1970). Loss of cyclic 3',5'-AMP dependent kinase and reduction of phosphorylase kinase in skeletal muscle of a girl with deactivated phosphorylase and glycogenosis of liver and muscle. *Biochem. Biophys. Res. Commun.*, **40**, 982

37. Hers, H. G. and van Hoof, F. (1968). Glycogen storage disease; type VI

glycogenosis, In *Carbohydrate metabolism and its disorders*. Dickens, F., Randle, P. J. and Whelan, W. J. (eds). **Vol. 2,** Chap. 6 (New York: Academic Press Inc.)

38. Appleman, M. M. (1962). Structural studies of glycogen phosphorylase. Dissertation. (Ann Arbor: University Microfilms Inc.)

39. McAdams, A. J., Hug, G. and Bove, K. E. (1974). Glycogen storage disease, types I to X: Criteria for morphologic diagnosis. *Hum. Pathol.*, **5,** 463

40. Tarui, S., Okuno, G., Ikura, Y., Tanaka, T., Suda, M. and Nishikawa, M. (1965). Phosphofructokinase deficiency in skeletal muscle; a new type of glycogenosis. *Biochem. Biophys. Res. Commun.*, **19,** 517

41. Hug, G., Schubert, W. K., Chuck, G. and Garancis, J. C. (1967). Liver phosphorylase: Deactivation in a child with progressive brain disease, increased hepatic glycogen and increased urinary catecholamines. *Am. J. Med.*, **42,** 139

42. Resibois-Gregoire, A. and Dourov, N. (1966). Electron microscopic study of a case of cerebral glycogenosis. *Acta. Neuropathol.*, **6,** 70

43. Lonsdale, D. and Hug, G. (1976). Normalization of hepatic phosphorylase kinase activity and glycogen concentration in glycogen storage disease type IX (GSD IX) during treatment with sodium dextrothyroxin. *Pediatr. Res.*, **10,** 368

19

Type VI glycogenosis: identification of subgroups
Th. de Barsy and B. Lederer

HISTORICAL

In 1959, Hers[1] reported the results of biochemical analysis of the livers of three patients, one girl and two boys, suffering from hepatomegaly. The livers of these patients were characterized by low activity of phosphorylase, normal activity of glucose-6-phosphatase and amylo-1,6-glucosidase and an excess of glycogen. The deficiency in phosphorylase was not complete and it could not be decided if the primary defect was due to phosphorylase or phosphorylase kinase. It was noted, however, that phosphorylase could not be activated by incubation in the presence of ATP and magnesium. Stetten and Stetten[2] have classified this group of patients as Type VI glycogenosis, sometimes also called 'Hers disease'.

Until recently[3,4], a precise determination of phosphorylase was technically difficult. The enzyme exists in two forms, one active *a*, the other inactive *b*, which are interconvertible under the action of phosphorylase kinase and phosphorylase phosphatase. A low phosphorylase activity in a biopsy could therefore be due to a defect of phosphorylase, a defect of phosphorylase kinase or an increased activity of phosphorylase phosphatase, as could result from hyperglycaemia at the time that the biopsy was taken. For this reason, a classification of cases based on the activity of liver phosphorylase was not feasible and it has been proposed to group in Type VI all cases of hepatomegalic glycogenosis in which the diagnosis of Type I, Type III or Type IV could be excluded on the basis of a normal glycogen structure and a normal activity of glucose-6-phosphatase and amylo-1,6-glucosidase[5, 6].

In 1966, Hug *et al.*[7] reported observations on a girl with hepatomegaly due to glycogenosis. The activity of phosphorylase in the biopsy of the liver was low and could not be increased upon incubation with ATP and magnesium, unless phosphorylase kinase was added. This was an indication, although indirect, that the low activity of phosphorylase was secondary to a defect in the activating enzyme, phosphorylase kinase. Later on, Huijing and Fernandes[8] reported a series of patients with a sex linked, transmitted phosphorylase kinase deficiency, demonstrated in leucocytes and erythrocytes. More recently, Lederer *et al.*[9] have developed a methodology that allows recognition of several kinds of Type VI glycogenosis based on the properties of phosphorylase and phosphorylase kinase in an haemolysate.

PHOSPHORYLASE AND ITS CONVERTER ENZYMES

Figure 19.1 shows the glycogenolytic cascade by which, upon stimulation of a membrane bound receptor by glucagon in the liver, or by epinephrine in the muscle, phosphorylase is activated and glycogen is degraded. The cascade includes the sequential activation of adenylate cyclase, of protein kinase, of phosphorylase kinase and of phosphorylase. In the muscle, the two forms of phosphorylase are easy to distinguish by the fact that phosphorylase *b* is completely inactive, but is fully activated by AMP. In contrast, it was believed that liver phosphorylase *b* is essentially inactive,

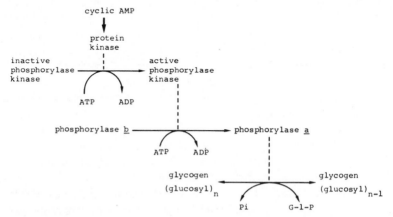

Figure 19.1   The schematic representation of the 'glycogenolytic cascade'

even in the presence of AMP[10]. Recently it has been established that, in the presence of several anions including sulphate and fluoride, phosphorylase b is partially active, unless caffein is added. This activity can be markedly stimulated by AMP. The kinetic properties of the a and b forms of liver phosphorylase are variable from species to species[3]. The properties of the human liver enzymes have been reported by Lederer and Stalmans[4] who have described the methodology for the separate determination of the phosphorylase a and of total phosphorylase. The saturation kinetics of human phosphorylase b with AMP and the effect of fluoride (0.15 mol/l) and of sulphate (0.5 mol/l) is illustrated in Figure 19.2. The salts increase

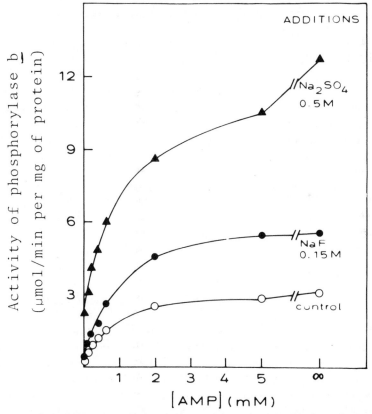

Figure 19.2 Effect of AMP on the activity of phosphorylase b. Purified phosphorylase b was assayed in the presence of 1% glycogen, 50 mmol/l glucose-1-phosphate, variable concentration of AMP and other additions as indicated. ∞ AMP indicates the activity at infinite concentration of AMP, as estimated from double reciprocal plots of the AMP effect (from Lederer and Stalmans[18])

the activity of the enzyme both in the absence of AMP and at saturating concentrations of the nucleotide.

Phosphorylase *b* is almost completely inhibited in the presence of caffein (0.5 mol/l)[4]. By using the properties of the two forms of the enzyme, a simple method for the assay of the *a* form and of the total (*a* + *b*) phosphorylase activity can be proposed. The assay of total phosphorylase allows unequivocally the recognition of hepatic glycogen phosphorylase deficiency.

Blood cells have been used also in the diagnosis of Type VI glycogenosis[11–15]. As mentioned above, the investigation of phosphorylase kinase in leucocytes has allowed recognition of a sex linked type of phosphorylase kinase deficiency[8]. More recently, Lederer *et al.*[9], using an haemolysate, were able to distinguish the two types of phosphorylase kinase deficiency, the sex linked and the autosomal recessive type of transmission.

Skin fibroblasts in culture have been investigated rarely. Koster *et al.*[16] reported that the activity of phosphorylase was normal in cultured fibroblasts from two patients suffering from a total deficiency of hepatic phosphorylase. The determination of phosphorylase kinase activity in cultured skin fibroblasts is difficult because the activity varies widely from experiment to experiment[17, 18]. Nevertheless, it was demonstrated that in two cases of sex linked[17, 18] and in one case of autosomal recessive[18] phosphorylase kinase deficiency, the activity of the enzyme was respectively about 40% and 60% of the controls but was much higher than that found in erythrocytes of the same patients. In this laboratory, we were able to show that the phosphorylase kinase activity in normal cells disappears progressively with the ageing of the culture[18, 19].

SYMPTOMS

Type VI glycogenosis is one of the milder forms. The general appearance of patients suffering from this disease is similar for the different subgroups[9, 15, 20–22]. During the first months of life, the patients are usually free of symptoms. Hepatomegaly develops slowly and is often discovered at the occasion of an intercurrent illness or a routine examination. Growth retardation is frequently observed. Muscular hypotonia is reported. Hypoglycaemic episodes occur, but are not the rule. Routine examination frequently reveals an elevation of blood lipids, cholesterol and transaminases. Ketosis is present in fasting periods but is age dependent and tends to disappear around the age of seven[23]. Hyperglycaemic response to glucagon is usually normal, but in some patients the response is slow or absent. Around puberty, hepatomegaly becomes less evident.

FREQUENCY

This is the most common type of glycogenosis and accounts for about half of the cases diagnosed in our laboratory (see Figure 19.3). In our experience, the sex linked deficiency of phosphorylase kinase is by far the most frequent, followed by the autosomal defect of the same enzyme and the partial phosphorylase deficiency. Complete phosphorylase deficiency is rare and difficult to demonstrate.

MORPHOLOGY

Liver morphology has been studied by light and electron microscopy[20, 24-26].

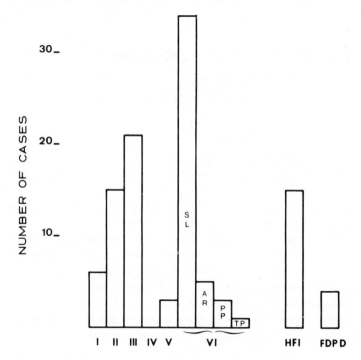

Figure 19.3 Distribution of the different types of glycogenosis, hereditary fructose intolerance and fructose-1,6-diphosphatase deficiency in 107 patients recently detected in this laboratory. The diagnosis was confirmed by biochemical study of liver, and/or erythrocytes and/or leucocytes. I: Type I; II: Type II; III: Type III; IV: Type IV; V: Type V; VI: Type VI; SL: sex linked transmission; AR: autosomal recessive transmission; PP: partial phosphorylase deficiency; TP: total phosphorylase deficiency; Hfi: hereditary fructose intolerance; FDPD: fructose-1,6-diphosphatase deficiency

By light microscopy, the general architecture of the liver may be well preserved or modified by fibrosis in widened portal tracts. Hepatocytes are swollen by the presence of PAS-positive material, digestible by α-amylase. Fat droplets are present but scarce.

On electron microscopic preparations, large areas of α-particles of glycogen are found in the cytoplasm of these cells, pushing other cytoplasmic elements against the nuclear and cell walls. In cases with fibrosis, collagen bundles are observed between the glycogen areas. Osmiophilic lipid droplets may be observed too. The other cellular constituents are normal except that the endoplasmic reticulum is less visible. Kupffer cells look normal. These morphological findings are common to Type III or Type VI glycogenosis. On the contrary, steatoses without excess of collagen, are more characteristic of Type I glycogenosis[26].

SUBGROUPS OF TYPE VI GLYCOGENOSIS

As already mentioned, fine enzymatic analysis of different tissues leads to the possibility of defining several subgroups.

Total phosphorylase deficiency

The activity of phosphorylase was undetectable in the livers of two brothers studied by Fernandes et al.[21] and of one girl investigated by Lederer and Stalmans[4].

In the patient of Fernandes et al.[21], the activity of phosphorylase kinase in the liver was not measured. The activity of phosphorylase was much reduced in the leucocytes but was normal in the cultured fibroblasts[16]. The administration of glucagon to these patients increased the concentration of cyclic AMP in the urine but failed to cause hyperglycaemia.

In the case reported by Lederer and Stalmans[4], the liver phosphorylase was measured by a method which was able to fully detect phosphorylase b. Liver phosphorylase kinase was measured and found to be normally active. The hyperglycaemic response to glucagon was normal.

Partial phosphorylase deficiency

This group includes the patients with a low activity of phosphorylase in the liver despite a normal activity of phosphorylase kinase. In a very few cases, phosphorylase kinase activity was measured directly in the liver[25, 27], whereas in others this activity was only demonstrated in the haemolysate[4]. In the haemolysate, the activity of phosphorylase was low and could not be greatly increased either by endogenous (Figure 19.4) or by exogenous phosphorylase kinase, suggesting that it was already in the *a* form.

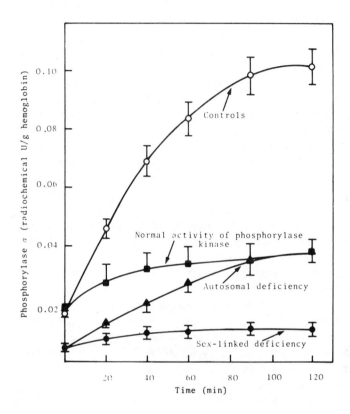

Figure 19.4 Activation of endogenous phosphorylase in haemolysates of patients with Type VI glycogenosis. The haemolysates were incubated at 20 °C in the presence of 0.1% glycogen and cyclic AMP (2 μmol/l). Normal subjects (O), patients suffering from phosphorylase kinase deficiency with sex linked mode of transmission ($n = 8$; ●) with autosomal mode of transmission ($n = 2$; ▲), or patient with partial phosphorylase deficiency ($n = 4$; ■). Data are means ± SEM (Lederer et al.[16])

Phosphorylase kinase deficiency

Two different types of inheritance are known for the deficiency of phosphorylase kinase, a sex linked transmission and an autosomal recessive transmission.

Sex-linked transmission   It was convincingly shown[8] that the deficiency of phosphorylase kinase can be transmitted by an X-linked gene. Twenty out of the 35 analysed patients, belonged to the same pedigree, which comprised more than 200 individuals. Thirty two cases were boys and three were girls, who showed mild clinical symptoms and were considered as heterozygotes. Their deficiency in phosphorylase kinase was demonstrated in leukocytes and erythrocytes. Other reports of sex linked phosphorylase kinase deficiency have indicated an almost complete defect of that enzyme in liver and normal activity in the muscle[9, 28, 29]. The deficiency can also be easily detected in an haemolysate. In contrast to normal subjects, there is practically no spontaneous activation of endogenous phosphorylase upon incubation of the haemolysate at 20 °C in the presence of glycogen and cyclic AMP (Figure 19.4). The deficiency of phosphorylase kinase can also be shown with purified muscle phosphorylase as a substrate.

According to Huijing[14], a low activity of phosphorylase kinase in leucocytes of the patients was due to decreased stability of the enzyme and was characterized by a low affinity for its substrate, phosphorylase *b*. The latter conclusion is not supported by the observation made by Lederer *et al.*[9] that, in haemolysates, the deficiency was as great when the enzyme was measured on the endogenous phosphorylase as in the presence of a 7500 times larger amount of substrate.

It is surprising that, in the absence of phosphorylase kinase, nearly all these patients react normally to glucagon. Fernandes *et al.*[23] suggested that the hyperglycaemic response to this hormone may be due to the formation of 5'-AMP by hydrolysis of cyclic AMP. Preliminary experiments performed in this laboratory[30], using anaesthetized mice, demonstrated that 15 min after the injection of glucagon (5 μg/g), the concentration of AMP in the liver rose from 0.1 mmol/l to 0.25 mmol/l. It is known that liver phosphorylase *b* is sensitive to AMP concentrations in this range of values. It seems therefore possible that a modification in the nucleotide concentration after glucagon may play a role in this hyperglycaemic response.

It is interesting to note that the activity of amylo-1,6-glucosidase was significantly increased in the haemolysate of these patients. Possible protection by a high amount of glycogen may be responsible for it.

The detection of heterozygotes has been tried by different authors. Huijing and Fernandes[8] considered that they could demonstrate, either directly or indirectly, some abnormality of phosphorylase kinase in leukocytes from all obligate heterozygotes. Lederer *et al.*[9] reported that in the haemolysate of three mothers of patients, the activity of phosphorylase kinase was respectively 30%, 58%, and 97% of the mean normal value, whereas in controls, the activity varies from 66% to 162% of the same value. Migeon and Huijing[17] have also reported that cultured fibroblasts from one mother had a normal activity of phosphorylase kinase, but that some isolated clones displayed an activity corresponding to the mutant range. This observation is in agreement with the Lyon hypothesis that heterozygotes for a sex linked deficiency are made up of two populations of cells, one normal, the other deficient.

Autosomal type of phosphorylase kinase deficiency Besides the sex linked type of transmission, evidence has been brought for an autosomal type of transmission. Indirect evidence for a deficiency of liver phosphorylase kinase in both sexes was first presented by Hug[7, 24], and has since been confirmed in other patients. In this laboratory, we had the opportunity to establish a defect in phosphorylase kinase in three pairs of siblings, either a brother and a sister or two sisters. The enzymatic activity in the haemolysate reached about 25% of the mean normal value and was similar in each pair of siblings (Figure 19.4). Phosphorylase could be completely activated in the presence of exogenous phosphorylase kinase. In the liver, phosphorylase kinase measured in two patients was almost inactive[19].

Other deficiencies

Besides these now well established enzymatic deficiencies, there are still patients difficult to classify. Thanks to the courtesy of Dr J. Fernandes, (Groeningen, Netherlands), we were able to demonstrate in the haemolysate of two unrelated boys with hepatomegaly that the activity of phosphorylase kinase was normal if measured on exogenous phosphorylase but very low (about 10% of the control value) on endogenous substrate. This suggested an anomaly in the affinity of the phosphorylase kinase for its substrate as already proposed[14] but it could not be confirmed in these patients: the K_m for the exogenous phosphorylase was not significantly different from that of the control. The very low activity of phosphorylase kinase was not modified by the addition of ATP in the incubation medium. On the other hand, the addition of phosphorylase kinase activated endogenous phosphorylase normally. No analysis of the liver could be performed.

In another 8 year old boy with asymptomatic hepatomegaly, activity of the phosphorylase kinase in the haemolysate was hyperactive (200% of the control value) when measured on exogenous substrates but was normal on endogenous phosphorylase. The diagnosis of glycogenosis rested on the clinical appearance of the child and a high level of glycogen in his erythrocytes (326 μg/g haemoglobin; the normal level being <50 μg/g haemoglobin). Liver tissue was not investigated.

TREATMENT

In this mild glycogen storage disease, treatment is mainly symptomatic and consists of an appropriate diet.

Recently, Londsdale and Hug[32, 33] reported that in four children with a low liver phosphorylase activity, the administration of 4 mg of D-thyroxin produced a decrease of the liver size and of the serum triglycerides associated with an increase of body growth, but without any modification in the phosphorylase activity. In a two year old girl suffering from liver phosphorylase kinase deficiency, the administration of 4 mg of D-thyroxin for 15 months produced disappearance of hepatomegaly, a drop in serum triglycerides and a normalization of the light and electron microscopic appearance of the liver. Moreover, the phosphorylase kinase activity in this organ increased from about 10% of the normal value before treatment, to a normal value after treatment. The glycogen content decreased from 8.1% to 3.8% of the wet weight. Results from our laboratory do not confirm all these findings. Thanks to the courtesy of Dr A. Winsnes (Oslo, Norway), hepatic tissue of a boy suffering from a phosphorylase kinase deficiency has been analysed before and after six months treatment with D-thyroxin. No significant difference in the phosphorylase kinase activity of the liver was observed, although the glycogen content decreased from 15.5% to 5.6% of the wet weight. The enlargement of the liver was not modified but the transaminases returned to normal values. In two other patients followed by Dr P. Durand (Genova, Italy), the same kind of treatment had no significant effect on the activity of phosphorylase kinase in the haemolysate, although the clinical status improved and hepatomegaly disappeared.

Acknowledgements

We are grateful to the physicians who provided us with the biological specimens and to Prof H. G. Hers for his continual interest and advice. This work was supported by the Fonds de la Recherche Scientifique Medicale and the US Public Health Service (Grant AM 9235). Th. de B. is 'Chercheur Qualifié' du FNRS.

References

1. Hers, H. G. (1959). Etude enzymatique sur fragments hépatiques. Applications à la classification des glycogénoses. *Rev. Int. Hépat.*, **9**, 35
2. Stetten, D. W. Jr. and Stetten, M. R. (1960). Glycogen metabolism. *Physiol. Rev.*, **40**, 505
3. Stalmans, W. and Hers, H. G. (1975). The stimulation of liver phosphorylase

b by AMP, fluoride and sulfate. A technical note on the specific determination of the *a* and *b* forms of liver glycogen phosphorylase. *Eur. J. Biochem.*, **54**, 341

4. Lederer, B. and Stalmans, W. (1976). Human liver glycogen phosphorylase. Kinetic properties and assay in biopsy specimens. *Biochem. J.*, **159**, 689

5. Illingworth, B. and Brown, D. H. (1964). Glycogen storage diseases, types III, IV and VI. In W. J. Whelan and M. P. Cameron (eds). *Ciba Foundation Symposium: Control of Glycogen Metabolism*, pp. 336–353 (Amsterdam: Elsevier Publishing Co.)

6. Hers, H. G. and van Hoof, F. (1968). Glycogen storage disease: Type VI glycogenosis. In F. Dickens, P. J. Randle and W. J. Whelan (eds). *Carbohydrate Metabolism and its Disorders.* **2**, pp. 166–168 (New York: Academic Press Inc.)

7. Hug, G., Schubert, W. K. and Chuck, G. (1966). Phosphorylase kinase of the liver: Deficiency in a girl with increased hepatic glycogen. *Science*, **153**, 1534

8. Huijing, F. and Fernandes, J. (1969). X-chromosomal inheritance of liver glycogenosis with phosphorylase kinase deficiency. *Am. J. Hum. Genet.*, **21**, 275

9. Lederer, B., van Hoof, F., van den Berghe, G. and Hers, H. G. (1975). Glycogen phosphorylase and its converter enzymes in haemolysates of normal human subjects and patients with Type VI glycogen storage disease. *Biochem. J.*, **147**, 23

10. Wosilait, W. D. and Sutherland, E. W. (1956). The relationship of epinephrine and glucagon to liver phosphorylase. II. Enzymatic inactivation of liver phosphorylase. *J. Biol. Chem.*, **218**, 469

11. Hülsmann, W. C., Oei, T. L. and Creveld, S. (1961). Phosphorylase activity in leucocytes from patients with glycogen storage disease. *Lancet*, **2**, 581

12. Williams, H. E. and Field, J. B. (1961). Low leucocyte phosphorylase in hepatic phosphorylase deficient glycogen storage disease. *J. Clin. Invest.*, **40**, 1841

13. Huijing, F. (1967). Phosphorylase kinase in leucocytes of normal subjects and of patients with glycogen storage disease. *Biochim. Biophys. Acta*, **148**, 601

14. Huijing, F. (1970a). Glycogen storage disease Type VI$_a$: low phosphorylase kinase activity caused by a low enzyme-substrate affinity. *Biochim. Biophys. Acta*, **206**, 199

15. Huijing, F. (1970b). Phosphorylase kinase deficiency. *Biochem. Genet.* **4** (**Suppl. 1**), 187

16. Koster, J. F., Fernandes, J. Slee, R. G., van Berkel, Th. J. C. and Hülsmann, W. C. (1973). Hepatic phosphorylase deficiency: a biochemical study. *Biochem. Biophys. Res. Commun.* **53**, 282

17. Migeon, B. R. and Huijing, F. (1974). Glycogen storage disease associated with phosphorylase kinase deficiency: evidence of inactivation. *Am. J. Hum. Genet.*, **26**, 360

18. Lederer, B. (1977). Etude biochimique de la glycogénose type VI. Thèse de doctorate en Sciences. Université Catholique de Louvain, 112 p.

19. Lederer, B., de Barsy, Th., Leroy, J. G. and Hers, H. G. (1974). Glycogen phosphorylase and its converter enzymes in cultured human fibroblasts. *Hoppe-Seylers Z. Physiol. Chem.*, **355**, 55

20. Lamy, M., Dubois, R., Rossier, A., Frezal, J., Loeb, H. and Blancher, G. (1960). La glycogénose par déficience en phosphorylase hépatique. *Arch. Fr. Pediatr.*, **17**, 14

21. Fernandes, J., Koster, J. F., Grose, W. F. A. and Sorgedrager, N. (1974). Hepatic phosphorylase deficiency. Its differentiation for other hepatic glycogenoses. *Arch. Dis. Child*, **49**, 186

22. Huijing, F. (1975). Glycogen metabolism and glycogen storage disease. *Physiol. Rev.*, **55**, 609

23. Fernandes, J. and Pikaar, N. A. (1972). Ketosis in hepatic glycogenosis. *Arch. Dis. Child.*, **47**, 41

24. Hug, G., Schubert, W. K. and Chuck, G. (1969). Deficient activity of dephosphophosphorylase kinase and accumulation of glycogen in the liver. *J. Clin. Invest.*, **48**, 704

25. Hug, G., Chuck, G., Walling, L. and Schubert, W. K. (1974). Liver phosphorylase deficiency in glycogenosis type VI: Documentation by biochemical analysis of hepatic biopsy specimens. *J. Lab. Clin. Med.*, **84**, 26

26. De Bruijn, W. C., Fernandes, J., Hubert, J. and Koster, J. F. (1975). Liver glycogenosis. A histochemical and ultrastructural study. *Pathol. Eur.*, **10**, 3

27. Drummond, G. I., Hardwick, D. F. and Israels, S. (1970). Liver glycogen phosphorylase deficiency. *Canad. Med. Assoc. J.*, **102**, 740

28. Morishita, Y., Nishiyama, K., Yamamura, H., Kodama, S., Negishi, H., Matsuo, M., Matsuo, T. and Nishizuka, Y. (1973). Glycogen phosphorylase kinase deficiency: a survey of enzymes in phosphorylase activating system. *Biochem. Biophys. Res. Commun.*, **53**, 833

29. Schimke, R. N., Zakheim, R. M., Corder, R. C. and Hug, G. (1973). Glycogen storage disease type IX: Benign glycogenosis of liver and hepatic phosphorylase kinase deficiency. *J. Pediatr.*, **83**, 1031

30. van den Berghe, G. (1974). Personnal communication

31. Lyon, M. (1961). Gene action in X-chromosome of the mouse (*Mus musculus*, L.). *Nature*, **190**, 372

32. Lonsdale, D. and Hug, G. (1976a). D-thyroxin induces phosphorylase kinase activity and normalizes glycogen concentration in the liver of a child with hepatic phosphorylase kinase deficient glycogenosis. *J. Cell Biol.*, **70**, 157a

33. Lonsdale, D. and Hug, G. (1976b). Normalization of hepatic phosphorylase kinase activity and glycogen concentration in glycogen storage disease type IX (GdD IX) during treatment with sodium dextrothyroxin. *Pediatr. Res.*, **10**, 368

Discussion

DISCUSSION OF GLYCOGEN STORAGE DISEASES

Clinical presentation and treatment

HERS: I would like to make some comments on the biochemistry of Type I glycogenosis, beginning with the surprising finding that liver glucose-6-phosphate is not increased. Considering the deficiency of glucose-6-phosphatase it must indicate that gluconeogenesis is somehow suppressed in these livers.

I have also been very interested in the cause of hyperuricaemia in this condition. It appears to be related to a fall in phosphate concentration in the liver and possibly a decrease of other metabolites, like GTP. Uric acid formation is regulated by the activity of inosine-5-phosphate (IMP) deaminase. IMP deaminase is not affected by glucose-6-phosphate, and anyway I have mentioned that this substance is not increased in Type I. The enzyme could be stimulated because of a low phosphate level in the liver. It may be postulated that the normally high concentration of phosphate in liver, about five times more than in blood, is reduced in Type I because of a lack of release from glucose-6-phosphate, and a failure to generate phosphate from stages of the gluconeogenesis pathway.

Hyperuricaemia develops in normal subjects following an intravenous fructose load and we believe this results from an accumulation of fructose-1-phosphate (F-1-P) because it is formed from fructose faster than it can be metabolized to either glucose or lactate. The patient with Type I is very sensitive to fructose intoxication and blood uric acid concentration is elevated even after oral fructose. This would be anticipated for several reasons. As mentioned previously, the potential for uric acid formation is greater because of enhanced IMP deaminase activity. In addition, there would be a slower utilization and thus a greater accumulation of F-1-P, because it cannot be metabolized through to glucose in the liver of Type I patients. For the same reason, relatively more lactate would be produced from F-1-P breakdown and hyperlactataemia reduces urinary excretion of uric acid. This would suggest that removal of fructose from the diet might result in lower blood uric acid concentrations.

NUKI (Cardiff): I should like to question Professor Hers' hypothesis regarding the origin of hyperuricaemia and the regulation of purine biosynthesis in Type I glycogen storage disease. There is now good evidence that in most situations where *de novo* purine biosynthesis is increased in man, this is regulated by the availability of phosphoribosyl pyrophosphate (PRPP). It seems to me that the increase in Type I glycogen storage disease is best explained by the conventional hypothesis, that PRPP is increased as a consequence of increased flow of metabolites through the pentose phosphate pathway. PRPP synthetase is sensitive to changes in phosphate concentration and, if phosphate concentration were decreased as postulated by Professor Hers, one would expect the rate of *de novo* purine synthesis to decrease rather than increase.

HERS: The point at which uric acid formation is regulated is speculative. We know for certain that fructose increases uric acid production and are convinced that this is secondary to deinhibition of the deaminase. Purine synthesis is increased, but it does not really matter if the primary disturbance is on the synthesis or the degradation of uric acid because if you stimulate degradation you deinhibit synthesis. Since a fructose load also increases synthesis I am not convinced that PRPP is the limiting factor.

DAVIDSON (Vancouver): We have used nocturnal nasogastric infusion as part of the therapy for Type I glycogen storage disease using a glucose polymer solution (Caloreen) because it has approximately one fifth of the osmotic effect of glucose solutions, thus avoiding delayed gastric emptying and erratic absorption. The smaller volumes infused prevent children wetting the bed or suffering recurrent nocturia. Our oldest patient is now eight and biochemical and clinical progress has been highly satisfactory over more than two years of treatment. His weight has improved from the third to the fiftieth centile and his height has improved by 19 cm and now approaches the 3rd centile. The liver size has decreased clinically and by isotope scan techniques. The least responsive measures have been blood uric acid and lactate. Although blood glucose levels could be maintained above hypoglycaemic levels by nasogastric glucose delivery rates as low as 0.25 (g/h)/kg, clinical progress deteriorated and blood lactate and uric acid levels rose with this dosage. Increasing the glucose delivery rate reversed this. We have concluded that nocturnal nasogastric feeding with a glucose polymer offers significant benefit to the patient. The optimal rate of nasogastric glucose delivery cannot be determined simply by observing blood glucose levels to ensure correction of hypoglycaemia, but requires measurement of clinical indices and attention to other biochemical parameters, such as blood lactate and uric acid.

O'BRIEN (Denver): Would Professor Fernandes comment firstly, on what he thinks is the biochemical basis of the neurological resistance to hypoglycaemia in Type I glycogen storage disease and secondly, on whether there might be a supplementary role for somatostatin in suppressing glucagon levels?

FERNANDES: To the first part of your question about adaption I have no answer but I should make the point that glucose-6-phosphatase deficient patients have shorter fasting periods than other patients with glycogen storage disease because they are unable to tolerate a normal nocturnal fast. They do not have time to develop ketosis except in a severe infectious crisis or during severe hypoglycaemia, when their lactic acid levels are extremely high and blood ketone levels are moderately elevated.

With regard to your question about somatostatin, I have no clear indication for the use of that in treatment now that we have possibilities for gastric drip feeding. It might be an additional means, but I have no experience of that.

STACEY: I agree with you about the lack of ketosis. Our children were acidotic but it was largely lactic acid and not ketones.

WICK (Basel): What is the importance of the high aminotransferases in Type III glycogenosis? Do you draw any conclusions about the management of such patients if blood levels of these enzymes are increased?

FERNANDES: They are very high, but I do not know what it means. There are two theories; one suggests that it is due to increased leakage and the other it is due to an increased expression of aminotransferase activity. It seems that the last possibility is most probable, but I have no proof and no personal studies of that.

BRENTON (London): May I ask Dr Stacey a question? His patients obviously did best while taking intravenous glucose, but as I understand it the dose within the 24 hour period was exactly the same as on the continuous nasogastric administration of glucose. The total glucose administration is not different and yet the growth results were very much better by the intravenous route. Were there any differences in the lactate levels between these two treatments which might explain why there was such a phenomenal growth on the intravenous route compared with the nasogastric route?

STACEY: The supplementary glucose was certainly the same, although the spontaneous food intake of course did vary. While on intravenous therapy she was extremely hungry, ate very well and became obese. Also during continuous nasogastric therapy, especially towards the end of it when she was on supplementary oral feeding, her glucose intake was reduced because of the problem of obesity. The lactate levels were much lower during the intravenous period than they were in the preceeding period, or in the oral 2 hourly therapy period that bracketed the intravenous period but the lactate levels were not lower during the continuous nasogastric therapy. Although lactic acid levels may have something to do with very rapid growth, good growth occurred with nasogastric therapy in spite of a similar range of lactate to that on oral glucose feeding.

FERNANDES: I have the impression that the growth of the patient is indeed dependent on the lactic acid overproduction, because we have observed that the patient with the highest lactate production in the urine has the severest growth retardation. Some children showed remarkable growth improvement and this was associated with a decrease in lactic aciduria and correction of the acid base balance.

BLASS (New York): One candidate for the substrate utilized by the brain in patients with hypoglycaemia, mild ketosis and lactic acidaemia is lactate itself. It is well established that lactate passes readily into the brain and that brain slices can oxidise lactate and thus maintain ATP levels. Normally the brain produces lactate, but in this abnormal situation there may be a net utilisation of lactate.

HERS: That also seems the most likely possibility to me.

STACEY: No-one has mentioned the role of portacaval shunting in these children. The reason that we started intravenous supplementation in our child was because of her terrible growth. A portacaval anastomosis was thought to be a reasonable thing to do, but everyone decided against it when she grew so well.

O'BRIEN: One of our cases grew well following a portacaval shunt, but in another the outcome was a disaster.

HUG: Perhaps we should try alternatives for lowering the serum lactate such as sodium difluoroacetate which I believe has been used in a trial for treatment of diabetes and has effectively lowered the lactate in over 70% of the cases.

STACEY: A high lactate is used for brain metabolism. With a low lactate level you grow better but you might suffer from hypoglycaemia. I just do not know what is the best thing to do.

BRENTON: May I add a warning about the possible hazards of exercise to patients with glucose-6-phosphatase deficiency. Older children with this disease may wish to cycle, swim or climb hills while on holiday. One of the patients described by Dr Stacey has been exercised by us on a static bicycle and even modest exercise for 30 minutes resulted in a fall of plasma glucose from about 4.5 mmol/l to 1.5 mmol/l.

Diagnostic problems

RYMAN: Can we agree among ourselves whether we are to continue to call Group 6 Group 6 with all its sub divisions, or whether we are to have Groups 8, 9, 10 and 11; because this seems to be a dilemma which many of us feel we ought to solve?

HUG: Gerti Cori suggested that one different enzyme defect ought to be assigned one different type. It seems logical to me to label these conditions in just that way as they are identified. Phosphorylase deficiency is something substantially different from phosphorylase kinase deficiency. It is just as different as would be glucose-6-phosphatase from debrancher enzyme deficiency. When the first patient was described with phosphorylase kinase deficiency it was just a logical extension of the table which we had at that time and logical to call it Type IX. We do not know the enzyme defect in Type VIII, but we can make an exception there as was previously made in the case of Type II. Before Hers demonstrated the acid α-glucosidase deficiency, Type II was an entirely clinical classification which was precise enough for specific diagnosis.

There are two principles. Firstly, if there is a different enzyme defect, then I would call it a different type following Cori's suggestion. Secondly, if there is a distinct clinical entity, even though the enzyme defect is now known, then we should accept that as another type.

de BARSY: I do not think it is necessary to separate the two different deficiencies of phosphorylase or phosphorylase kinase. The two enzymes are so closely related that it is not necessary to give two names for patients who are clinically entirely similar. I suggest that we maintain Type VI with sub groups because this is not so important to clinicians and is purely an enzymatic problem.

HERS: I agree with Dr Hug that there are many more forms than numbers up to now, but I do not agree with his views on the classification. There are many cases in which there is no clear biochemical defect but there is an excess of glycogen. If numbers were given to all these cases I do not know where we should be now. The situation is so complicated that we prefer to wait until such time as several similar cases have been published. Among the best new entity which has not been quoted in this symposium are the ones that we call pseudoglycogenoses. These are children who behave like Type I in every respect and the physician is quite sure about his diagnosis, and yet there is normal glucose-6-phosphatase activity. We do not know the primary enzymatic defect but at some time in the future these cases will be given a classification number.

CHALMERS (Harrow): Why use classification numbers for glycogen storage disease rather than the actual enzyme deficiency? Why not use the enzyme deficiency as a name?

RYMAN: We would have so many conditions without names that would be unclassified that the position would be impossible.

HERS: I think Dr Chalmers is suggesting that we at least call those where we know the enzyme defect by the name of the enzyme deficiency.

BLAU (London): Use of the deficiency of the specific enzymes for nomenclatures may not be an unequivocal answer to the problem. In the mucopolysaccharidoses the deficiency of the iduronidase turned out to be common to the clinically different entities of Hurler and Scheie syndromes.

HUG: May I ask Professor Hers why we see so little glycogen in the muscles in McArdle's syndrome? In Type V there is a total absence of phosphorylase and I would expect the glycogen to accumulate because the degradative enzyme is not there, but it doesn't. In none of our cases is the glycogen level above 4% and most of them are around about 2%.

HERS: I think this indicates that muscle has some further regulatory mechanism that prevents a large increase in glycogen in some patients. Presumably through inhibition of synthetase phosphatase by glycogen in muscle. In Type III the accummulation in muscle rarely gets much higher than 3–5% and it is only in Type II that very high concentrations are found, but that is intralysomal.

HUG: The abnormal lysosomes in Type II are explained by Hers' demonstration of the α-glucosidase deficiency in the muscle, but by low magnification light microscopy and also by electron microscopy there is an excess of cytoplasmic glycogen. Why does it not get degraded by the phosphorylase pathway, if all that is wrong is a deficiency of a lysosomal enzyme?

HERS: We are not sure that the glycogen which you see is outside the membrane. If it is outside the lysosomes I have no good answer.

RYMAN: There is some interesting published work suggesting that high molecular weight glycogen is engulfed by lysosomes. Maybe it has to be of a particular high molecular weight and this glycogen may not be acceptable to the phosphorylase system.

HERS: I have doubts concerning the conclusion that high or low molecular weight glycogen could be inside or outside lysosomes because technically it is such a difficult experiment.

HUG: May I make two practical points with respect to prenatal diagnosis? In Type I it has been shown that the amniotic fibroblasts in culture do not show glucose-6-phosphatase activity but the epithelial cells do. The amniotic fluid in all our cases showed α-glucosidase activity, even when the fetus had Type II glycogenosis.

HERS: Confusion has existed in the literature for 25 years between true glucose-6-phosphatase which is entirely a hepatic or kidney enzyme and any other phosphatase in a tissue that would also act on glucose-6-phosphate or glycerophosphate or glucose-1-phosphate, or any phosphoric ester.

In Type II glycogen storage disease, Dr Hug implied that he had to look for several hours under the electron microscope to find glycogen loaded lysosomes in amniotic fluid cells. If the child really is Type II do we need to look for so long? Dr de Barsy has experience with fibroblasts of heterozygotes with a few loaded lysosomes so if they are so rare might the fetus be a heterozygote rather than a homozygote?

HUG: In the 20 or more cases that we have done there have been five which were diagnosed on the basis of these inclusions. One was a single inclusion in one cell and occasionally there might have been half a dozen. I can make this diagnosis based on this appearance and in the heterozygote fibroblasts I have never seen anything abnormal. We have done fibroblast cultures and liver and muscle biopsies on parents, but we could not find any electron microscopic evidence of abnormal lysosomes in those tissues.

RYMAN: I would like to ask Dr de Barsy about the haemolysates of erythrocytes or leucocytes which he uses. Is there a danger that you are handling a different cell population which may be reflected in the changes in K_m which you see? If you take a leucocyte preparation you have all sorts of cells and if you take an erythrocyte population you have all age groups.

de BARSY: With leucocytes I agree. We do not find leucocyte preparations very useful and prefer to use erythrocytes which are a much more homogeneous population. Our erythrocytes are washed three times and there is no contamination by leucocytes. I agree with you about the different ages of cells within the population but I am not sure it would make any difference.

NUKI: Do all the experts agree that the hepatic type of glucose-6-phosphatase is really only detectable in liver tissue and in the kidney as Professor Hers has suggested. What about intestine and platelets?

HERS: There is no specific glucose-6-phosphatase except in liver, kidney and intestine and enzyme assays should not be done on any other tissue.

BESLEY (Edinburgh): It has been claimed that glucose-6-phosphatase activity can be measured in placenta and that this tissue can be used in prenatal diagnosis.

HERS: I do not think so.

RYMAN: This is all the same problem of methodology which Professor Hers has mentioned. You have to correct for the non-specific phosphatase activity.

BRENTON: Could I ask Dr Hug what he thinks one should tell an 18 year old boy with classic glucose-6-phosphatase deficiency about his future?

HUG: That is almost impossible to answer because the answer needs to be individualized. In such a situation I tend to go on the positive side saying that you have this condition but you can live with it. You have a future. There is no gain in my way of thinking to try and point out every single bad thing that can happen to these people and in anticipation wreck their lives right now, even if they have tragedy down the road. If I am going to be a fool when he finds out that it doesn't work out quite that way, I can take the brunt of that.

BRENTON: What kind of problems are your patients over the age of 18 years running into?

HUG: An inordinately large number of them are susceptible to development of hepatoma. There may be heterogeneity there, but cirrhosis is not the problem. Gout is a problem, vascular disease might be, but on the whole most of our patients in this group have done well on conventional treatment. I have been impressed with the comments on nasogastric feeding, although personally I have never used it, but I would not hesitate to do so. I would certainly not do a portacaval shunt in any of these cases.

FERNANDES: The summary in answer to your question is that they will get nephropathy, hepatoma and gout and perhaps (but we so not know sufficent about it) arteriosclerosis.

SECTION SEVEN

Genetic Aspects of Diabetes

20

Clinical studies of the inheritance of diabetes mellitus

R. Tattersall

Diabetes mellitus is a common and economically important disorder. The maturity onset type (also called insulin independent or Type II diabetes) affects 1–2% of the population depending on the age structure and exact diagnostic criteria used. Juvenile onset (also called insulin dependent or Type I) diabetes has an incidence in Europe of about 13 per 100 000 per year[1] and there is evidence to suggest that its incidence has been steadily increasing in the half century since the discovery of insulin[2]. The micro and macro vascular complications affect almost every organ system and make the disease a major public health problem. In the developed world, diabetes is the third leading cause of death[3] and the commonest cause of blindness under the age of 65[4]. The palliative nature of present treatment highlights the importance of research into its aetiology and prevention.

Mode of inheritance

It has been known for centuries that diabetes often runs in families but until the last decade it would have been difficult to find two workers in the field who agreed on anything other than this simple fact. The first scientific investigations of the inheritance of diabetes were carried out in the early 1930s by Allan[5] and Pincus and White[6]. They devised methods for pooling pedigrees and testing the findings against various Mendelian hypotheses. These studies confirmed the increased prevalence of diabetes among relatives of diabetics and both groups concluded that their findings were most compatible with a single recessive gene. Further work over the next 30 years merely led to increasing confusion. Almost every pattern of Mendelian inheritance was proposed but either rejected or devalued by the need to invoke various degrees of reduced penetrance to explain inconsistencies between the observed and expected findings.

In spite of wide spread disagreement among geneticists, many workers accepted the autosomal recessive hypothesis as a fact. Apart from leading to erroneous genetic counselling, this assumption also led to faulty deductions in research. If all cases of diabetes were inherited as an autosomal recessive, then all offspring of two diabetic parents would necessarily carry the diabetic genotype and be either already diabetic or, if they had normal carbohydrate tolerance, pre-diabetic. Much effort was expended in investigating offspring of two diabetic parents in the hope of finding abnormalities which would represent the very early features of diabetes. Some minor abnormalities were indeed found but none of them have thrown any light on the pathogenesis of diabetes. It has been pointed out that one cannot assume that 'slight' changes, for example in glucose tolerance, are the same as 'early' changes[7]. Recent research (discussed below) has shown that not all offspring of two diabetic parents or even identical twins of diabetics will develop diabetes, so that the term pre-diabetes should only be used in retrospect after a patient has actually developed the disease.

It is important to consider briefly the reasons why diabetes has proved to be such a nightmare for geneticists[8]. The disease is common and has a marked variation in age at onset and severity, two factors which increase the difficulty of genetic analysis. The variable age of onset meant that, in the absence of a marker of the pre-diabetic state, it was impossible to be sure that clinically unaffected relatives would remain so. Most data submitted for genetic analysis were obtained by questionnaire and seriously under estimated the prevalence of the disease among relatives. The use of glucose tolerance tests with unequivocal criteria of abnormality could increase the number of affected relatives as much as five fold[9]. No amount of statistical sophistication could ever compensate for basic inadequacies in the data. A further problem was the difficulty of understanding why diabetes should be so common since, unlike the sickle cell gene, it does not appear to confer any survival advantage. The final difficulty was that it was impossible to be sure that diabetes was a single disease.

Multifactorial inheritance[10] offered a neat mathematical solution to the apparently insoluble problem but was instinctively rejected by clinicians as improbable. Genetic heterogeneity, the existence of two or more fundamentally different entities with the same phenotype, was being increasingly recognised as a common phenomenon in the 1950s and 1960s[11] and was acknowledged by several geneticists as a ready explanation of the problem of the inheritance of diabetes.

GENETIC HETEROGENEITY

The possible existence of genetic heterogeneity in diabetes was proposed by Sir Archibald Garrod in his Croonian lecture as long ago as 1908[12] but was largely forgotten because of the insistence of many clinicians in lumping all cases of diabetes together. Certain distinct types were of course known: for example the glucose intolerance which occurs with acromegaly and chronic pancreatitis. However, patients with these types of diabetes were few and were thought to be distinct from 'genetic' or 'idiopathic' diabetes on the ground that they did not develop complications in spite of being hyperglycaemic. This erroneous impression arose from the short duration of carbohydrate intolerance in most cases of secondary diabetes and it is now clear that hyperglycaemia of any cause can result in typical microvascular complications, even proliferative retinopathy[13].

Genetic heterogeneity in terms of a difference between insulin dependent and insulin independent diabetes was strongly championed by R. D. Lawrence[14] although a major conceptual stumbling block was the existence of pedigrees in which the two types coexisted, or appeared to.

Several lines of clinical evidence had already indicated unequivocally that diabetes mellitus was genetically heterogeneous before studies of HLA antigens and islet cell antibodies (discussed in the next chapter by Dr Thomsen and his colleagues) provided the final proof. The evidence will be reviewed under the following headings:

(1) Genetic disorders associated with glucose intolerance.
(2) Diabetes in experimental animals.
(3) Twin studies.
(4) Family studies.
(5) Conjugal diabetes.

Genetic disorders associated with glucose intolerance

The association of glucose intolerance with a number of distinct genetic syndromes due to mutations at different loci was the major line of evidence cited by Rimoin in 1967 to support his theory of genetic heterogeneity in diabetes[15]. In a recent review, Rimoin[16] was able to collect over 30 distinct genetic disorders, many inherited as simple Mendelian traits which are associated with carbohydrate intolerance. Both typical insulin dependent and typical maturity onset diabetes occur among these disorders. For example, in the recessively inherited syndrome of diabetes mellitus, diabetes insipidus, optic atrophy and high tone nerve deafness (DIDMOAD syndrome)[17] the diabetes is typically ketosis prone and clinically and biochemically indistinguishable from that of any other juvenile diabetic. Even within this rare disorder there may also be heterogeneity since some families have only diabetes mellitus and optic atrophy while others have the full syndrome. Other apparently typical cases of infantile onset diabetes can be distinguished by associated abnormalities such as multiple epiphyseal dysplasia in the Wolcott–Rallison Syndrome[18]. A careful search in diabetic clinics might disclose further examples of distinct autosomal recessively inherited syndromes with diabetes as an integral feature.

More or less typical maturity onset diabetes occurs in the absence of obesity with haemochromatosis, isolated growth hormone deficiency and in a single pedigree with photomyoclonus, nerve deafness, nephropathy and progressive neurological deterioration[19]. Carbohydrate intolerance with obesity and not requiring insulin, even in young patients, is found in a wide variety of inherited disorders such as Alström's syndrome and the Prader–Willi syndrome. Here the carbohydrate intolerance is presumably a result of obesity rather than of an inherited abnormality of the pancreas such as appears probable in the DIDMOAD syndrome.

Certain unusual types of insulin resistant diabetes are clearly separate from both the juvenile and maturity onset forms. For example, in 1956 Mendenhall[20] described three siblings with severe insulin resistance, ketosis, enlarged genitalia, acanthosis nigricans and pineal hyperplasia. The mechanism of insulin resistance in this disorder is not clear, although it was counteracted by hypophysectomy in the only other case of the syndrome ever reported[21]. Other cases of insulin resistant diabetes with acanthosis nigricans are due to either a congenital or acquired absence of insulin receptors[22].

Although these conditions are collectively rare, they not only illustrate the heterogeneity of diabetes but also indicate the wide variety of pathogenic mechanisms which can theoretically lead to carbohydrate intolerance.

Diabetes in animals

Diabetes is not confined to man and has been reported in almost every animal species including foxes, dolphins, turtles and goldfish. It is also frequent in laboratory rodents which have been most extensively studied because of their convenience. The syndromes in these animals are extraordinarily varied. Inheritance may be by simple Mendelian dominant or recessive genes or polygenic with the simplest explanation in the Chinese hamster being a combination of four separate genes[23]. Obesity and hyperinsulinism in animals such as the New Zealand obese (NZO) mouse lead to a condition similar to maturity onset diabetes while others such as the spontaneously diabetic Wistar rat have islet cell destruction with insulinopenia and ketosis, a syndrome which is in some ways similar to that in juvenile onset diabetes[24].

Investigation in laboratory rodents has shown how the effects of a 'diabetogenic' gene can be modified by the prevailing genetic background. The db mutation on the C57BL/KsJ background on which it was originally developed produces severe insulin deficiency and ketosis, whereas the ob mutation in the closely related C57BL/6 strain produces obesity and hyperinsulinaemia. Transfer of the obese (ob) gene onto the original genetic background of the db gene (C57BL/KsJ) produces severe insulin deficiency whereas the db gene on the original background of the ob gene (C57BL/6) produces hyperinsulinism and mild hyperglycaemia[25]. The prevailing genetic background in man, although difficult to investigate, may be important and may explain the differing susceptibilities of various races to diabetes.

Although animal studies do not tell us anything about the genetics and aetiology of human diabetes, they are of considerable interest in indicating the extent of possible heterogeneity even in 'simple' animal models and also in drawing our attention to mechanisms which could be applicable in man.

Twin studies

Twins provide a convenient model for deciding the contribution of heredity to human disease. Monozygotic (MZ) twins are derived from the splitting of a single fertilized ovum and thus have identical genetic complements whereas dizygotic (DZ) twins are the product of fertilization of two separate ova and are genetically no more alike than siblings. Although MZ twins tend to be brought up more closely than fraternal twins, both types are assumed to be exposed to the same environment. Any excess of concordance in the monozygotic as opposed to dizygotic pairs is likely to be due to genetic factors. The results of this type of study in diabetes have confirmed the importance of inherited factors since they show a concordance rate of 45–96% in monozygotic twins compared to only 3–37% in dizygotic pairs.

Studies of monozygotic twin pairs with a diabetic proband are more informative since they indicate more clearly what is not inherited. If diabetes depended on genetic factors alone (like haemophilia, for example) one would expect to find 100% concordance in MZ pairs. In the original twin series from King's College Hospital[26], there were a total of 96 twin pairs, 65 concordant and 31 discordant, giving an overall concordance rate of 68%. Differences became apparent when the pairs were divided into two groups according to whether the index twin developed diabetes under or over the age of 40 years; a fortunate division since it produced an almost complete separation into pairs where the index twin had insulin dependent diabetes (age of onset under 40) and those with maturity onset diabetes (age of onset over 40). The concordance rate in the maturity onset twins approached 100% whereas in the insulin dependent pairs it was less than 50%. This finding suggested that maturity onset diabetes is almost completely determined by inheritance whereas environmental or non-genetic factors play a part in the juvenile onset form.

These conclusions have been confirmed by others and by an expanded series from King's College Hospital[7]. Follow up of the unaffected members of the discordant pairs has shown no evidence of progressive decrease in either glucose tolerance or insulin reserve. After ten years of discordance the rate of becoming concordant is only 3%[27], suggesting that diabetes in the affected members of discordant pairs has a different aetiology from that in concordant pairs.

One important feature of these observations is that they indicated an unequivocal difference between juvenile and maturity onset diabetes. Furthermore, they suggested that juvenile onset diabetes was, in part at least, of non-genetic origin. This conclusion raises the possibility of intervention to prevent beta cell destruction.

Too much importance must not be attached to the exact concordant/discordant ratios. One cannot say as Rubinstein and coworkers have done[28] that a 50% concordance rate indicates that the hypothetical 'diabetogenic' gene has a 50% penetrance. The method by which twin series are collected introduces an ascertainment bias in favour of concordance. Concordant pairs, having two diabetics, have a double chance of being ascertained so that the frequency of discordance is likely to be seriously underestimated.

Family studies

One of the observations which led many clinicians to believe that juvenile and maturity onset diabetes had a similar genetic background was the frequency with which diabetic children appeared to have a grandparent or other relative with maturity onset diabetes. Maturity onset diabetes is a common condition with a prevalence of 1–2% and it is inevitable that it will occur by chance in the families of insulin dependent patients. These families will be both more aware of an already diagnosed diabetic and also more likely to uncover a latent one with their urine testing equipment. Macdonald[29] investigated the parents and grandparents of 50 children with diabetes and 50 controls and found an equal prevalence of maturity onset diabetes among the parents and grandparents. Similar findings were reported by Lestradet and coworkers[30]. More recent studies using HLA antigens as markers of the type of diabetes have shown that, in families with an insulin dependent (Type I) proband, there is a significant excess of other family members with the same type of diabetes whatever their age at onset[31]. Confusion in previous studies has resulted from a failure to distinguish between patients who are *insulin dependent* and patients who merely take insulin, a problem clearly recognised by Simpson[32] who suggested that *propositi* in family studies should be classified on the basis of their phenotype rather than age at onset.

Further subdivision of diabetes in the young on the basis of phenotypic differences led to recognition of the syndome of maturity onset type diabetes of the young (MODY). Three unusual families were described in which most patients developed diabetes under the age of 20 but showed no tendency to ketosis or progression in severity of carbohydrate intolerance. They could be managed without insulin indefinitely. In spite of a mean duration of diabetes of 22 years, 90% had no evidence of microvascular complications[33]. Diabetes in the original three families seemed to be inherited as an autosomal dominant and this was confirmed in further studies by Tattersall and Fajans[9] who also showed a clear difference between the inheritance of MODY and classical juvenile onset diabetes. Non-insulin requiring diabetes may account for up to 15% of all cases diagnosed under 20 years of age[34] and there is now evidence of considerable heterogeneity in this as in other types of diabetes[7].

Conjugal diabetes

Analysis of the frequency and types of diabetes of offspring of marriages of two diabetic parents could have answered many questions about the inheritance and possible heterogeneity of diabetes. In practice the results have been disappointing and conflicting. The percentage of abnormal siblings has varied from 3–67%. This discrepancy results from a number of factors:

(1) Criteria of abnormality have differed with some investigators con-

sidering only clinical diabetes while others have used glucose or steroid primed glucose tolerance tests.

(2) Methods of ascertainment have varied. Only if ascertainment is through the parents will there be a lack of bias. If the families are ascertained through a diabetic child, there will be a bias in favour of an excess of diabetics and, if through a non-diabetic child, a bias in favour of unaffected offspring and families.

(3) The various series have differed substantially in racial composition and body weight of offspring.

Of the five series which are suitable for analysis, it is clear that not all marriages between diabetic parents necessarily produce affected offspring[35]. At least a quarter have no diabetic children, suggesting that in these marriages the parents have different types of diabetes and that neither has a dominantly inherited form. The vast majority of reported marriages are between two maturity onset diabetics and the children develop the same type of disease. If the only difference between juvenile onset and maturity onset diabetes was one of gene dosage then one might have expected conjugal maturity onset diabetics to produce large numbers of juvenile onset diabetic children. That they do not is strong evidence in favour of a genetic difference between the two types of diabetes. Virtually nothing is known about the genetic risks of a marriage between two juvenile onset diabetics since no series has ever been collected.

CONCLUSION

For the first 40 years after the discovery of insulin, clinicians remained obstinate lumpers and regarded diabetes mellitus as a single genetic disorder with variable phenotypic manifestations. This dogma led to the nightmare situation in which geneticists attempted, with little success although much ingenuity, to fit heterogenous and often rather poor data into various Mendelian moulds. It is now clear that diabetes is no more a single disorder than anaemia and a high blood sugar no more indicative of a single pathogenesis than a low haemoglobin.

References

1. Christau, B., Kromann, H., Andersen, O. O., Christy, M., Buschard, K., Arnung, K., Kristensen, I. H., Peitersen, B., Steinrud, J. and Nerup, J. (1977). Incidence, seasonal and geographical patterns of juvenile-onset insulin-dependent diabetes mellitus in Denmark. *Diabetologia*, **13,** 281

2. North, F. A., Gorwitz, K. and Sultz, H. A. (1977). A secular increase in the incidence of juvenile diabetes mellitus. *J. Pediatr.*, **91,** 706

3. Report of the National Commission on Diabetes to the Congress of the United States. Vol. I: The Long-Range Plan to Combat Diabetes. (1976). *D.H.E.W. Publication,* **No. (NIH),** 76–1018

4. Kohner, E. M. (1977). Diabetic Retinopathy. *Clin. Endocrinol. Metab.,* **6,** 345

5. Allan, W. (1933). Heredity in diabetes. *Ann. Intern. Med.,* **6,** 1272

6. Pincus, G. and White, P. (1933). On the inheritance of diabetes mellitus. I. An analysis of 675 family histories. *Am. J. Med. Sci.,* **186,** 1

7. Pyke, D. A. (1977). Genetics of diabetes. *Clin. Endocrinol. Metab.,* **6,** 285

8. Neel, J. V., Fajans, S. S., Conn, J. W. and Davidson, R. T. (1965). Diabetes mellitus, In: *Genetics and the Epidemiology of Chronic Diseases. PHS Publication No. 1163,* (Washington: Government)

9. Tattersall, R. B. and Fajans, S. S. (1975). A difference between the inheritance of classical juvenile-onset and maturity-onset diabetes of young people. *Diabetes,* **24,** 44

10. Falconer, D. S. (1967). The inheritance of liability to disease with variable age of onset with particular reference to diabetes mellitus. *Ann. Hum. Genet,* **31,** 1

11. McKusick, V. A. (1969). On Lumpers and Splitters, or the nosology of genetic disease. *Perspect. Biol. Med.,* **12,** 298

12. Garrod, A. E. (1908). Inborn errors of metabolism. *Lancet,* **2,** 1

13. Walsh, C. H. and Malins, J. M. (1978). Proliferative retinopathy in a patient with idiopathic haemochromatosis. *Br. Med. J.,* **2,** 16

14. Lawrence, R. D. (1957). Types of human diabetes. *Br. Med. J.,* **1,** 373

15. Rimoin, D. L. (1967). Genetics of diabetes mellitus. *Diabetes,* **16,** 346

16. Rimoin, D. L. (1976). Genetic syndromes associated with glucose intolerance. In W. Creutzfeldt, J. Köbberling and J. V. Neel (eds.). *The Genetics of Diabetes Mellitus,* pp. 43–63 (Berlin: Springer)

17. Page, M. McB., Asmal, A. C. and Edwards, C. R. W. (1976). Recessive inheritance of diabetes: the syndrome of Diabetes Insipidus, Diabetes Mellitus, Optic Atrophy and Deafness. *Q. J. Med.,* **45,** 505

18. Wolcott, C. D. and Rallison, M. L. (1972). Infancy-onset diabetes mellitus and multiple epiphyseal dysplasia. *J. Pediatr.,* **80,** 292

19. Herrmann, C., Augilar, M. J. and Sacks, O. W. (1964). Hereditary photomyoclonus associated with diabetes mellitus, deafness, nephropathy and cerebral dysfunction. *Neurology* (Minneap.), **14,** 212

20. Mendenhall, E. N. (1956). Familial hypertrophy of pineal body, hyperplasia of the adrenal cortex and diabetes mellitus. *Am. J. Clin. Pathol.,* **26,** 283

21. West, R. J., Lloyd, J. K. and Turner, W. M. (1975). Familial insulin resistant diabetes, multiple somatic abnormalities and pineal hyperplasia. *Arch. Dis. Child,* **50,** 703

22. Kahn, C. R., Flier, J. S., Bar, R. S., Archer, J. A., Gorden, P., Martin, M. M. and Roth, J. (1976). The syndromes of insulin resistance and acanthosis nigricans: insulin receptor disorders in man. *N. Engl. J. Med.,* **294,** 739

23. Gerritsen, G. C., Blanks, M. C., Schmidt, F. L. and Dulin, W. E. (1976). Environmental influences on the manifestation of diabetes mellitus in Chinese hamsters. In W. Creutzfeldt, J. Köbberling and J. V. Neel (eds). *The Genetics of Diabetes Mellitus,* pp. 165–187 (Berlin: Springer)

24. Nakhooda, A. F., Like, A. A., Chappel, C. I., Murray, F. T. and Marliss, E.

B. (1977). The spontaneously diabetic wistar rat: metabolic and morphologic studies. *Diabetes*, **26,** 100

25. Coleman, D. L. and Hummel, K. P. (1973). The influence of genetic background on the expression of the obese (ob) gene in the mouse. *Diabetologia*, **9,** 287

26. Tattersall, R. B. and Pyke, D. A. (1972). Diabetes in identical twins. *Lancet,* **2,** 1120

27. Pyke, D. A., Theopanides, C. G. and Tattersall, R. B. (1976). Genetic origin of diabetes: re-evaluation of twin data. *Lancet,* **2,** 464

28. Rubinstein, P., Suciu-Foca, N. and Nicholson, J. F. (1977). Genetics of juvenile diabetes mellitus – a recessive gene closely linked to HLA D and with 50% penetrance. *N. Engl. J. Med.*, **297,** 1036

29. Macdonald, M. J. (1974). Equal incidence of adult-onset diabetes among ancestors of juvenile diabetics and non-diabetics. *Diabetologia*, **10,** 767

30. Lestradet, H., Battiselli, J. and Ledoux, M. (1972). L'Heredite dans le diabete infantile. *Diabete Metab.*, **20,** 17

31. Irvine, W. J., Toft, A. D., Holton, D. E., Prescott, R. J., Clarke, B. F. and Duncan, L. J. P. (1977). Familial Studies of Type I and Type II idiopathic diabetes mellitus. *Lancet*, **2,** 325

32. Simpson, N. E. (1962) The genetics of diabetes: A study of 233 families of juvenile diabetics. *Ann. Hum. Genet.*, **26,** 1

33. Tattersall, R. B. (1974). Mild familial diabetes with dominant inheritance. *Q. J. Med.*, **43,** 339

34. Gorwitz, K., Howen, G. G. and Thompson, T. (1976). Prevalence of diabetes in Michigan school-age children. *Diabetes*, **25,** 122

35. Tattersall, R. B. (1976). Diabetes in the offspring of conjugal diabetic parents. In W. Creutzfeldt, J. Köbberling and J. V. Neel (eds). *The Genetics of Diabetes Mellitus*, pp. 188–193 (Berlin: Springer)

21

HLA antigens and diabetes

M. Thomsen, J. Nerup, M. Christy,
O. Ortved Andersen, M. Kromann, P. Platz,
L. P. Ryder and A. Svejgaard

It has become increasingly evident that the major histocompatibility complexes (MHCs) which have been found in all vertebrates studied so far, have other functions than creating difficulties for transplant surgeons. From studies in experimental animals and in man, it has been discovered[1] that the MHC contains (1) genes controlling antigens on cell surfaces, (2) genes controlling some components of the complement cascade, and (3) genes controlling the immune response against certain antigens, the Ir genes.

The MHC of man is called HLA, and in recent years it has been associated with a multitude of diseases, the aetiology of which was hitherto more or less unknown. One of them is juvenile onset diabetes mellitus, in which HLA has been shown to be a major genetic factor, although environmental factors also play a considerable role.

In this survey, the HLA system and some of its biological functions are summarized, and its association with diabetes mellitus is discussed including our own investigations and some from the literature. Fuller discussions of the HLA system and its association with diseases have been published by Svejgaard et al.[2], and Dausset and Svejgaard[3].

The genes of the HLA region are usually inherited 'en bloc'. Only in about 2% of meioses are crossovers found between A and D locus. As shown in Table 21.1, the antigens of the HLA are polymorphic and the number of different possible pheno-types is astronomical. Many of these are not as rare as expected from the frequencies of the different HLA genes as there is a strong linkage disequilibrium between the different alleles. This is probably the case not only for the genes we can recognize, but also for all the hundreds or even thousands of other genes located within the HLA region.

TABLE 21.1   HLA antigens

HLA-A1	HLA-B5		HLA-Cw1	HLA-Dw1
HLA-A2	HLA-B7		HLA-Cw2	HLA-Dw2
HLA-A3	HLA-B8		HLA-Cw3	HLA-Dw3
HLA-A9	HLA-B12	HLA-Bw41	HLA-Cw4	HLA-Dw4
HLA-A10	HLA-B13	HLA-Bw42	HLA-Cw5	HLA-Dw5
HLA-A11	HLA-B14	HLA-Bw44	HLA-Cw6	HLA-Dw6
HLA-A25	HLA-B15	HLA-Bw45		HLA-Dw7
HLA-A26	HLA-B17	HLA-Bw46		HLA-Dw8
HLA-A28	HLA-B18	HLA-Bw47		HLA-Dw9
HLA-A29	HLA-B27	HLA-Bw48		HLA-Dw10
HLA-Aw19	HLA-B37	HLA-Bw49		HLA-Dw11
HLA-Aw23	HLA-B40	HLA-Bw50		
HLA-Aw24	HLA-Bw4	HLA-Bw51		
HLA-Aw30	HLA-Bw6	HLA-Bw52		HLA-DRw1
HLA-Aw31	HLA-Bw16	HLA-Bw53		HLA-DRw2
HLA-Aw32	HLA-Bw21	HLA-Bw54		HLA-DRw3
HLA-Aw33	HLA-Bw22			HLA-DRw4
HLA-Aw34	HLA-Bw35			HLA-DRw5
HLA-Aw36	HLA-Bw38			HLA-DRw6
HLA-Aw43	HLA-Bw39			HLA-DRw7

Internationally recognized antigens of the five different segregant series (HLA-A, B, C, D, and DR). HLA-D and DR loci may be identical

HLA AND DISEASE

The association between HLA and diseases can be investigated by population studies and family studies.

Population studies

Population studies are the simpler. A number of unrelated patients with a given disease are typed and the frequencies of the different HLA antigens compared with the frequencies in a normal population of same ethnic origin. The strength of the association between a given HLA antigen and the disease is expressed as the relative risk, which indicates the frequency of the disease in a group of individuals carrying the antigen relative to a group lacking it. Even if the relative risk deviates from one, the statistical significance has to be taken into consideration. Chance deviations are to be expected as a large number of antigens are usually tested for. Often it is necessary to investigate a large number of patients or to pool the results from different surveys to confirm an association. As the association between disease and HLA usually varies in different ethnic groups, pooling of data has to be made carefully. For instance, there are considerable differences between populations in the northern and southern part of Europe regarding association between HLA and juvenile diabetes mellitus.

Family studies

Even if population data show no association with HLA, it is still possible that family studies will show linkage with HLA. Such studies require families where more than one member is affected, and are often difficult as varying penetrance and age at onset has to be taken into account. Furthermore, families with accumulated cases represent biased samples as they may carry more disease susceptibility genes than families with only one patient. Despite these drawbacks, much information can be obtained from family studies. When population studies show association with the HLA markers, the genetics of the disorder may be elucidated and risk factors for relatives with and without the HLA markers can be estimated.

DIABETES MELLITUS

Diabetes mellitus is a heterogeneous disease group (see Tattersall, this volume). Only insulin dependent diabetes (IDD) has been shown to be associated with HLA. The first report of an association was made by Singal and Blajchman[6], who found an increase of HLA-B15 on a small group of patients. This finding was contradicted by the report of Finkelstein et al.[7]. In 1974 Nerup et al.[8] proved a definite association with HLA-B15 and with HLA-B8 and this was soon confirmed by Cudworth and Woodrow[9] independently. HLA-B18 was found with an increased frequency, especially in France, but the association with B15 was not observed[10].

In 1975 we demonstrated the association with IDD to be closer with HLA-D antigens[11], namely Dw3, which is in linkage disequilibrium with B8, and Dw4, which is in linkage disequilibrium with B15 and possibly also with

B18. HLA-B7 is decreased in IDD, and Dw2, which is in linkage disequilibrium with B7, has not been found in any of our patients. The frequency of Dw2 in the normal population is approximately 25%.

Family studies have shown that disease susceptibility usually follows certain HLA haplotypes. In a family with six cases of diabetes in three generations, the disease was linked to the same HLA haplotype and this can best be explained by dominant susceptibility[11]. In sibship studies, where more than one sib is affected, our data does not yet allow conclusions regarding dominant versus recessive susceptibility. Of 32 diabetic sibpairs, 12 were HLA identical, 16 had identical haplotypes, and four were nonidentical. In the studies of Rubinstein et al.[12], a recessive inheritance was suggested as most of the affected sibpairs were HLA-identical. In some of the sibships which were not HLA-identical, a crossover was claimed because the sibs were HLA-D identical but HLA-A,B,C different. A very high recombination frequency in diabetic families has been postulated by these investigators, but neither we nor other groups have been able to confirm this.

Earlier, we suggested[2] that susceptibility to insulin dependent diabetes was due to two different HLA linked genes which act in concert (over-dominance). The basis for this was the observation that HLA-B8/B15 heterozygotes have a higher risk of developing IDD than other individuals, including those apparently homozygous for B8 or B15. When it became clear that HLA-D factors were more closely associated with IDD than HLA-B, we undertook a prospective study of all newly diagnosed cases during one year in the greater Copenhagen area, covering a third of the Danish population. Table 21.2 shows the frequencies of HLA-Dw2, 3, and

TABLE 21.2   HLA-D antigen frequencies in unrelated patients with insulin dependent diabetes

HLA-D	Group I (retrospective)	Group II (prospective)	Group III (familial)	Controls
Dw2	0/20 (0.0)	0/73 (0.0)	0/25 (0.0)	89/345 (25.8)
Dw3	26/52 (50.0)	32/73 (43.8)	14/25 (56.0)	88/334 (26.3)
Dw4	32/79 (40.5)	41/73 (56.2)	18/25 (72.0)	67/345 (19.4)

The figures are number of positive/number investigated and percentages in brackets.
Group I is retrospectively ascertained patients, Group II prospectively ascertained patients, and Group III is familial cases (cases with two or more affected members of a sibship). Only the eldest affected sib is counted. The frequency of Dw4 is significantly lower in Group I than in groups II and III ($p = 0.04$ and $p = 0.006$, respectively)

4 in this group, an earlier retrospective group[11] of IDD from an outpatient clinic, and a sample of sibpairs (only the eldest affected sib). Dw2 is absent from all groups. Dw4 is significantly more frequent in the prospective group and the familial cases than in the retrospective group. This could be explained by technical difficulties in the typing, but we do not consider it likely as the same typing cells and many controls have been used throughout. The difference between group 1 and 2 can be explained by biased sampling as the retrospective group contains more patients with later onset of IDD.

We tried to establish the HLA-D genotypes in group 2 and 3 by typing for eight different HLA-D antigens (HLA-Dw1–8) and family studies. When we were in doubt about the patients being homo- or heterozygous for Dw3 or Dw4, the patients' lymphocytes were used as stimulators in MLC with HLA-Dw3 and Dw4 homozygous cells as responders. In the prospective group (group 2), patients were subdivided according to an onset before or after the age of 16. Detailed data are published elsewhere[13] and show firstly that Dw4 is found most frequently in patients with age at onset before 16 ($p = 0.02$), whereas Dw3 is equally common in both groups. This supports the suggestion that Dw3 and Dw4 act by different mechanisms.

Secondly, Dw3/4 heterozygotes are more frequent in familial cases than in the prospective series ($p = 0.03$). Thus, familial cases represent a special sample of all cases of IDD which has a greater frequency of disease susceptibility factors than the remainder.

Finally, we have found that HLA-Dw3/4 heterozygotes have the highest risk of developing diabetes followed by Dw4 and Dw3 homozygotes. The lowest risk was found in Dw4 and Dw3 heterozygotes. This indicates an interaction between Dw3 and Dw4 when present together and some dose effect for each of those genes.

Autoimmunity

Autoimmune phenomena are frequently found in IDD. One week after diagnosis 71% of B8 negative patients were found to have islet cell antibodies (ICA) but only 50% of B8 positives. After some time, ICA gradually disappears in patients not carrying B8, whereas they are still present in even higher frequency in those bearing B8. Other autoimmune phenomena can often be found in patients with IDD, e.g. thyroid, and adrenal antibodies. In Graves' disease and idiopathic Addison's disease B8 and Dw3 are increased[11]. In Addison's disease a significant increase of adrenal autoantibodies was found in Dw3 positive compared with Dw3 negative patients (96% and 40%, respectively).

Mechanisms

No conclusive evidence exists regarding the mechanisms which confer susceptiblity to IDD. The theory most favoured by us is the existence of immune response genes acting abnormally in the diseased patients. The Ir genes probably influence the co-operation between different subsets of lymphocytes and macrophages, and autoimmune phenomena may be due to a lack of suppressor T cells. As B8 and Dw3 are common denominators for diseases with autoimmune phenomena, it may be that abnormal Ir genes are in strong linkage disqeuilibrium with Dw3.

Another possibility to explain disease associations is interaction between HLA and hormones and hormone receptors[14]. As B15 and Dw4 are not particularly associated with autoimmune phenomena, such a mechanism might be operating for diabetic patients with these antigens.

A number of other theories can explain the association between HLA and disease and it is possible that more than one mechanism can operate in the widely differing diseases which have been associated with HLA.

SUMMARY

Insulin dependent diabetes is positively associated with HLA-Dw3 and -4, and negatively associated with Dw2. Association with HLA-B antigens is secondary to this. HLA-D genotyping in insulin dependent diabetes indicates that the disease is heterogeneous and that Dw3 and Dw4 operate via different mechanisms in conferring susceptibility.

Acknowledgements

The study was aided by grants from the Nordic Insulin Foundation, the Danish Medical Research Council and the Danish Blood Donor Foundation. The extremely skilful secretarial assistance of Elly Andersen is greatly acknowledged.

References

1. Snell, G. D., Dausset, J. and Nathenson, S. (1977). *Histocompatibility*, p. 401 (New York: Academic Press)
2. Svejgaard, A., Platz, P., Ryder, L. P., Nielsen, L. Staub and Thomsen, M. (1975). HL-A and disease associations – a survey. *Transplant. Rev.*, **22**, 3
3. Dausset, J. and Svejgaard, A. (1977). *HLA and Disease*, p. 316 (Copenhagen: Munksgaard)
4. Thomsen, M., Ryder, L. P. and Svejgaard, A. (1976). Typing for MLC determinants, methods and applications. *Scand. J. Immunol.*, **5**, (**Suppl. 5**), 157

5. Bodmer, J. G. (1978). Ia antigens. *Br. Med. Bull.*, **3**, 233
6. Singal, D. P. and Blajchman, M. A. (1973). Histocompatibility (HL-A) antigens, lymphocytotoxic antibodies and tissue antibodies in patients with diabetes mellitus. *Diabetes*, **22**, 429
7. Finkelstein, S., Zeller, E. and Walford, R. L. (1972). No relation between HL-A and juvenile diabetes. *Tissue Antigens*, **2**, 74
8. Nerup, J., Platz, P., Andersen, O. O., Christy, M., Lyngsøe, J., Poulsen, J. E., Ryder, L. P., Nielsen, L. Staub, Thomsen, M. and Svejgaard, A. (1974). HL-A antigens and diabetes mellitus. *Lancet*, **2**, 864
9. Cudworth, A. G. and Woodrow, J. C. (1975). HL-A system and diabetes mellitus. *Diabetes*, **24**, 345
10. Nerup, J., Cathelineau, Cr., Seignalet, J. and Thomsen, M. (1977). HLA and endocrine diseases. In J. Dausset and A. Svejgaard (eds). *HLA and Disease*, pp. 149–167 (Copenhagen: Munksgaard)
11. Thomsen, M., Platz, P., Andersen, O. Ortved., Christy, M., Lyngsøe, J., Nerup, J., Rasmussen, K., Ryder, L. P., Nielsen, L. Staub and Svejgaard A. (1975). MLC typing in juvenile diabetes mellitus and idiopathic Addison's disease. *Transplant. Rev.*, **22**, 125
12. Rubinstein, P., Suciu-Foca, N. and Nicholson, J. F. (1977). Genetics of juvenile diabetes mellitus. *N. Engl. J. Med.*, **297**, 1036
13 Svejgaard, A., Christy, M., Nerup, J., Platz, P., Ryder, L. P. and Thomsen, M. (1978). HLA and autoimmune disease with special reference to the genetics of insulin-dependent diabetes. In N. R. Rose, P. E. Bigazzi and N. L. Warner (eds.), *Genetic Control of Autoimmune Disease*, p. 101 (North Holland/New York: Elsevier)
14. Svejgaard, A. and Ryder, L. P. (1976). Interaction of HLA molecules with non-immunological ligands as an explanation of HLA and disease associations. *Lancet*, **2**, 547

22

Juvenile diabetes and optic atrophy

S. M. M. Sheriff, J. G. Tetley and
C. R. Maddock

A familial condition characterized by juvenile diabetes mellitus (DM), optic atrophy (OA), nerve deafness (D), diabetes insipidus (DI) and central nervous system defects is appearing in the medical literature with increasing frequency. These clinical features are found in variable combinations. The syndrome is either referred to as Wolfram–Tyrer syndrome[1] after two independent early observers[2,3], or as DIDMOAD syndrome[4], an acronym depicting some of its most commonly expressed features. Other features have been reported including heredo-familial ataxias, dilatation of the urinary tract and sideroblastic anaemia. Despite the diversity of expression of the syndrome, there is a similarity in the pattern of clinical presentation among affected individuals of the same family.

Table 22.1 indicates the main findings in the condition and attempts to classify and disentangle the clinical features, some of which are common to other clinical entities. The group of disorders labelled A are those most commonly reported. Those labelled A1 are also reported frequently but are secondary to features in Group A. The features in Group A2 have also been reported in conjunction with one of more of the disorders mentioned in Group A but occur in fewer families.

A recent review of 88 cases indicates that the most frequently recognised

TABLE 22.1   Wolfram–Tyrer syndrome (DIDMOAD)

Group	Clinical observations	References	Remarks
A	juvenile diabetes mellitus (DM) optic atrophy (OA) diabetes insipidus (DI) bilateral nerve deafness (D)	5, 6, 7, 8	Clinical features most frequently reported by independent observers presenting in combination or singly in cumulative sequence
A1	atony of bladder hydroureters colour blindness	4, 9, 18	Disorders resulting from pre-existing DI and OA respectively
A2	heredo-ataxia (unspecified) Friedreich's ataxia sideroblastic anaemia	10, 11, 12, 13	Clearly defined syndromes repeatedly found in association with one, two or three of the features in group A
B	obesity infantilism menstrual disturbances atrophic uterus testicular atrophy cataract, ptosis anosmia EEG abnormality thermoregulatory failure blunted plasma cortisol response to pyrogen infusion thyroid disorder aminoaciduria (predominantly alanine)	6, 7, 8	Additional, less frequently described features, mainly consistent with partial hypothalamic dysfunction or disordered central nervous system function
C	retinitis pigmentosa Refsum's disease Alström's disease Laurence Moon Biedl syndrome Rosenberg Chutorian syndrome Nyssen–van Bogaert syndrome	14, 15, 16	Other hereditary syndromes also associated with visual and hearing defects, to be distinguished from Wolfram–Tyrer syndrome either by absence of juvenile diabetes mellitus or differing patterns of clinical evolution. Sometimes inheritance patterns differ

components of the syndrome are juvenile diabetes mellitus (99%), optic atrophy (98%), bilateral nerve deafness (39%) and diabetes insipidus (32%)[5]. Not all four features are necessarily found in any one individual, but the most frequent combinations among affected siblings are DM with OA, DM with DI or lone DM. DI with OA alone, lone DI and lone OA are not considered to be a partial expression of the syndrome[4] though there may be a stage in the clinical evolution of cases where only one feature is recognisable.

CASE REPORT

The patient was born on 28.9.73, the firstborn daughter of healthy unrelated Indian parents. There was no relevant family or perinatal history. At the age of 8 months the parents suspected deafness. At 17 months sensorineural deafness was confirmed by Professor I. G. Taylor of Manchester but no cause was recognized. Hearing aids were prescribed.

At 18 months the child was admitted to hospital with a severe upper respiratory tract infection. Routine urine tests revealed glycosuria. A fasting blood glucose level was more than 11 mmol/l (200 mg/100 ml). Treatment with 2 units of soluble insulin twice daily was begun.

At the age of 22 months she appeared anaemic. Haemoglobin was 6.1 g/dl with a normal total and differential white cell count. Blood film showed macrocytosis, anisocytosis and poikilocytosis. Haemoglobin was 12.5 g/dl at 14 months. Serum iron, iron binding capacity, folate and B_{12} values were normal. Haemoglobin electrophoresis was normal. Bone marrow showed some frank megaloblasts. The anaemia responded partially to treatment with folic acid.

At 33 months, nystagmus was observed. The optic discs were pale and some small level pigmentary aggregations were present at both maculae. There was no diabetic retinopathy. Gross astigmatism and slight convergent squint were noted in addition. The vitreous was clear.

At 35 months, haemoglobin was 9.8 g/dl, MCV 94 fl, MCHC 33%, white cell count 11.2×10^9 cells/l, neutrophils 54%, lymphocytes 44%, monocytes 1%, erythroblasts 1%, reticulocytes 1.6%. Blood film showed normochromic red cells, anisocytosis, poikilocytosis, target cells and macrocytosis. Marrow biopsy showed a cellular marrow with little stainable iron. Erythropoiesis was normoblastic although a few precursors showed megaloblastoid changes. About 70% of red cell precursors were abnormal sideroblasts and one half of these were ring forms. They were PAS negative. Granulocyte precursors and megakaryocytes were normal. The appearances were those of sideroblastic anaemia.

Folic acid (5 mg) on alternate days and pyridoxine (20 mg) daily were prescribed.

The diabetes remained controlled with Isophane Insulin (4 units daily) and 120 g carbohydrate diet. At 57 months of age the child's physical and neurodevelopmental progress was satisfactory for a partially hearing child. Height and weight were on the 50th centiles.

Comment on case

This case shows the rarely reported feature of sideroblastic anaemia. This type of anaemia is found most frequently in elderly patients usually secondary to some other disease but may be a sex linked hereditary disorder in male children or young adults. Reviewing 70 cases of sideroblastic anaemia, MacGibbon and Mollin[12] found only one male with associated optic atrophy, deafness and diabetes. Two siblings described by Byrd and Cooper[17] were also males. Sideroblastic anaemia associated with diabetes mellitus, optic atrophy and heredo-ataxia but without deafness has been described in a 23 year old woman and her 18-year old brother[13].

This patient is unique as she has shown more features of the syndrome at an earlier age than others previously reported and is the first female to demonstrate both sideroblastic anaemia and deafness. The diagnosis of optic atrophy in our case is not yet completely proven and reliable visual acuity still not established. The macular lesions are consistent with the observations of others in this syndrome[6, 18].

AETIOLOGY

The cause of such an intriguing constellation of clinical features has provoked much speculation. Beyond doubt, the condition is inherited as an autosomal recessive. Pedigrees repeatedly demonstrate affected siblings of both sexes with normal parents and among such parents there is a high proportion of consanguineous marriages[4, 19]. Assuming the fully developed syndrome to be manifest in homozygotes and the heterozygous state to be clinically expressed as lone DM, the ratio of affected subjects to siblings with lone DM is consistent with this Mendelian inheritance pattern[20].

There is no agreement yet regarding the underlying pathology. Early observers recognized that the optic atrophy was certainly not a consequence of diabetes mellitus as visual symptoms sometimes preceeded the onset of diabetes[9]. A number of features suggest a nervous system lesion in the region of the hypothalmus and the supraoptico hypophyseal tract but neuroradiological investigations have not shown any consistent abnormality. Autopsy information is scanty. One report described a normal hypothalamus, thalamus, substantia nigra and red nucleus. The optic nerves, chiasma and optic tracts showed only slight gliosis and loss of myelin. There was no active demyelination[5]. Another report of a patient dying with Laurence Moon Biedl syndrome mentions the presence of a small hypophysis and mild hydrocephalus[21].

Gunn et al.[22] postulated a relationship between neurological defects and diabetes mellitus on the basis that neural crest epithelial elements (APUD cell system) migrate into the developing sympathetic chain and adrenal medulla, from C cells in the thyroid and contribute to the pancreatic islets. This embryological origin of the islet cells is not currently accepted[23] and this thesis does not explain the sideroblastic anaemia occasionally reported in Wolfram–Tyrer syndrome.

INCIDENCE

There is no satisfactory information about the incidence of this syndrome. In a diabetic clinic only one out of 150 juvenile diabetics was recognized to have the condition[22]. Even this low frequency probably overestimates the incidence in the general population[20].

The racial distribution has some practical consequences as the haematological features may be confused with thalassaemia[13]. Most case reports originate from Western Europe, Scandinavia, USA and Canada. On the other hand African – Arabic parents from Tanzania[4] and, in our case, Indian parents have also had affected children. These observations suggest that the gene is probably world wide and not confined to Caucasian parentage.

CLINICAL PRESENTATION

The order of appearance of the various features is unpredictable but affected siblings usually follow a similar pattern and have a similar degree of handicap. The patient may appear first in a specialist clinic for hearing, visual or neurological defects, but the commonest presenting symptoms are those of thirst and polyuria, common to both diabetes mellitus and diabetes insipidus. Either DM or OA is most likely to be recognized before the age of 12 years[4], but in those families where Friedreich's ataxia is also manifest, DM and OA may not be recognized until the third decade[11, 24]. The earliest age at which relevant symptoms are recognized will depend on the observations of parents and the timing of medical investigations.

Long time intervals may elapse between the onset of DM and that of OA.

In a review by Marquardt the average interval was about four and a half years; the longest interval was fourteen years[8].

Bilateral nerve deafness

The degree of hearing loss may be confined to higher frequencies and cause no handicap. Many of the reported cases of deafness were only recognized when tested by pure tone audiometry[5]. Assessment of hearing defects in pre-school children may be difficult, requiring special experience and techniques to detect minor abnormalities.

Diabetes insipidus

Although polyuria and polydipsia may be the presenting symptoms DI may remain asymptomatic and may be easily overlooked in the presence of poorly controlled DM. Eight hour water deprivation tests with plasma and urine osmolarity studies, and urinary vasopressin levels (by radio-immuno assays) may prove the diagnosis of unsuspected DI[4]. Investigation for DI should only be performed if DM is adequately controlled.

Diabetes mellitus

Although DM in young subjects usually has an explosive onset requiring urgent medical management, it may present with intermittent glycosuria and hyperglycaemia before treatment with insulin is required[9, 22]. In some instances presymptomatic patients have shown an abnormal glucose tolerance curve with poor insulin response. Insulin levels in serum have not risen after tolbutamide treatment[22].

Optic atrophy

There is difficulty in assessing visual acuity precisely in early childhood. Ophthalmoscopic findings may be inconclusive in the early stages, but in older subjects impairment of colour vision may be recognized in association with, or preceeding confirmatory tests of impaired visual acuity or field defect[18].

PROGNOSIS

Diabetes mellitus is the component affecting life expectancy and does not differ in character or severity from that found in other diabetic patients of the same age. Deaths from ketoacidosis have occurred.

Blindness is the most severe and most frequently recorded handicap. Progression of OA to eventual loss of useful sight seems to be the usual outcome. This handicap is typically preceded by progressive concentric contractions of the visual fields[4,9]. Deafness has produced a handicap severe enough to oblige only three subjects out of eighty eight to attend a special school. The earlier in life that deafness is recognized the more likely is it to be progressive. High frequency loss predominates but in most instances hearing loss is not severe[5].

DI may be completely or only partially relieved by specific treatment with pitressin or chlorpropamide. Dilatation of the urinary tract occurs only in cases with DI and has been shown to be reversible if the polyuria is controlled[4,8]. Dilatation of the urinary tract has predisposed to urinary tract infection which in one instance led to death[5].

Information on sexual development and reproductive ability is sparse. Several reports refer to poor sexual development for age but usually the external genitalia appear normal. Cordier[25] mentions one patient who had three pregnancies which ended in still births at eight months gestation. Successful reproductive performance of an affected man or woman has not yet been positively reported.

IMPORTANCE OF DIAGNOSIS

The clinician has a duty to recognize any condition which has an autosomal recessive inheritance. There must be an inevitable delay in diagnosis of Wolfram–Tyrer syndrome when the different clinical manifestations are widely separated in time, particularly if the onset of DM is delayed. If the patient is aged 20 years or less, simple investigations for DI, DM, OA, D (water deprivation test, blood sugar two hours after food, visual acuity and audiometry) are worthwhile after the onset of one of these four components. In children of pre-school age, where D and OA are more difficult to assess and an adequate eight hour water deprivation test practically more difficult, much will depend on individual circumstances and the relative importance of making an early diagnosis for the sake of genetic advice.

The responsibility for diagnosis in the first born is perhaps most burdensome when such serious handicaps as blindness, deafness and life-threatening heredo-ataxia are involved yet intelligence is spared, as may well be the case in Wolfram–Tyrer syndrome.

In countries where genetic counselling is valued and available, small families are often completed within the span of a few years. This syndrome may unfold too slowly to allow opportunity for advice to the parents of the one in four hazard of further children of their marriage inheriting the disorder. Computerized axial tomography of the brain, fibroblast culture or HLA analysis have not yet been shown to contribute towards diagnosis and there is no recognized marker which allows prenatal or early postnatal diagnosis. No known dietary or therapeutic measures are at present available which will protect an affected subject from the onset of one or more of the disabilities.

References

1. Sorsby, A. (1973). Some newer genetic entities. In A. Sorsby and S. Miller (eds), *Modern Trends in Ophthalmology*, pp. 89–91. (London: Butterworth)
2. Wolfram, D. J. (1938). Diabetes mellitus and simple optic atrophy among siblings: report of four cases. *Mayo Clin. Proc.*, **13**, 715
3. Tyrer, J. (1943). A case of infantilism with goitre, diabetes mellitus, mental defect and bilateral primary optic atrophy. *Med. J. Aust.*, **2**, 398
4. Page, M. McB., Asmal, A. C. and Edwards, C. R. W. (1976). Recessive inheritance of diabetes: the syndrome of diabetes insipidus, diabetes mellitus, optic atrophy and deafness. *Q. J. Med.*, *New Series XLV*, **179**, 505
5. Cremers, C. W. R. J., Wijdereld, P. G. A. B. and Pinckers, A. J. L. G. (1977). Juvenile diabetes mellitus, optic atrophy, hearing loss, diabetes insipidus, atonia of the urinary tract and bladder and other abnormalities (Wolfram Syndrome). *Acta Paediatr. Scand.*, (Suppl.) 264
6. Rose, C., Fraser, G. R., Friedmann, A. I. and Kohner, E. M. (1966). The association of juvenile diabetes mellitus and optic atrophy: clinical and genetical aspects. *Q. J. Med.*, *New Series XXXV*, **139**, 385
7. Ikkos, D. G., Fraser, G. R., Matsouki-Gavra, E. and Petrochilos. M. (1970). Association of juvenile diabetes mellitus, primary optic atrophy and perceptive hearing loss in three sibs, with additional idiopathic diabetes insipidus in one case. *Acta Endocrinol. (Kbh)*, **65**, 95
8. Marquardt, J. L. and Loriaux, D. L. (1974). Diabetes mellitus and optic atrophy with associated findings of diabetes insipidus and neurosensory hearing loss in two siblings. *Arch. Intern. Med.*, **134**, 32
9. Stevens, P. R. and Macfadyen, W. A. L. (1972). Familial incidence of juvenile diabetes mellitus, progressive optic atrophy and neurogenic deafness. *Br. J. Ophthalmol.*, **56**, 496
10. Ashby, D. W. and Tweedy, P. S. (1953). Friedreich's ataxia combined with diabetes mellitus in sisters. *Br. Med. J.*, **1**, 1418
11. Thoren, C. (1962). Diabetes mellitus in Friedreich's ataxia. *Acta Paediatr. Scand.*, 135 (Suppl.), 239
12. MacGibbon, B. H. and Mollin, D. L. (1965). Sideroblastic anaemia in man. Observations on seventy cases. *Br. J. Haematol.*, **11**, 59
13. Järmerot, G. (1973). Diabetes mellitus with optic atrophy – thalassaemia-like sideroblastic anaemia and weak isoagglutinins. A new genetic syndrome? *Acta Med. Scand.*, **193**, 359
14. André-van Leeuwen, M. and van Bogaert, L. (1949). Hereditary ataxia with optic atrophy of the retrobular neuritis type and latent Pallido-Luysian degeneration. *Brain*, **72**, 340

15. van Bogaert, L. and Martin, M. (1974). Optic and cochleovestibular degenerations in the hereditary ataxias. I Clinico-pathological and genetic aspects. *Brain*, **97,** 15
16. Konigsmark, B. W., Knox, D. L., Hussels, I. E. and Moses, H. (1974). Dominant congenital deafness and progressive optic nerve atrophy. *Arch. Ophthalmol.*, **91,** 99
17. Byrd, R. B. and Cooper, T. (1961). Hereditary iron loading anaemia with secondary haemochromatosis. *Ann. Intern. Med.*, **55,** 103
18. Rorsman, G. and Söderström, N. (1967). Optic atrophy and juvenile diabetes mellitus with familial occurence. *Acta Med. Scand.*, **182,** 419
19. Anonssakis, C., Liakakos, D., Vlachos, P., Zervos, N. and Simonetos, G. (1975). Le syndrome familial associant in diabète sueré juvénile et une atrophie optique primitive. A propos de trois observations. *Pediatrie*, **30,** 179
20. Fraser, F. C. and Gunn, T. (1977). Diabetes mellitus, diabetes insipidus and optic atrophy. An autosomal recessive syndrome. *J. Med. Genet.*, **14,** 190
21. Fraccano, M. and Gastaldi, F. (1952). La patologia della sindrome de Laurence-Moon-Biedl. *Folia. Hered. Pathol.*, **2,** 177
22. Gunn, T., Bortolussi, R., Little, J. M., Andermann, F., Fraser, F. C. and Betmonte, M. M. (1976). Juvenile diabetes mellitus, optic atrophy, sensory nerve deafness and diabetes insipidus – a syndrome. *J. Pediatr.*, **89,** 565
23. Coupland, R. E. (1978). Personal communication.
24. Podolsky, S., Pothier, A. and Krall, L. P. (1964). Association of diabetes mellitus and Friedreich's ataxia. *Arch. Intern. Med.*, **114,** 533
25. Cordier, J., Reny, A. and Raspiller, A. (1970). Atrophie optique familiale et diabéte juvénile. *Rev. Otoneuroophthalmol.*, **42,** 269

Discussion

DISCUSSION ON DIABETES

BLASS (White Plains): What was the evidence for autosomal recessive inheritance in Dr Maddock's child?

MADDOCK (Sutton-in-Ashfield): The evidence is based on the work of other people as this case is the first born child of the marriage. The parents are both healthy with respect to diabetes and optic atrophy.

TATTERSALL (Nottingham): It is fairly conclusively established in the literature that this is an autosomal recessive condition. There is a tremendous excess of consanguinity, certainly in both families reported by Page when he coined the term 'the DIDMOAD syndrome'.

There is a considerable amount of heterogeneity in this syndrome because there are some families in whom optic atrophy and diabetes go together and in which you never get the diabetes insipidus and high tone nerve deafness. It is difficult when you get additional problems like sideroblastic anaemia, to discover whether that is chance or really an associated abnormality. On one of your slides you mention a 'psychic' abnormality. Could you clarify please?

MADDOCK: In the cases described there was one family where the affected siblings all showed some sort of disorder of an emotional nature but could not be given a recognized psychiatric label.

O'BRIEN (Denver): Would you comment on the natural history of the deafness and loss of vision in this group of patients?

MADDOCK: In the literature deafness is not very often a severe component of this group of disorders and in many cases has only been recognized by pure tone audiometry. In the instance that we had, this was the earliest sign of the disorder. As regards the blindness, our child was not very severely affected, but, from the literature, this seems to be much more worrying. Progressive loss of vision sometimes occurs with concentric restriction of the visual fields; it is the most frequently encountered disability.

TATTERSALL: All the patients I have seen have been effectively blind by the age of 16 years. They developed severe tunnel vision and severe optic atrophy. In the families reported by Page which I look after, almost all the patients went blind. Dr Maddock is absolutely right; there is usually high tone nerve deafness, which is only detected on audiometry.

UNKNOWN PARTICIPANT: Does it make any difference if they have retinitis pigmentosa or optic atrophy?

TATTERSALL: Retinitis pigmentosa in diabetes is in the land of Alstrom's syndrome and Refsum's syndrome. Diabetes is a complication of Refsum's syndrome. There have been families reported in which the two appear to go together.

STACEY (London): For some time immunization with live mumps virus has been going on in various parts of the world. Is there any good evidence that this is increasing the incidence of juvenile diabetes?

TATTERSALL: I think there is fairly good evidence that the incidence of juvenile diabetes has increased. Whether it has anything to do with mumps virus I wouldn't be prepared to hazard a guess. Certainly mumps virus has come back into prominence because work at the National Institute of Health in Bethesda has shown within the last year that mumps virus is cytotoxic to human B cells grown in culture. Some people would suggest that as many as 2% of all cases of juvenile diabetes are due to mumps of the pancreas. I don't know whether Dr Thomsen would be prepared to comment?

THOMSEN (Copenhagen): The problem about the rising incidence is that there is nothing to compare it with. No-one has any accurate figures for 20–30 years ago. The marvellous study carried out in Copenhagen, which can only really be done in a relatively small city, showed an overall incidence of 13.2/100 000 per year. There was a very big difference between two areas, the lower social class area had a much higher incidence.

MOORE (Dublin): From Dr Tattersall's evidence there appears to be many children on insulin who are really suffering from maturity onset diabetes of the young and might do better on tablets. Is there any way, short of the very detailed antibody studies of Dr Thomsen, that might distinguish these children at an early age?

TATTERSALL: The problem is that you can only recognize whether a patient will do well in retrospect. It always annoys me when insurance companies talk about mild and severe diabetes, by which they mean severe diabetics are on insulin and mild diabetics are not. Everyone who works in a diabetic clinic has patients who have been on insulin for 50 years and have had no complications, which, if words mean anything, must be mild diabetes. You can also find people who have never been on insulin, who have gone blind, had legs amputated and had heart attacks. Once again, I think that is severe diabetes. Now, I am about to publish several cases of young people, diagnosed in their early twenties, who have been treated with tablets but who have gone blind before the age of 30 of proliferative retinopathy. My own personal view is that insulin is a very good drug and that tablets are absolutely useless in the treatment of childhood diabetes. I have no doubt that if my child got diabetes I would put him onto insulin and I would not withhold it from any child.

Index